LANGUAGE ACQUISITION ACROSS NORTH AMERICA

CROSS-CULTURAL AND CROSS-LINGUISTIC PERSPECTIVES

CULTURE, REHABILITATION, AND EDUCATION SERIES
SERIES EDITOR
Orlando L. Taylor, Ph.D.

Language Acquisition Across North America:
Cross-Cultural and Cross-Linguistic
Perspectives
By Orlando L. Taylor, Ph.D.,
and Laurence Leonard, Ph.D.

Bilingual Speech-Language Pathology:
An Hispanic Focus
Edited by Hortencia Kayser, Ph.D.

Integrating Language and Learning for
Inclusion: An Asian/Pacific Focus
Edited by Li-Rong Lilly Cheng, Ph.D.

LANGUAGE ACQUISITION ACROSS NORTH AMERICA

CROSS-CULTURAL AND CROSS-LINGUISTIC PERSPECTIVES

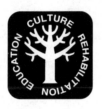

EDITED BY

ORLANDO L. TAYLOR, Ph.D.
DEAN, GRADUATE SCHOOL OF ARTS AND SCIENCES
PROFESSOR OF COMMUNICATION SCIENCES AND DISORDERS
HOWARD UNIVERSITY
WASHINGTON, D.C.

AND

LAURENCE LEONARD, Ph.D.
RACHEL E. STARK DISTINGUISHED PROFESSOR
AUDIOLOGY AND SPEECH SCIENCES
PURDUE UNIVERSITY
WEST LAFAYETTE, INDIANA

SINGULAR PUBLISHING GROUP, INC.
SAN DIEGO • LONDON

Singular Publishing Group, Inc.
401 West A Street, Suite 325
San Diego, California 92101-7904

Singular Publishing Ltd.
19 Compton Terrace
London N1 2UN, UK

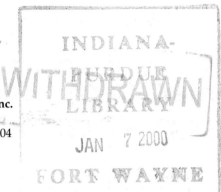
Singular Publishing Group, Inc., publishes textbooks, clinical manuals, clinical reference books, journals, videos, and multimedia materials on speech-language pathology, audiology, otorhinolaryngology, special education, early childhood, aging, occupational therapy, physical therapy, rehabilitation, counseling, mental health and voice. For your convenience, our entire catalog can be accessed on our webside at *http://www.singpub.com*. Our mission to provide you with materials to meet the daily challenges of the ever-changing health care/educational environment will remain on course if we are in touch with you. In that spirit, we welcome your feedback on our products. Please telephone (**1-800-521-8545**), fax (**1-800-774-8398**), or e-mail (*singpub@singpub.com*) your comments and requests to us.

Typeset in 10/12 Palatino by Thompson Type
Printed in the United States of America by Bang Printing

Library of Congress Cataloging-in-Publication Data
Language acquisition across North America : cross-cultural and cross-linguistic
   perspectives / edited by Orlando L. Taylor and Laurence Leonard.
       p.   cm. — (Culture, rehabilitation, and education series)
   Includes bibliographical references and index.
   ISBN 1-56593-862-3 (softcover : alk. paper)
       1. Language acquisition.   2. Afro-American children—Language.
   3. North America—Languages.   I. Taylor, Orlando L., 1936–   .
   II. Leonard, Laurence B.   III. Series.
   [DNLM: WS 105.5.C8L2852 1998]
   P118.L2538   1998
   401'.93'097—dc21
   DLC
   for Library of Congress   98-28126
                                                                         CIP

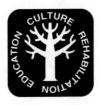

CONTENTS

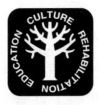

FOREWORD

This book is the third in a series of books on "Culture, Rehabilitation and Education in Culturally and Linguistically Diverse Populations." The series is the first major effort to present a comprehensive, interdisciplinary documentation of the literature on the impact of culture on rehabilitation in a variety of fields, especially in the field of communication disorders.

The series focuses on a wide array of disciplines in response to the rapidly changing environments in which health care, rehabilitation, and education are offered, particularly in the United States. Increasingly, these services are provided in an interdisciplinary manner in which professionals work in teams and in collaboration with one another to address the needs of the whole person.

On the eve of a new millennium, issues pertaining to racial, ethnic, linguistic, and cultural diversity permeate virtually all disciplines within the social, behavioral, and rehabilitation sciences, as well as the field of education. The research literature has increasingly reflected these issues, and professional practice reveals growing sensitivity to the culturally based differences and needs that often characterize humankind.

Demographic changes are often cited as the primary reason for attending to cultural matters in social science, rehabilitation, and education. These changes are real. Such factors as modern transportation, the quest for economic improvement, differences in birth rates, political realities, and social needs, among many others, have produced demonstrable changes in the make-up of the population of many nations around the world and within the 50 states of the United States.

In the United States, for example, approximately one-third of the population will be comprised of African Americans, Hispanics, Asian Americans, Native Americans, and other people of color around the turn of the century. Already upwards of 40% of the school-age population come from these groups. Indeed in some states—California and Texas—these groups will comprise the majority of the total population during the first decade of the twenty-first century. They already do in the public school populations of most urban school systems. Similar, although less dramatic, trends have been reported in many countries in Europe and elsewhere.

An even more compelling reason for addressing the issues of culture and culture diversity within the social sciences, rehabilitation, and education is the fact that all behavior—normal as well as disordered—is acquired and sustained within the context of culture. This is particularly true in the area of speech and language behavior where the particular language(s) and dialect(s) acquired and used by individuals for communicative purposes are influenced directly by the cultural context in which children acquire language and in which adults function in their daily lives. It is precisely because of these facts that professional practice in fields that focus directly or indirectly on language and communicative behavior must consider the cultural issues.

In this book, the authors explore a variety of topics associated with the acquisition of language among a select group of children in the United States and Canada. They provide in-depth discussions of the cultural and familial contexts in which language is acquired within these groups and the developmental milestones that characterize the development of various aspects of language structure and communicative competence. Readers will note many unique aspects of language acquisition among children from these groups, as well as many areas of similarity despite often dramatic differences in the target languages and cultures in which they mature. The latter fact serves to remind us that, despite observable differences in many aspects of the human condition, we are all members of the same human family!

Other books in this series have focused on in-depth analyses of topics pertaining to educational and rehabilitation issues in Hispanic and Asian-Pacific populations. Future books will focus on other distinct groups.

The primary goal of the series is to provide a scholarly context for the preparation of new professionals and for professional practice in the rehabilitation and education fields. In addition, it is hoped that the books in the series will inform future research in these disciplines in years to come.

Orlando L. Taylor, Ph.D.
Series Editor

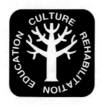

PREFACE

Statements to the effect that there are thousands of languages and dialects spoken in the world usually evoke images of distant lands and exotic cultures. Yet, North Americans can enjoy a rich variety of languages and cultures without leaving their continent. Some of the languages with the fewest speakers in North America were among the first to be spoken on this continent, such as Cree, Navajo, and Inuktitut. Others, such as Vietnamese, Thai, and Korean, are relatively new to North America, but their speakers brought with them a rich culture that is already thriving on these shores.

Although the languages spoken in North America—and the dialects of those languages—vary greatly in number of speakers, many serve as a first language for children born on this continent. This fact brings both advantages and responsibilities. Because language development is an active field of inquiry in North America, the accessibility of native speakers of diverse languages and dialects affords the researcher the opportunity to learn more about both developmental universals as well as crosslinguistic differences in development. This is especially useful for languages that are not objects of formal study elsewhere in the world.

The responsibility stems from the fact that a small percentage of children in any language or dialect group will experience great difficulty in acquiring that language. An informed evaluation of their language-learning problems will require knowledge of how typically developing children acquire that language or dialect. Comparisons of the child's language development with that of the dominant and better studied languages of the continent can provide only limited information about the child's status. For example, a child with a language disorder who is acquiring a language with a rich set of grammatical suffixes will seem as capable as typically developing children acquiring English in the use of grammatical endings (see Leonard, 1998). Yet, this strength is an illusion, based on the fact that English-speaking children are notoriously late in acquiring these kinds of grammatical forms.

Without a clear sense of the course of typical development in the child's own language, it would be most difficult to chart the proper course for clinical or educational services.

In this volume we try to narrow the gap between North American language demographics and published information on children's development of these diverse languages and dialects. The emphasis is on typical development; other volumes in the series focus on clinical and educational issues (see Cheng, 1995; Kayser, 1995). It was not possible to include all of the languages spoken in North America. There are many languages that deserve coverage, and we do not pretend that those included have any privileged status. In some cases, a language has been included principally because we know a great deal about how it is acquired by children. In spite of the gaps, we made efforts to select languages and dialects from a variety of language families and ethnic groups. We feel that the contents of this volume will provide readers with a representative, if not comprehensive, view of the language landscape in North America.

Many of the children whose first language is discussed in this volume will acquire a second language during childhood. We do not discuss issues of second language learning here. The field of second language (or L2) acquisition has now reached levels of sophistication that, in our opinion, cannot be adequately reflected in the one or two chapters that we would be able to include in a book such as this one. However, we feel that we have contributed to the larger issue by providing detailed information on particular languages and dialects. It seems to us that there must be a clear understanding of a child's first language or dialect before the child's acquisition of a second language can be properly studied or facilitated.

The book begins with chapters that argue for the importance of studying different cultural groups and languages to arrive at a better understanding of language development. In these foundation chapters, many of the constructs employed in this type of study are introduced. We then turn to African American English, which is the focus of three separate chapters, devoted to cultural factors, semantic development, and the development of grammar.

In the chapters that follow—chapters on Spanish, French, Inuktitut, and Korean—the authors begin with demographic information about the use of the language in North America as well as a brief discussion of cultural considerations. A sketch of the structure of the language is then provided, followed by the relevant language acquisition data.

Although the book is organized for the usual cover-to-cover reading, we hope that it enjoys a life beyond the first reading by serving as a useful reference for child language specialists or speech-language pathologists who plan to see children from a particular language or cultural group. Before the final version of the manuscript even went to press—and after having read each chapter at least a couple of times—we ourselves have had occasion to consult individual chapters for facts of which we were in need.

We would like to thank Sadanand Singh and Marie Linvill at Singular Publishing for encouraging us to produce this volume, which is the third in the Culture, Rehabilitation, and Education Series. Thanks are also extended to Debra Garrett for her contributions to the early formulation of the book. Special thanks go to the authors for their willingness to write chapters in spite of other commitments. We hope they are pleased with the finished product.

REFERENCES

Cheng, L. (1995). (Ed.). *Integrating language and learning for inclusion: An Asian-Pacific focus.* San Diego: Singular Publishing Group.

Kayser, H. (1995). (Ed.). *Bilingual speech-language pathology: An Hispanic focus.* San Diego: Singular Publishing Group.

Leonard, L. (1998). *Children with specific language impairment.* Cambridge, MA: MIT Press.

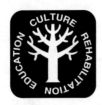

CONTRIBUTORS

Shanley E. M. Allen, Ph.D.
Research Fellow
Max Planck Institute for
    Psycholinguistics
Nijmegen, The Netherlands

Lisa M. Bedore, Ph.D.
Research Associate
Developmental Psycholinguistics
    Laboratory
San Diego State University
San Diego, California

Soonja Choi, Ph.D.
Associate Professor
Department of Linguistics and
    Oriental Languages
San Diego State University
San Diego, California

Martha B. Crago, Ph.D.
Associate Professor
    Communication Disorders
    and Sciences
Associate Vice-Principal,
    Graduate Studies
McGill University
Montreal, Canada

Josée Fortin, Ph.D.
Associate Researcher
Hôpital Sainte-Justine
Department of Speech and
    Language Pathology
University of Montreal
Montreal, Quebec, Canada
Professor of Speech Pathology
Université Laurentian
Master's Program in
    Speech-Language
    Pathology
Sudbury, Ontario, Canada

Laurence B. Leonard, Ph.D.
Professor
Department of Audiology and
    Speech Sciences
Purdue University
West Lafayette, Indiana

Thomas Roeper, Ph.D.
Professor
Linguistics Department
University of Massachusetts
Amherst, Massachusetts

Harry N. Seymour, Ph.D.
Professor and Chair
Department of Communication
    Disorders
Adjunct Professor of Linguistics
University of Massachusetts
Amherst, Massachusetts

Ida J. Stockman, Ph.D.
Professor of Speech-Language
    Pathology
Audiology and Speech Sciences
Michigan State University
East Lansing, Michigan

Orlando L. Taylor, Ph.D.
Dean, Graduate School of Arts
    and Sciences
Professor, Communication
    Sciences and Disorders
Howard University
Washington , D.C.

Michele Clarke Walker, Ph.D.
Lecturer, Department of Hearing
    and Speech Sciences
University of Maryland
Baltimore, Maryland
Adjunct Assistant Professor
Department of Communication
    Sciences and Disorders
Howard University
Washington, D.C.

PART I

FOUNDATIONS

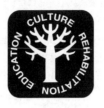

CHAPTER 1

THE STUDY OF LANGUAGE ACQUISITION ACROSS LANGUAGES

LAURENCE B. LEONARD, PH.D.

This chapter discusses some of the ways in which languages differ and how these differences can influence the nature, sequence, and rate of children's language acquisition. We first review some of the major typological differences between languages. Then we discuss other factors that distinguish languages and how these factors might directly influence a child's relative ease or difficulty in learning a language. We conclude with a discussion of alternative ways of comparing children's language acquisition across languages, as well as some of the hazards that must be avoided in making such comparisons.

Many of the characteristics highlighted in this chapter are seen in the languages spoken in North America. As a result, this material might also serve as a useful preview of some of the more detailed linguistic descriptions that appear in the chapters to follow. Because not all languages spoken in North America could be included in this volume (e.g., Mandarin Chinese, Thai), we also review characteristics of some of these languages here in the hope that such information will be useful to those who work with (or otherwise study) children speaking these languages.

The ideas expressed in this chapter owe much to the pioneering work of Slobin (1973, 1985), whose descriptions of how language learning is shaped by the nature of the target language constitute the foundation for the crosslinguistc study of children's language development. The important proposals of Peters (1985), Bates and MacWhinney (1987), MacWhinney (1987), and Pinker (1984) have also been influential and some of their thinking is reflected here, as well.

⊐

LANGUAGE TYPOLOGY: A LOOK AT SOME OF THE DISTINCTIONS

MORPHOLOGICAL UNIFORMITY

Languages differ in the uniformity of their inflectional morphology. A language is uniform if nouns, verbs, and adjectives must always have inflections or, conversely, if these word classes are always bare stems, that is, never inflected. An example of the first type of morphological uniformity is seen in Italian. One says *dormo* "I sleep," *dormi* "you sleep," *dormiranno* "they will sleep," *dormivamo* "we used to sleep," but one cannot say *dorm*. An example of the second type of uniformity is seen in Mandarin Chinese. In this language, there are no inflections for person, number, gender, and case. Verb tense is expressed primarily by adverbials such as "yesterday." Although Italian and Mandarin are very different, they share the characteristic of treating inflections in a consistent manner—inflections are always present or never present.

In contrast, other languages lack uniformity and are viewed as having a mixed system. English is a good example of such a language. Inflected forms such as *jumping, jumped,* and *jumps* are used, but so are bare stems, as in *I jump, you jump, they jump, I saw him jump,* and so on.

Differences in uniformity have developmental ramifications. In a language such as Italian, young children's early errant productions of nouns and verbs will have inflections, albeit the wrong ones. They might say *scrive* "he or she writes" when they should say *scrivono* "they write," but they will not say *scriv*. This is not to say that young children understand the precise grammatical function of each inflection they produce; it is possible that, early on, *scrive* is an unanalyzed, memorized form in a child's linguistic system. However, a bare stem will not be produced, presumably because one is never heard.

For languages with a mixed inflectional morphology, the degree to which nouns, verbs, and adjectives are inflected will dictate the nature of young children's errors. In English, bare stems are much more frequent than inflected forms and errors are almost always bare stems (*run* for *runs; Mommy car* for *Mommy's car*). However, in Russian, a language that permits bare stems but in only a limited number of grammatical contexts, errors can take the form of using an inflection where a bare stem was required. For example, a feminine accusative suffix is often used with singular masculine nouns occupying a sentence position requiring accusative case. Such nouns should remain as bare stems.

Some languages with a uniform inflectional morphology permit null subjects. That is, subjects need not be expressed, if from the conversational or nonlinguistic context the referent is clear. Some of the Romance languages such as Spanish and Italian have this property. Languages from other language families that permit null subjects include Mandarin and Japanese. Null objects are also permitted in certain languages, such as Korean and Japanese. When young children produce sentences without subjects and objects, therefore, one must be careful in attributing the absence of these elements to developmental limitations. The children might be following the dictates of their ambient language in this regard. For example, although young English-speaking children often omit subjects, Italian-speaking children do so even more frequently.

INFLECTIONAL LOAD

Languages differ in the number of grammatical notions that might be expressed by an affix. For example, in Spanish the verb inflection -*o* expresses, simultaneously, present tense, first person, and singular. In Swedish, a verb is inflected for present tense (with the form -*r*), but not for person or number. One might assume that a child's job of discovering the grammatical function of the inflection is easier in the second case.

Languages such as Spanish are said to have a fusional inflectional morphology because several features (e.g., tense, number, and person), are "fused" into a single affix. Other languages express multiple features by making use of an agglutinating morphology. Here, several different affixes are attached to a verb in sequence with each affix conveying a different feature. The first affix might express tense, the second might express number, and so on. Turkish, Hungarian, Tamil (spoken in India and Sri Lanka), Korean, and Japanese are among the languages with an agglutinating morphology. Although a child learning a language of this type must contend with several affixes in sequence, the learnability problem is more easily surmounted, because the child need only hypothesize a single grammatical function for each affix rather than two or three functions operating in combination.

WORD ORDER

Languages also differ in the degree to which word order can vary. English is typically described as a language with rather rigid word order, with variation from the subject-verb-object (SVO) order reserved for only a few constructions. Yet, Mandarin is more rigid in its SVO word order than English. Even *wh*-questions and yes-no questions employ the same order as declaratives.

In languages in which word order variations often occur, languages differ in the operations necessary to support the word order changes. For example, in Italian, sentence components referring to pragmatically salient (e.g., newly introduced) information can move to the front of the sentence (OSV, VSO) and remaining constituents retain their original order. But in German and Swedish (and a few other Germanic languages), when pragmatically salient information is moved to the front of the sentence, the verb must also move in front of the subject and occupy second position in the sentence. This is true also if adverbials are placed at the beginning of the sentence. For example, if "yesterday" is used in the beginning of a German sentence, the verb, not the subject, must immediately follow, as in Example 1.

(1) gestern fand die Frau die Kinder

    yesterday found the woman the children

    "yesterday the woman found the children"

It seems likely that flexibility in word order is related to the relative importance of grammatical morphology in a language. It is probably no coincidence that languages that rely heavily on grammatical morphology possess relatively flexible word order, whereas in a language with a relatively sparse morphology such as English, word order is quite rigid. Indeed in a language with no agreement inflections at all—such as Mandarin—word order is the least flexible.

The dominance of grammatical morphology or word order in a language probably influences the language learner. Children learning English appear to register the strong word order regularities of the language and rarely deviate from the SVO pattern in their own speech. Armed with word order to express basic sentence relations, young English-speaking children have less motivation in the early stages of language use to bother with, say, the present third singular inflection or the distinction between nominative and accusative case. If the child is quite consistent in expressing subject + verb and verb + object utterances, for example, the utterance *me get* is fairly recognizable as an attempt at the former. Of course, the price paid for focusing so much on word order is that, relative to children learning languages such as Italian and Spanish, English-speaking children will be rather slow in their development of grammatical morphology.

GRAMMATICAL DISTINCTIONS THROUGH INFLECTIONS VERSUS SYNTACTIC STRUCTURE

Languages differ in whether notions such as reciprocity, causality, and reflexivity are expressed primarily through verb morphology or through syntactic constructions and the addition of specific lexical items. For example, in English, to express reciprocity, specific lexical items are employed in combination with the verb (e.g., "We write *each other* everyday"). To express causality, a particular syntactic construction is employed (e.g., "We will have a letter written") or a verb that is distinct from its noncausative counterpart is called on (e.g., "We *dictated* the letter").

In Hebrew, such notions are part of the verb morphology. Hebrew verbs consist of a root plus a pattern. The root conveys the core meaning and the pattern conveys the notions that modify this meaning— notions such as reciprocity and causality. For example, the root for the meaning "write" consists of the (often discontinuous) consonant sequence *k-t-v*.[1] The patterns are formed through the insertion of vowels between the consonants of the root and the addition of syllabic prefixes. For example, *kotvim* is from the pattern employed for intransitives ("they are writing") and simple transitives ("they are writing a letter"). The form *mitkatvim* comes from the pattern used for reciprocal acts ("they are writing each other"); causative acts ("they are dictating a letter") are expressed by still another pattern, as seen in *maxtivim*. It can be seen that the velar stop *k* changed to the velar fricative *x* in the last example. Such changes are dictated by phonological rules and do not represent a change in the core meaning of the root.

---

[1] Phonetic symbols are used rather than Hebrew script for clarity of presentation.

ERGATIVITY

Some languages are ergative where, for example, the subject of an intransitive verb is assigned the same case as the object of a transitive verb. Ergative languages include Hindi, Warlpiri (spoken in Central Australia), and Inuktitut. The task of figuring out the parallels between the subjects of one type of verb and objects of another could be complicated by two other properties already mentioned—word order variability and the use of null subjects or objects. It is not difficult to imagine the protracted period that might be necessary for a child to solve this problem if, say, subjects of transitive verbs were often omitted and (as is seen in ergative languages) objects were often placed in the same position occupied by subjects of intransitive verbs.

FORM CLASS BOUNDARIES

Languages differ in the degree to which adjectives and verbs overlap in grammatical function. In Mandarin, stative verbs convey many notions (e.g., is/are cold, sweet) that are expressed by adjectives in languages such as English. In Japanese, tense is marked on adjectives as well as verbs.

HONORIFICS

Some languages possess honorifics, that is, a grammatical means of marking the social standing of the speaker relative to the listener. Among European languages, several show a distinction between familiar and formal address. This distinction occurs in direct address and is reflected in the choice of pronoun forms used. The inflection of the verb will also differ, if the pronoun referring to the addressee is the grammatical subject. For example, in French, the familiar and formal forms for "you sell" are *tu vends* and *vous vendez*, respectively.

In languages such as Japanese and Korean, the honorific system is much more elaborate. There are verb inflections reflecting varying degrees of politeness and distinctions in grammatical marking for referring to persons of higher social status even when these persons are not present in the speaking situation.

TONE

Although changes in pitch level are used in most languages to express affect, some languages employ systematic changes in pitch, that is, tone contrasts, for linguistic purposes. In many of these languages, such as Mandarin Chinese and Thai, tone is employed for lexical contrast. Typically, tones are distinguished according to pitch level (e.g., high, low tone) and direction of movement (e.g., falling, rising, level). A few languages make use of tone for morphosyntactic purposes. For example, in Bini (a language spoken in Nigeria), a monosyllabic verb expressing a habitual action is produced with a low tone, but the same verb expressing an action in the past is produced with a high tone.

ᒳ

OTHER PROPERTIES OF LANGUAGES THAT INFLUENCE LEARNING

Thus far we have seen that languages differ not only in the number of notions that are expressed in the grammar, but also in the types of notions expressed. Investigators have proposed that some grammatical notions are more readily hypothesized by language learners than others. Notions such as number marking on nouns are usually hypothesized quite early by children, probably because such notions are semantically salient. That is, children can discover the basis for a grammatical distinction by observing the referents of the utterance (e.g., seeing one dog called *dog* and several dogs called *dogs*). One can easily see how children could learn that noun inflections make distinctions of number more quickly than they could learn that verb inflections make distinctions between witnessed events and events heard about but not actually observed. In the latter case, the child might have no knowledge of whether the speaker was present during the event being described.

However, semantic salience cannot explain differences in children's ease or difficulty in learning many other grammatical notions. For example, children seem to acquire verb inflections that agree with the person or grammatical gender of a subject more readily than they acquire an inflection that agrees with an object in definiteness (as exists in Hungarian). Findings of differences in ease of learning have led some investigators to rank notions in terms of "grammaticizability." However, at this point, the rankings are primarily descriptive; we don't yet know the basis for why some notions are more readily hypothesized than others when all else is equal. It is certainly true that relative ease of learning can be predicted by the number of languages in the world that express a particular notion. However, the factors that account for the appearance of a notion in many languages are probably the same ones that account for early learning.

The qualifier "when all else is equal" used in the preceding paragraph is essential. Often all else is not equal. Earlier in the chapter, it was noted that in some languages—those with a fusional inflectional morphology—a single inflection marks two or three notions simultaneously, such as person, number, and gender, whereas other languages employ a distinct inflection for each of these notions. Learning in the latter case is facilitated, because children can hypothesize one notion at a time until the right one is discovered. In the case of fusional languages, the children must hypothesize and reject each notion taken singly and then (correctly) hypothesize the combination of these notions.

There are other factors that influence ease of learning. Although some are bound up with language typology, others seem to operate independently of typological considerations. A brief discussion of some of these factors follows.

SYNCRETISM

Languages differ in the degree and patterns of syncretism that are seen in their morphology. Syncretism is the use of the same morpheme to express distinct features. For example, in English, copula *are* is used for second person singular as well as first, second, and third person plural. In Spanish, the copula shows a unique form for each permutation of features (*soy, eres, es, somos, sois, son*).

The pattern of syncretism can be important for the language learner. For example, in Hebrew, third person singular past tense verb inflections are distinguished according to gender, but third person plural past tense uses the inflection *-u* for both genders. Given that the referents for which *-u* is used share most features (third person in the past), the child might have less difficulty learning the use of this form than if the same form were used for, say, third person feminine plural and third person masculine singular.

We should probably note cases where syncretism exists in the ears and minds of children learning a language even where it might not exist in the adult system. In French, the first, second, and third person singular present verb forms (e.g., *parle, parles, parle; finis, finis, finit; vends, vends, vend*) are pronounced in the same way even though distinctions are made in the orthography.

HOMOPHONY ACROSS PARADIGMS

The homophony inherent in syncretism is not the only case in which we see morphemes sharing the same phonetic form. In English, for example, the inflection -s is used for noun plurals and also verbs in the present third person singular. Because these two functions belong to different paradigms (for noun and verbs, respectively) any learnability challenge they pose would probably be in the very early stages of acquisition, before the children have reached the point of determining the precise grammatical function of these inflections. For example, it seems likely that very young children use the appearance of inflections to help them identify grammatical categories such as noun and verb and to associate these categories with particular sentence positions. No understanding of the precise meaning of the inflections is necessary at this early point; these forms are merely flags that can be associated with one or another category. Given this assumption, it can be seen that this process might proceed more slowly if there is considerable homophony in the inflections from different paradigms.

Homophony could be somewhat problematic in a language with an agglutinating morphology, because a child must learn the order in which inflections from different paradigms (e.g., tense, gender, number) are sequenced. The paradigm represented might be more difficult to discover if there is considerable homophony. This might be one reason why the inflectional morphology of Turkish—a language with relatively little homophony—seems to be easier for children than the inflectional morphology of Hungarian, where homophony is more frequent.

REDUNDANCY

In some languages, a grammatical notion is expressed through the application of the same morpheme in more than one place. For example, in Hebrew, the definite prefix *ha-* appears not just once in the noun phrase as in its English equivalent *the*, but rather with the noun and all modifiers, as in Example 2.

(2) ha-iparon ha-adom

the red the pencil

"the red pencil"

Another type of redundancy is seen in constructions that require two components to convey a notion. For example, for notions such as "not see anybody" and "don't do anything," indefinite pronouns are used along with the negative particles. Languages differ in how such indefinite pronouns are marked. In standard English, there is a disjoint relationship; a negative indefinite pronoun (as in "You understand nothing" and "You see nobody") must be changed if a negative particle appears in the same sentence ("You don't understand anything" and "You don't see anybody"). However, in many languages, use of a negative particle requires a corresponding negative indefinite pronoun. Thus, in Italian, *Non capisci niente* and *Non vedi nessuno* is, literally, "(you) don't understand nothing" and "(you) don't see nobody," respectively. In African American English, the same coordination between negative particles and indefinite pronouns is seen.

REGULARITY

There are two senses of regularity and languages can vary according to each. One type of regularity is the degree to which there are exceptions to the usual way of marking a grammatical distinction. In English, for example, there are many verbs whose past tense forms deviate from the typical *-ed* suffix rule. There are numerous examples of irregular noun plurals in Arabic, which might be one explanation for why noun plurals are acquired later in Arabic than in other languages.

The other sense of regularity is the uniformity of the paradigms of the language. In standard English, the present tense verb paradigm contains only one overt form, the third person singular inflection *-s*. In African American English, on the other hand, the absence of an overt third singular form renders the present tense verb paradigm more regular.

RELIABILITY

The presence of a grammatical construction or morpheme may typically call for a particular interpretation, but this signal may be far from perfect. Although Italian word order is considered SVO, placement of the subject relative to the verb is not a reliable cue. Exceptions frequently occur, making the grammatical inflection the more dependable cue on which to rely.

RANGE OF RULE APPLICATION

Languages differ in the range of application of their rules. The use of simple present tense is a good example. In English, simple present tense is restricted to habitual activities ("She goes to the store every Saturday") or stative verbs ("He likes this car"). In Italian, in contrast, simple present tense is also used for overt actions in the present and actions to be performed in the near future. Consequently, English-speaking children will have far fewer opportunities to hear instances of third person singular use than will children learning Italian.

SENTENCE AND WORD POSITION

A well-known principle of language learning was labeled "pay attention to the ends of words" by Slobin (1973). This principle was based on the observation that suffixes appear to be acquired by children earlier than prefixes, to the extent that the grammatical function of these forms across languages could be equated. Position effects also seem to operate when free-standing prenominal forms are compared to noun suffixes. For example, in German, case is marked on prenominal articles, whereas in Polish case is marked via word-final inflections. It appears that the latter are acquired earlier than the former. In Swedish, prenominal articles are used for the indefinite, but suffixes attached to the ends of nouns are used for the definite, as in Example 3.

> (3) en kanin "a rabbit"   ett lejon "a lion"
>
>   kaninen "the rabbit"   lejonet "the lion"

Definite suffixes are learned earlier than the indefinite articles and seem to be acquired at an earlier age than the definite article *the* is acquired by English-speaking children.

     Some languages employ a different pronominal form, depending on whether the form refers to a person or object already identified clearly by the discourse (or physical context). Italian is one such language, as can be seen in Examples 4 and 5.

> (4) Gina lo vede
>
>   Gina him sees
>
>   "Gina sees him"

(5) Gina vede lui

Gina sees him

"Gina sees him" (not someone else)

It can be noted that the form (*lo*) used in Example 4 appears in front of the verb, whereas the form (*lui*) used in Example 5 appears after the verb. In English, pronouns serving these two functions are not only identical in form, but they also occupy the same sentence position. Italian-speaking children acquire forms such as the one in Example 4 at later ages than English-speaking children acquire the English pronominal equivalents.

WORD LENGTH AND PROSODIC DEMANDS

In many languages, children's early utterances are described as consisting of single words. These single-word utterances usually reflect phonological limitations; it is rare for young children to produce early words that sound adult-like. One of the most important phonological limitations is a tendency to omit syllables from multisyllabic words. Typical pronunciations of *banana* and *telephone* are *nana* and *tefon*, for example. The consequences of syllable reduction will vary from language to language. For English-speaking children, the discrepancies between the adult form and the child's form will not be as great as in certain other languages.

This can be confirmed by inspecting the composition of children's early lexicons in different languages. For example, the words constituting nouns that first appear in young English-speaking children's speech based on the *MacArthur Communicative Development Inventory* (Fenson et al., 1993) average 1.55 syllables in length. In contrast, the corresponding words for the Italian version of this inventory (Caselli & Casadio, 1995) average 2.77 syllables. Only 2 one-syllable words appeared on the Italian list (both borrowed words), whereas there were 122 one-syllable words for English. Omissions of syllables is therefore a much more likely occurrence in Italian.

The number of syllables in a word is not the only factor. The prosodic and morphological properties of the language also play a role. Many young children are limited to strong-weak syllable sequences in their word productions (Gerken, 1996). For English-speaking children at the two-word utterance stage of development, this is not a significant impediment, as so many words are either one-syllable words or two-syllable words with the strong-weak syllable pattern (e.g., *baby, mommy, apple*).

Thus, an utterance such as *open letter* might not be clear in terms of tense and number, but the intended lexical items are quite clear. On the other hand, an utterance produced by an Italian-speaking child at the same point in development might take a form such as *pato telli*, in which the listener can be relatively certain that the action took place in the past and the object noun is plural, but the precise action performed and object acted on are less certain. K'iche', a Mayan language spoken in Guatamala, is an example of a language in which the prosody renders verb inflections more salient than the stems to which they are attached (see Pye, 1983).

⊔

COMPARISONS ACROSS LANGUAGES

Crosslinguistic comparisons of children's language development can yield important information. First, they might point to universals of acquisition shared by all children, regardless of target language. Second, they can be helpful to practitioners who are in a position of evaluating children whose language is other than the dominant language in a community. It would be helpful to know, for example, that a 3-year-old Spanish-speaking child residing in an English-speaking community is not necessarily functioning at age level, even though he or she is producing verb inflections. Although English-speaking children are only in an early phase of verb inflection use at this age, children acquiring Spanish can be expected to use verb inflections from the outset of verb use.

On the other hand, in some languages, certain inflections that are relatively early attainments in English (e.g., noun plurals) are quite demanding in other languages. An Arabic-speaking child will produce incorrect plural forms relatively often; however, the plural system is considerably more complicated in Arabic than in English. A practitioner's knowledge of the differences between plural use in the two languages is, therefore, very useful.

Unfortunately, crosslinguistic comparisons can be tricky. Even questions that seem straightforward are, on close inspection, rather thorny. For example, assume we wish to compare two languages in terms of the typical age at which two-word utterances emerge. In English, such utterances are often combinations of subject and verb, verb and object, verb and name of location (e.g., *put table* for "I'll put it on the table"), object name and adjective (e.g., *big shoe*), and so on. In languages such as Spanish and Italian, null subjects are permitted; therefore, subject and verb combinations won't play a significant role in the emergence of two-word utterances. And, in Korean and Inuktitut—languages that allow objects as well as subjects to be omitted—even verb + object combinations won't be as influential as in English. Furthermore, as is shown in a later chapter, much of grammar in Inuktitut is accomplished through the combination of several morphemes within the same word. A one-word utterance can express notions comparable to utterances several words in length in English. Thus, the idea of two-word combinations as an important developmental milestone is not really relevant for Inuktitut.

One might suppose that a solution to the problem of comparing such disparate languages is to match children from the two languages in terms of the average number of morphemes used in their utterances. It might be assumed that an Inuktitut-speaking child should produce two-morpheme utterances at about the same time that English-speaking children produce them. Of course, for English, early two-morpheme utterances will be two words in length, whereas for Inuktitut they would probably be one-word utterances.

Unfortunately, such a basis for matching is also wrought with difficulties. The chief problem is that, in many languages, it is not clear how many morphemes a given inflection or function word should be considered to possess. For example, in the Italian utterance *vedo macchine* "(I) see cars," it is not clear if the verb inflection *-o* represents three morphemes (present tense, first person, singular) or just one. Similarly, the noun inflection *-e* could be taken to reflect feminine and plural or only a single morpheme. The consequences of making any decision are probably clear. The more generous rendering would treat the utterance *vedo macchine* as consisting of seven morphemes. If such utterances were typical of the average length of a child's utterances, the child would be compared to an English-speaking child who says things like *I wanna see some cars* and *Can I see these big cars?* Even the greater number of syllables in Italian words does not make up the difference in the number of syllables likely to be produced in the utterances of children from these two languages.

Another illustration of the complicated nature of crosslinguistic comparisons can be seen if we ask the question of whether children develop out of the telegraphic stage earlier in some languages than in others. As we have seen, in many languages, all lexical categories must be inflected. For these languages, the trick is determining not when inflections are added but when the word endings that were present all along can be interpreted to reflect productive analyzed inflections rather than part of an unanalyzed whole.

For certain languages, crosslinguistic comparisons can be made if children from the two languages are matched according to mean length of utterance (MLU) measured in words rather than morphemes. For example, in both English and Spanish, articles and copula forms are separate words, whereas verb and noun inflections are bound morphemes and hence not counted in this measure. Even with these general similarities, it is not safe to assume that children with similar MLUs in the two languages are comparable. Some additional criteria should be met. For example, MLU in words should systematically increase with age in each language, at least through the preschool years. Furthermore, children with similar MLUs in the two languages should be similar in age.

Many languages are simply too different to use MLU in words as a basis for matching. An alternative is to match children in the two languages on the basis of standard scores on tests of language ability. Of course, the tests in each language must have sufficient psychometric strength to provide confidence that the scores are reliable and valid. Just as important, the tests should purport to assess the same dimensions of language and the tasks employed should be similar. An example of a good match would be if each test contained subtests for vocabulary comprehension through picture pointing, vocabulary production through picture naming, grammatical comprehension through picture pointing, and grammatical production through sentence imitation. In this case, crosslinguistic comparisons between children of similar age with similar standard scores seem highly reasonable. Any differences that are observed can probably be taken to reflect genuine differences between the properties of the two languages rather than inadvertent selection of children whose language abilities in the respective languages are not on the same level.

The challenges of comparing children across languages are many. However, the enterprise is worth the effort. Through greater appreciation of how languages vary, our understanding of the language acquisition process will deepen, and our efforts at assisting children with language learning difficulties will be better informed.

⊓

REFERENCES

Bates, E., & MacWhinney, B. (1987). Competition, variation, and language learning. In B. MacWhinney (Ed.), *Mechanisms of language acquisition* (pp. 157–193). Hillsdale, NJ: Lawrence Erlbaum.

Caselli, M. C., & Casadio, P. (1995). *Il primo vocabolario del bambino: Guida all'uso del questionario MacArthur per la valutazione della communicazione e del linguaggio nei primi anni di vita.* Milan, Italy: FrancoAngeli.

Fenson, L., Dale, P., Reznick, S., Thal, D., Bates, E., Hartung, J., Pethick, S., & Reilly, J. (1993). *The MacArthur Communicative Development Inventories: User's guide and technical manual.* San Diego: Singular Publishing Group.

Gerken, L. (1996). Prosodic structure in young children's language production. *Language, 72,* 683–712.

MacWhinney, B. (1987). The competition model. In B. MacWhinney (Ed.), *Mechanisms of language acquisition* (pp. 249–308). Hillsdale, NJ: Lawrence Erlbaum.

Peters, A. (1985). Language segmentation: Operating principles for the perception and analysis of language. In D. Slobin (Ed.), *The crosslinguistic study of language acquisition: Vol. 2. Theoretical issues* (pp. 1029–1064). Hillsdale, NJ: Lawrence Erlbaum.

Pinker, S. (1984). *Language learnability and language development.* Cambridge, MA: Harvard University Press.

Pye, C. (1983). Mayan telegraphese: Intonational determinants of inflectional development in Quichè Mayan. *Language, 59,* 583–604.

Slobin, D. (1973). Cognitive prerequisites for the development of grammar. In C. Ferguson & D. Slobin (Eds.), *Studies of child language development* (pp. 175–208). New York: Holt, Rinehart and Winston.

Slobin, D. (1985). Crosslinguistic evidence for the language-making capacity. In D. Slobin (Ed.), *The crosslinguistic study of language acquisition: Vol. 2. Theoretical issues* (pp. 1157–1256). Hillsdale, NJ: Lawrence Erlbaum.

LAURENCE B. LEONARD, Ph.D.

Laurence B. Leonard, Ph.D., is Rachel E. Stark Distinguished Professor in the Department of Audiology and Speech Sciences at Purdue University. His publications focus on children with specific language impairment as well as typically developing children. Dr. Leonard's major interests concern the manner in which language impairment is expressed in children who speak different languages, and the interactions between phonology/prosody and morphosyntax.

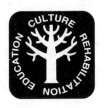

CHAPTER 2

CULTURAL ISSUES AND LANGUAGE ACQUISITION

ORLANDO L. TAYLOR, Ph.D.

Children's acquisition of the language of the families and communities in which they mature is a universal human process. Although some children in all cultures fail to successfully negotiate this process for a variety of physical, social, or psychological reasons and, thereby, are categorized as having a language disorder, the overwhelming proportion of the world's children acquire the basic language systems of their families and communities. While the *milestones* of the acquisition process are related to the language system being acquired, the acquisition *process* seems to be remarkably similar for all children, irrespective of race, culture, or family socioeconomic status.

Many theories have been advanced over the years to explain this marvelous universal process (e.g., Crystal, 1997). For example, some theorists have posited a learning model in which children are thought to acquire language through a process of imitation and reinforcement of the adult language system spoken in their environments. Indeed, much of the phonology and vocabulary of children's language around the world are reflective of the language systems spoken in their adult environments. Recent research suggests, however, that imitation and reinforcement models are unable to account for children's unique grammatical rules *or* their inability to imitate certain grammatical utterances from adults, even when prompted to do so.

Other theorists (e.g., Lenneberg, 1967) have posited a biological, or innate, basis of language and language acquisition. In the innateness models, language acquisition is viewed as a maturation process as opposed to a learned process. Indeed, because of the universal nature of language and perhaps the language acquisition process, Lenneberg argued that language was *unlike* other learned phenomena, inasmuch as learned phenomena, tend to reflect great variation within species instead of universal attributes. As the language acquisition process seems to have many universal properties, one is given pause to accept totally a learning model of acquisition. Yet, on the other hand, innateness models fail to account for how children use their biological hardware to predictably acquire the language system(s) to which they have been exposed—and only those systems!

The generative grammarians of the 1960s, headed by Noam Chomsky, provided an alternative model that takes into account both the biological and learned dimensions of language acquisition. They argued that, although children are born with an innate propensity for language *and* an ability to "discover" a set of underlying rules for generating language (i.e., a language acquisition device, or LAD), children nonetheless require access to a language system from the environment in order to develop hypotheses for a grammar to generate utterances that have meaning and appropriateness within their environments. Over time and after a series of trials and errors based on the utterances generated from LADs, an approximation of the adult grammar is thought to be realized by children as illustrated in Figure 2–1.

No matter which theory of language acquisition one espouses, one cannot ignore that children mature within the context of caregivers, whether they are parents, siblings, family members, or other individuals within the child's community. These caregivers, no matter who they are, provide a linguistic and communicative environment for the maturing child that is reflective of the range of meanings, values, perceptions, and beliefs of the cultures of which they are a part. It is for this reason that culture has to be paramount in a thoughtful discussion of language acquisition.

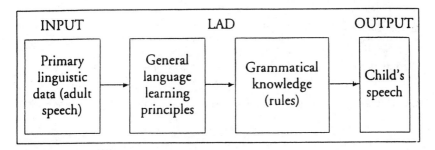

FIGURE 2-1
A schematic of LAD. (From *The Cambridge Encyclopedia of Language* [2nd ed., p. 236], by Crystal, D., 1997. Cambridge [UK]: Cambridge University Press. Copyright 1997 by Cambridge University Press. Reprinted with permission.)

⌐

THE NATURE OF CULTURE

Saville-Troike (1986) defined culture as the collectivity of shared rules for appropriate behavior (including verbal and nonverbal communication) learned and used by individuals as a consequence of being members of the same group or community, as well as the values and beliefs that underlie overt behaviors that themselves are shared products of group membership. In addition to such phenomena as the creation of institutions and family practices (see Table 2–1), culture defines—at least by inference—what an individual needs to know to be a functional member of a community and to regulate interactions with other members of their communities and with individuals from other cultures. Children acquire their language system within this context.

Several general principles seem to undergird cultures around the world. Three of the more important for our purposes are:

1. Cultures are dynamic and are in a constant state of evolution. The cultural context in which children acquire language in one generation may be different in the next generation. For example, the advent of television has had a major impact on the language acquisition environments of children where television access is a part of the culture. This is especially

TABLE 2–1
Questions to ask about cultures.

Family Structure	Who is considered as belonging to the family?
	What are the rights, roles, and responsibilities of the family members?
Life Cycle	What are the important stages, periods, and transitions in life?
	What behaviors are inappropriate or unacceptable for children at various ages?
Roles	What roles are available to whom?
	How are roles acquired?
Interpersonal Relationships	How do people greet each other?
	Who may disagree with whom?
	How are insults expressed?
Communication	What languages and dialects are spoken?
	What are the characteristics of speaking "well"?
	What roles, attitudes, and personality traits are associated with particular aspects of verbal and nonverbal behavior?
	How much emotional intensity is desirable in speech?
Decorum and Discipline	How do people behave at home and in public?
	What means of discipline are used?
Religion	What religious roles and authority are recognized?
	What should an outsider not know or acknowledge knowing?
Health and Hygiene	How are illness and death explained?
	How are specific illnesses treated?
	What are thought to be causes of disabilities and who should treat them?
Food	What is eaten, in what order, and how often?
	What are the rules for table manners, including offering foods, handling foods, and discarding foods?
Holidays and Celebrations	What holidays are observed? For what purpose?
	Which holidays are important for children?
	What cultural values are instilled in children during the holidays?
Dress and Personal Appearance	What significance does dress have for social identity?
	What is the concept and value of beauty and attractiveness?
	What attributes are considered undesirable?

TABLE 2–1 *(continued)*

Values	What traits and attributes in oneself or others are important?
	Which values are undesirable to have?
	What attributes in the world are important?
History and Traditions	How are history and tradition passed on to the young?
	How do cultural understandings of history differ from "scientific" facts or literate history?
Education	What are the purposes of education?
	What kinds of learning are favored?
	What teaching and learning methods are used in the home?
	What are parental expectations for boys versus girls?
Work and Play	What behaviors are considered "work"? "Play"?
	What kinds of work are prestigious? Why?
Time and Space	What is considered "on time"?
	What is the importance of punctuality?
	How important is speed of performance?
	How are groups organized spatially by age, gender, and role?
Natural Phenomena	Who or what is deemed responsible for rain, thunder, floods, and hurricanes?
	Are behavioral taboos associated with natural phenomena?
Pets and Animals	Which animals are valued and for what reasons?
	What animals are considered appropriate or inappropriate as pets?
Art and Music	What forms of art and music are most highly valued?
	What forms of art and music are considered appropriate for children to perform or appreciate?
Expectations and Aspirations	Do parents expect and desire assimilation of children to the dominant culture, and language, or dialect?
	What cultural values are expected to be maintained despite the degree of formal education?

Source: Based on material from *A Guide to Culture in the Classroom,* by M. Saville-Troike, 1978. Rosslyn, VA: National Clearinghouse for Bilingual Education.

true for North American cultures; however, television did not become a major factor in child language acquisition until the 1950s.

2. Cultures are *not* mutually exclusive of one another, indeed they enjoy a good deal of overlap. As a result, generalizations about the language acquisition process that may be true for one culture, may be true also for another culture. Indeed cultural similarity may exist for two cultures in totally different parts of the world or for two or more cultures that have no history of intercultural contact, whatsoever. For example, the extended family is a setting in which language is acquired by some cultures within the United States (e.g., the traditional African-American culture); however, the extended family environment is one that characterizes many other cultures throughout the world.

3. There is considerable variation *within* cultures, often associated with such phenomena as gender, age, education, and exposures of its individual members to other cultures. Thus, any generalization about a culture is likely to be erroneous at best and the seedlings for creating a stereotype at worse. It is for this reason that it is very difficult to make a single set of generalizations about language acquisition behavior for a particular group, although there may well be a set of *tendencies* that may characterize a large portion of that group.

Hamayan and Damico (1991) have suggested several continua along which cultures might reflect variation (Table 2–2). As shown, these continua include such attributes as language, cognitive style, roles of individual members, and rules governing interactions. Many, if not most, of these attributes may have an impact on language acquisition in children.

North America contains great cultural—and linguistic—diversity. On this continent, like all others, there are many cultures and language systems within the environment that children might acquire if they are exposed to them. Depending on the particular cultural context in which language is to be acquired, as well as the particular language system being acquired, there is the very real possibility that culturally specific nuances may be found in the language acquisition patterns for different groups of children. In short, despite the notion of universals, very real and important differences might well occur across groups. We explore some of these possibilities—and realities— in later chapters.

TABLE 2–2
Continua along which cultural preferences might be determined.

Attributes	Continua	
Movement	Active _____	Passive
Space	Close _____	Distant
Time	Strict time schedule _____	No strict time schedules
Interactions	Polychronic _____	Monochronic
Goal/Structures	Cooperative _____	Competitive
Gender/Role	Inequality _____	Equality
Role	Group _____	Individual
Locus of Control	External _____	Internal
Perceptual Style	Field-Dependent _____	Field-Independent
Cognitive Style	Intuitive _____	Reflective
Language Patterns	Mismatch _____	Match
Language Loss	Extensive _____	Minimal
Code Switching	Frequent _____	Infrequent
Language Variance	Nonstandard _____	Standard

Source: From Limiting Bias in the Assessment of Bilingual Students (p. 131), by E. V. Hamayan and J. S. Damico, 1991. Austin, TX: PRO-ED. Copyright 1991 by PRO-ED. Reprinted with permission.

⌐

CULTURE, LANGUAGE, AND COMMUNICATION

Central to the notion of a cultural basis for language acquisition are the notions of *speech community* and *communication competence*. These notions are derived from the field of communication ethnography.

According to Hymes (1966), the pioneer of the ethnography of communication, ethnographic approaches focus on the *patterning of communicative* behavior as one aspect of culture, as it functions within the context of the total culture of a group, and as it relates to other aspects of culture. This approach considers *language as a socially situated cultural form*, while simultaneously recognizing the necessity to analyze linguistic codes and the cognitive processes underlying them among speakers and listeners. The ultimate goal of ethnography is to understand how language actually functions in the lives of individuals and cultural groups. A central question of the ethnography of communication is: What does a speaker need to know to communicate appropriately within a particular speech community, and how does he or she acquire this knowledge? According to Hymes, such knowledge, together with whatever skills are needed to make use of it, is termed *communicative competence.*

The knowledge subsumed under the concept of communication competence involves both linguistic and sociolinguistic rules. In addition, communication competence includes the cultural rules and knowledge that form the bases for the content and context of communicative events and interactive processes. These notions suggest that a comprehensive theory of language acquisition must consider how children acquire both the rules governing the surface structure features of the adult language, as well as the cultural norms for language use.

Hymes (1966) claims further that a *speech community* consists of a collection of individuals who learn, share, and utilize a particular set of linguistic codes that serve to represent the universe of meanings characteristic of that culture. Persons may share the same language code, but still not belong to the same speech community. For example, although both Parisians and many Canadians in the province of Quebec speak French, the variations of speech spoken by these two groups separate them into different speech communities. And, of course, the speakers of the creolized variety of French spoken by the Cajuns in Louisiana in the southern United States constitute yet another speech community.

Within any speech community, subgroups may exist. These subgroups may be marked by the speaking of a variety (dialect) of the language spoken within the larger speech community. Some of these dialects may be traced to historical and social forces within a geographical region (e.g., Appalachian English and New York City English in the United States), with others directly associated with the linguistic and social histories of a particular group (e.g., African American English or Ebonics). If dialect variations are so great within a language that they are rendered largely unintelligible to the larger speech community, a case can be made that their speakers are no longer members of a subgroup of a speech community, but indeed they form their own speech communities. For example, the linguistic codes spoken within the islands of the Chesapeake Bay (e.g., Tangier Island, Smith Island, etc.) are so unique—and often unintelligible—to outsiders, that they might be considered as separate speech communities.

Children acquiring language are inevitably thrust into at least one speech community during the acquisition years. It is the language of that speech community that presumably impacts most directly on the child's

LAD and helps to determine which language and the variety of that language that he or she is likely to acquire as their first language (L1).

In the past two decades, a rich literature has emerged to describe many American English social dialects in the United States , especially those spoken by many African Americans. Much of the standard language acquisition literature has failed, however, to describe children's language acquisition norms from the vantage point of these linguistic communities.

Although dialects of a language are generally intelligible to individuals outside of the dialect community of its speakers, they tend to reflect variations in almost every aspect of language—phonology, vocabulary, semantics, prosody, pragmatics, grammar, and so on. Although it is often the case that the concept of *dialect* is thought to be isomorphic with the concept of *nonstandard* language, such notions are incorrect. Linguists view *any* variety of a language as a dialect, including those varieties that happen to acquire the designata as "standard." It is simply the case that more prestigious varieties of languages— especially those that become the codes of education and of books—are perceived as the standard variety, or the standard dialect. In this sense, therefore, every child is presented with a dialect of a language and it is that dialect (or dialects, if several are presented) that becomes the adult model onto which LAD is applied.

North America is a continent—like all others—that reflects enormous diversity in culture and language. Not only are there several national languages spoken—Spanish in Mexico, English in the United States and Canada, and French in some parts of Canada—but numerous other languages and dialects are spoken in all three countries. These languages range from millions of Spanish speakers in the United States to many Native American, Native Canadian, and Native Mexican languages spoken by native peoples, to numerous regional and social dialects and to the numerous languages brought to the Americas by immigrant populations. To say that North America is linguistically diverse is to state the obvious. It is this multilingual environment into which children acquire language in North America. The scholarly imperative, of course, is to determine, to the extent possible, the elements of language on the continent that conform with universal principles, as well as those attributes that are language specific. To date, our scholarship has regrettably focused on the language acquisition patterns of middle class Standard English speakers in the USA and Canada and often erroneously generalized to the total North American population as *normal* language acquisition for all children. In recent years, however, considerable scholarship has documented language and communication acquisition in culturally and linguistically diverse children. Much of this research is reported elsewhere in this volume.

As an indication of the great diversity of language spoken in North America, one might examine recent reports of language use in the United States. According to these reports, although English is the dominant language within the United States, there are numerous other languages spoken in the homes of children throughout the country. This means, of course, that the basic social-cognitive language to be acquired by many children is a language other than English.

Specifically, the National Association of Bilingual Education (*Education Week*, April 15, 1998) reports that since 1980, the number of language-minority Americans in the United States has increased at more than four times the rate of overall population growth. Because these groups are, on average, younger than native English speakers, the number of language-minority children has increased even faster. According to the 1990 Census, nearly one of every six school-aged youth regularly spoke a language other than English in their homes. In 1994–1995, there were an estimated 3.2 million limited English proficient (LEP) students in U.S. elementary and secondary schools, nearly 7% of total enrollment. Some states have felt an even more dramatic impact. In California in 1997, for example, it was reported that 36% of K–12 students spoke a language other than English at home and 24% were LEP, a population that has more than doubled in 10 years.

Figure 2–2 illustrates the sharp increase in the non-English speaking population in the United States. As shown, considerable growth in the number of non-English speakers has occurred in the southwestern and northeastern sections of the United States. Many of these children acquire both languages—English and the non-English home language—simultaneously during the language acquisition process.

Although many national or official languages may be spoken within a society, the language acquired by a child is likely to be the one spoken in the home or within the community setting of the major caregivers. In those cases where children acquire more than one language at the same time during the language acquisition years, Crystal (1997) observed that the millions of such children begin their schooling at the same level of language development as their monolingual counterparts.

Likewise, there are many varieties of English spoken in the United States. Although Ebonics received most of the public attention in recent years, numerous regional and social dialects are spoken in the United States. This phenomenon, of course, is true all over the world. For example, there is low German and high German in Germany, received English and Cockney in Great Britain, and standard English and patois in Jamaica.

The estimated percentage of people with a non-English background in the U.S. The first figure is based on a 1976 Survey of Income and Education (after F. Grosjean, 1982); the second is based on the 1990 census. The highest figures are in the northeast (around New York and its hinterland) and in the southwest (where the main influx of Spanish speakers has taken place). The past 20 years has seen a steady increase in the states of the south and along the west coast, most dramatically in California and Florida (Louisiana is the only southern state where the trend is in the opposite direction); most other states show stability or a decrease.

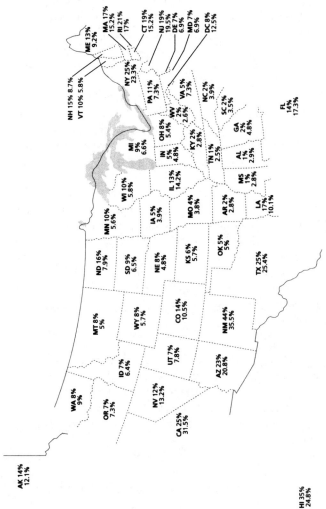

FIGURE 2-2

The percentage of non-English speakers in the United States, 1976 to 1990. (From *The Cambridge Encyclopedia of Language* [2nd ed., p. 363], by D. Crystal, 1997. Cambridge [UK]: Cambridge University Press. Copyright 1997 by Cambridge University Press. Reprinted with permission.)

🔓

CULTURE AND CAREGIVER-CHILD INTERACTIONS

A critical dimension of the language acquisition process revolves around the parenting styles employed by parents or by the adult/sibling/community environment in which a child matures. Heath (1989) cited an array of behaviors in adult–child interactions that may characterize cultural beliefs about the way children develop. For example, she noted that in cultures that believe children "grow up," adults do not intervene with highly specific verbalizations of the here and now or with requests or recounts of shared events.

Conversely, Heath (1989) reported that in cultures where adults believe that children are "raised," adult intervention actions are characterized by verbalizations of step-by-step features, requests of children to recount what is already known to have been experienced by both adults and children, and assertions by adults themselves as primary actors or agents.

Citing numerous researchers and making observations from the African, Canadian, Japanese, Melanesian, Polynesian, and from several cultures within the United States (notably Cajun, middle class white, Mexican American and African American), van Kleeck (1994) made observations about several major aspects of cultural variation that may impact directly on the sociocultural milieu in which a child might acquire language. Recalling an earlier point, it is interesting to note that there is considerable overlap reported in the parenting styles of families all over the world. The five major aspects are:

1. **Social Organization Issues and Interaction**—Who talks to small children, in what contexts and about what topics (Schieffelin & Eisenberg, 1984)? What is the role of siblings in the child rearing and language learning processes? What are the rules governing turn-taking, that is, dyadic versus multiparty during conversations?

2. **The Value of Talk**—What is the amount of talk (and silence) that is valued during interactions? What is the role of talk in teaching children? To what extent is talk considered an indicator of knowledge? Depending on culture, there may be vast differences in the amount of talk provided to children by their families. However, the most important fact to remember in

considering these reports is that children in each of these diverse cultures manage to acquire the language of their environments irrespective of the amount or reported caregiver talk!

3. **Status in Interactions**—Who initiates adult–child interactions? Who directs interactions? Who adapts to whom during interactions? Who carries the burden of understanding during conversations? In nuclear families, the stimulant is typically the mother or the father. In non-nuclear family settings, however, the stimulant is often someone other than an adult, often an older child. In view of the rapidly changing social environments of parenting in North America, it is very likely that changes will also occur in the patterns associated with adult–child and other forms of caregiver–child interactions. In any case, because of great internal variations within cultures, it is highly unlikely for a single description of adult–child interactions for a culture to be applicable for all members of that culture.

4. **Beliefs About Intentionality**—How are the intentions of others determined? When does intentionality begin?

5. **Language Teaching Beliefs**—What are the beliefs concerning the need for direct teaching of language to children? What are beliefs concerning the role of observation in language acquisition? To what extent does the culture believe that multiple approaches are desirable in presenting the culture's language to children?

The classic view in language acquisition theory is that interactions between adults and children form the foundations for the sociocultural context in which a child acquires language. Vygotskii (1962) asserted that as a result of these social and cultural interactions, children come to acquire a set of concepts and thoughts. Over time, verbal and non-verbal symbols are acquired to represent these thoughts and concepts, along with a set of rules for using them—all within the context of cultural norms.

Although the family is thought to be the usual social institution for presenting the behaviors, norms and expectations for children to acquire with respect to language (Anderson & Battle, 1993), the structure of the family and the roles of different family members may vary considerably from culture to culture. For example, extended family environments consisting of several cohorts of individuals, such as grandparents, children of various ages, grandchildren, cousins, nieces/nephews, aunts/uncles, and so on—and residing in the same residence or within close proximity— may provide a wider range of interactions across ages and relationships than in families where the interactions are largely between parents and their children.

Crago (1992) suggested that differences across cultures in caregiver–child discourse affects the quality of the processes of language acquisition. Moreover, cultural perceptions toward children influence adults' assumptions of children's abilities and value to the community. For example, Westby (1986) stated that although one society may seek and respond to gestural and linguistic nuances demonstrated by infants to determine their desires and needs, another culture may anticipate these needs and not allow them to influence the nature of adult–child interactions.

Westby (1986) also cited several specific cultural differences in parenting styles across cultures that may have a direct impact on language acquisition. For example:

- Anglo mothers reportedly are inclined to rely on vocalizations and repositioning when interacting with an infant. Hopi Indian mothers, by contrast, reportedly are inclined to rely more on such tactile movements as bouncing and juggling the infant during interactions (Callaghan, 1981).
- Sibling child rearing is a frequent characteristic of many cultures. (In North America, this phenomenon may become more of a norm as the single parenthood population increases.)
- Some Asian cultures are reported as being inclined to view infants as being born independent, with the culture responsible for developing the child's interdependence on the family and society. Western cultures, by contrast, reportedly are inclined to view the child as being born a dependent being, with the culture responsible for teaching independence and autonomy (Kagan, Kearsley & Zelazo, 1978).

Of course, these reported styles must be viewed with considerable caution in view of the earlier observation that there is considerable variation within cultures. In addition, because modern technology— notably television—has brought cultures into greater contact with one another (particularly Western cultures with the remainder of the world), it is very possible that traditional patterns of child rearing around the world are undergoing considerable changes. In any event, despite whatever differences that may, in fact, exist across cultures, Taylor and Clarke (1994) asserted that a major universal of all language acquisition caregivers, no matter who they are, is that they introduce and provide cues to children about accepted linguistic and communicative behavior within a culture. Moreover, they provide support, guidance, and reinforcement to complement the language learning process.

In addition to the nature of the language and communicative system to be acquired by children and the nature of caregiver–child interactions, culture influences other aspects of language acquisition. For example, culture may influence the preferred cognitive styles involved in language learning. Thus, in those cultures that are field independent (Ramirez & Price-Williams, 1974; Witkin, 1967), or analytical, in nature, the language acquisition process may be characterized by a focus on the finite elements of language, for example, sounds and words. Moreover, the interactions may be characterized by explicit statements of specific "rules" to be employed in acquiring and using language. In such cultures, language acquisition in children may be viewed as a deductive process.

Conversely, children who come from more field-dependent or object-oriented cultures may focus more on social interactions and the dynamics of social relationships as opposed to explicit exhortations on finite elements of the language to be acquired or of the underlying rules governing utterances. In this type of culture, children may be expected to induce or discover rules of communication as a result of having the benefit of these social interactions.

Cognitive style might also influence the discourse strategies employed by parents in the child rearing process and also by the developing child. For example, children who develop language within a culture that has a high preference for a field-independent cognitive style may also tend to cultivate a Topic Centered narrative style. By contrast, children who develop language within a culture that has a high preference for a field-dependent cognitive style may tend to cultivate a Topic Association narrative style.

According to Michaels (1981), Topic Centered (literate strategy) narratives are linear presentations of tightly structured discourse on a single topic or a series of closely related topics that have (1) temporal orientation, (2) thematic focus, coherence and progression, and (3) topic elaboration. These narratives presume little shared knowledge between speakers and listeners, therefore, they involve more "telling" than "sharing."

By contrast Topic Associating (oral strategy) narratives are a series of associated segments that are *implicitly* linked to a topic, but that have no explicit theme. They typically begin with a set of background statements, then shift across segments that are implicitly linked, although temporal orientation, location, and focus of segments often shift from one segment to another. Linkages across segments are left for the listener to infer on a presumption of shared knowledge. These narratives tend to have less detail than Topic Centered narratives and contain more "sharing" than "telling."

With these notions of culture, language, and communication in mind, let us now examine in succeeding chapters what the research literature tells us about language acquisition among select groups of children in North America.

⊔

REFERENCES

Anderson, N. B., & Battle, D. E. (1993). Cultural diversity in the development of language. In Delores Battle (Ed.), *Communication disorders in multicultural populations* (pp. 158–185). Boston: Andover Medical Publishers.

Callaghan, J. W. (1981). A comparison of Anglo, Hopi and Navajo mothers and infants. In T. M. Field, A. M. Sostek, P. Vietze, & P. H. Leiderman (Eds.), *Culture and early interactions.* Hillsdale, NJ: Lawrence Erlbaum.

Crago, M. B. (1992). Ethnography and language socialization: A cross-cultural perspective. *Topics in Language Disorders, 12,* 28–39.

Crystal, D. (1997). *The Cambridge encyclopedia of language* (2nd ed.). Cambridge (U.K.): Cambridge University Press.

Hamayan, E. V., & Damico, J. S. (1991). *Limiting bias in the assessment of bilingual students.* Austin: PRO-ED.

Heath, S. B. (1989). The learner as cultural member. In M. Rice & R. Schiefelbusch (Eds.), *The teachability of language* (pp. 333–350). Baltimore: P. H. Brookes.

Hymes, D. (1966). *On communicative competence.* Paper presented at the Research Planning Conference on Language Development Among Disadvantaged Children, Yeshiva University, New York.

Kagan, J., Kearsley, R. B., & Zelazo, P. R. (1978). *Infancy: Its place in human development.* Cambridge (MA): Harvard University Press.

Lenneberg, E. (1967). *Biological foundations of language.* New York: John Wiley and Sons.

Michaels, S. (1981). "Sharing time": Children's narrative styles and differential access to literacy. *Language in Society, 10,* 423–442.

Ramirez, M., & Price-Williams, D. (1974). Cognitive styles of children of three ethnic groups in the United States. *Journal of Cross-Cultural Psychology, 5,* 212–219.

Saville-Troike, M. (1978). *A guide to culture in the classroom.* Arlington, VA: National Clearinghouse for Bilingual Education.

Saville-Troike, M. (1986). Anthropological considerations in the study of communication. In O. Taylor (Ed.), *Nature of communication disorders in culturally and linguistically diverse Populations* (pp. 47–79). Austin, TX: PRO-ED.

Schieffelin, B., & Eisenberg, A. (1984). Cultural variation in children's conversations. In R. L. Schiefelbusch & J. Pickar (Eds.), *The acquisition of communicative competence.* Baltimore: University Park Press.

Taylor, O. L., & Clarke, M. (1994). Culture and communication disorders: A theoretical perspective. *Seminars in Speech and Language, 15,* 103–114.

van Kleeck, A. (1994). Potential bias in training parents as conversational partners with their children who have delays in language development. *American Journal of Speech-Language Pathology, 3,* 67–78.

Vygotskii, L. S. (1962). *Thought and language.* Cambridge, MA: MIT Press.

Westby, C. E. (1986). *Cultural differences in caregiver-child interaction.* Unpublished manuscript.

Witkin, H. A. (1967). A cognitive styles approach to cross-cultural research. *International Journal of Psychology,* 233–250.

🏳

SUGGESTED READINGS

Battle, D. (1993). *Communication disorders in multicultural populations.* Boston: Andover Press.

Taylor, O. (1986). *Nature of communication disorders in culturally and linguistically diverse populations.* Austin, TX: PRO-ED.

Saville-Troike, Muriel (1989). *The ethnography of communication: An introduction.* New York: Basil Blackwell.

ORLANDO L. TAYLOR, PH.D.

Orlando L. Taylor, Ph.D., is Dean of the Graduate School of Arts and Sciences and graduate Professor of Communication Sciences and Disorders at Howard University in Washington, DC. Taylor's numerous publications have focused principally on the rich linguistic and communicative diversity of the United States, with a particular focus on the language and culture of African Americans. His work has led to the development of new theories and practices related to distinguishing between language differences and language disorders and to teaching standard American English to children who acquire vernacular dialects of English as their first language.

Dr. Taylor is currently president of the National Communication Association. He received his doctoral degree from the University of Michigan. Purdue University awarded him an honorary doctorate degree in 1994.

PART II

THE ACQUISITION OF AFRICAN AMERICAN ENGLISH

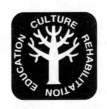

CHAPTER 3

THE ACQUISITION OF AFRICAN AMERICAN ENGLISH: SOCIAL-COGNITIVE AND CULTURAL FACTORS

MICHELE CLARKE WALKER, Ph.D.

The acquisition of African American English (AAE) is influenced by several variables. These variables include, but are not limited to, interactions within the family and broader environment, cognitive styles of learning, gender, age, occupation, and socioeconomic status. AAE has been referred to as a vernacular form of English, with a name that is continually evolving and has included labels such as Black English Vernacular, Black Vernacular English, African American Vernacular English, Black English, and Ebonics. Particular attention has been paid to the degree that AAE varies from Standard American English (SAE).

The language development process experienced by African American children who use AAE has for several years prompted great concern. The children who embrace this form of English have frequently performed below normative groups on several standardized assessments, including tests of speech and language development, regardless of the language/dialect used in testing (Pena & Quinn, 1997).

This chapter has been designed to outline current data-based research that is relevant to the speech and language development of African American speakers of AAE. Highlighted within this effort are sociocultural factors that contribute to the development of AAE in young speakers. Future research needs are also discussed. Elsewhere in this book Ida Stockman addresses semantic development and Harry Seymour and Thomas Roeper discuss the development of grammar.

⊔

FACTORS THAT CONTRIBUTE TO LANGUAGE DEVELOPMENT

Massey (1996) highlighted several questions that are important to the study of language acquisition in African American children that deserve consideration in the examination of the current research, namely:

- What triggers language development?
- What social and cultural variables initiate and propel the process of language acquisition?
- What defines typical language development and use?
- How do we know if a child's language development is on target?

Factors that influence language acquisition and development include, child–caregiver, child–family, child–community, and child–peer interactions occurring within the sociocultural context. These interactions provide the foundation for cultural and linguistic development (Taylor & Clarke, 1994). A developing child learns to imitate the models available to him or her in these interaction dyads which, in turn, promote the acquisition of verbal and nonverbal communication. Just as in other groups, an African American child acquires and develops language within the context of his or her culture. The child is exposed to words, symbols, contexts, emotions, literature, and songs that convey meanings and reinforce principles relevant to the child's culture.

It is worthwhile to examine cultural factors that influence language acquisition and development in African American AAE users to determine patterns of behavior, similarities to SAE users, and idiosyncratic patterns. Such information is useful to the clinician contemplating the need for therapeutic intervention for an AAE speaker and, thus, facilitates more appropriate placement. Further, such an investigation adds to our knowledge of language development and the factors that influence the way different children respond to identical stimuli.

SOCIOECONOMIC STATUS

Contrary to frequent implications found within the literature, African Americans are not members of a homogeneous cultural group (Clarke, 1997; Taylor & Clarke, 1994). Diversity is evident in several aspects of this culture and includes differences in linguistic use and proficiency. Socioeconomic status, genetic predisposition, educational accomplishment, family constellation, religious affiliation, and cognitive styles of learning (in addition to other factors) are each important to the development of language. Any combination of these factors can potentially contribute to the diversity in the language more than any one factor (Terrell & Terrell, 1993). For example, some groups, typically the educated, middle class, embrace SAE. Other groups of African Americans, typically the urban, working class, may embrace AAE. According to Stockman and Vaughn-Cooke (1986), lower income White and Black children use nonstandard forms more frequently than their middle class peers. Several members within the African American culture (middle and working class) are able to competently utilize both language or dialect systems interchangeably to meet their communicative needs, as is appropriate to the social context, which may include audience (e.g., race, level of authority), purpose (e.g., casual conversation, lecture) and conversational intentions (e.g., to teach, to inquire) (Saferstein, 1991; Terrell & Terrell, 1993). Under these circumstances, the speakers utilize bidialectal capabilities to meet their communicative needs.

THE HOME ENVIRONMENT

A child who successfully participates in his or her speech community is considered to be communicatively competent. This child acquires linguistic and grammatical elements of the "home" dialect in addition to developing sensitivity towards the context, function, and meaning of the interactional patterns (Garcia, 1992). The family nucleus assists in this acquisition and instructs the child regarding the fundamental linguistic precepts embraced by the culture. However, the child is not always prepared to enter into a different linguistic environment.

According to Taylor and Payne (1994), when an individual's native language or dialect differs from the official language (or dialect), that individual may learn the official language, but continue to retain characteristics of the first language. The degree to which an individual may utilize both systems is critically related to the level of proficiency in the first language (L1) and the age at which the second language (L2) was acquired (Hymes, 1966). L1 is typically the language found within the home and cultural group of which the child is a member. An individual may have a wide variety of exclusive experiences with the L1 language system until he or she enters the school environment or seeks clinical assistance. If the language of the school or clinic is not the child's L1, the child may experience difficulty meeting the linguistic demands of the new situation. Problems may be seen completing homework assignments successfully, taking topical examinations, responding to questions, and engaging in conversational exchanges with peers, teachers, and speech-language clinicians.

Adaptations and accommodations to L2 may be difficult to accomplish. The level of importance L1 has within its culture, the level of interest an individual has in learning L2, and the opportunities provided to the individual to learn and become proficient in L2 greatly influence successful transition to a different language system.

When African American speakers who use AAE as their L1 enter the school system, they frequently experience transitional difficulties when attempting to learn and embrace SAE. This is because SAE is the official language of the academic setting and seldom accommodates AAE form and use. A child who has been exposed to SAE in the home will inherently have a more successful transition to the academic linguistic system than a child who has been primarily exposed to AAE. However, it is possible for a child to utilize both systems successfully, although the level of success is temporally influenced.

COGNITIVE STYLES OF LEARNING

Hansen and Stansfield (1980) defined cognitive styles as psychological phenomena used to describe individual differences in the way a person perceives, organizes, analyzes, and recalls information and experiences. Cognitive styles appear to influence patterns of learning, thinking, and social interaction. Cognitive styles of learning appear to be influenced by culture (Hunt, 1993; Taylor & Clarke, 1994) and appear to impact how children learn language (Hale, 1994; Nichols, 1987).

Field dependence and field independence are terms used to label differences in processing information and in the use of internal and external frames of reference. Field dependence defines an individual's interpersonal orientation (Hunt, 1993) and embraces global, synthetic thought patterns. These individuals depend less frequently on internal (processing) mechanisms and prefer to relate to external sources, such as other persons. Field-dependent individuals are influenced by affective variables in learning (Creason, 1992) and tend to be socially oriented. They typically initially perceive elements and ideas holistically and only later break them into component parts. According to Lee (1987), individuals who exhibit a field-dependent cognitive style preference tend to rely on context to create and support their language meaning.

Field independence is defined by a capacity to employ internal referents as guides to behavior (Goodenough & Witkin, 1977). These individuals tend to be task- or object-oriented and pay little attention to the external or social environment when attempting to achieve a goal. Field-independent individuals tend to learn inanimate and impersonal material with greater ease than material involving social content and exhibit greatest incidental memory for information that is directly relevant to an assigned task.

No one person or group exclusively exhibits any one cognitive style; however, preferences may be evident from early preschool years. Most studies of cognitive styles in African Americans have concentrated on the working class and concluded that this group exhibits field-dependent preferences. Just as is true for other cultural groups, African Americans (from working class backgrounds) can exhibit preferences for field independence and field dependence. There is evidence that children who are exposed to the academic environment become increasingly field independent with age (Witkin, Oltman, Raskin, & Karp, 1971). The distinction between field independence and field dependence does not denote differences in ability, but rather differences in execution (Taylor & Clarke, 1994). Adapting to an academic environment that embraces field-independent precepts increases the transitional difficulties that AAE-speaking field-dependent children experience.

🔁

A RETROSPECTIVE ON SPEECH AND LANGUAGE ACQUISITIONAL RESEARCH

Although language acquisition research within other groups has been longstanding and consistent, empirical and ethnographic research describing the speech and language skills of African American children has been sparse. In fact, acquisition research within the African American population was not initiated until the mid-to-late 1970s (Stockman, 1986). Little research has been conducted, although African Americans are officially the largest minority group within the United States (U.S. Bureau of Census, 1994) and are represented in large numbers within clinical and special education settings. Research in this area has been sparse for three primary reasons. First, it is difficult to prioritize the areas of need; second, most researchers are not familiar enough with the African American culture to provide accurate information on language acquisition and development within this population; and third, some researchers are uninterested in this area of study.

As acquisition research has been limited, needs assessment research has also been an area of concern within the literature. According to Craig (1996), past research on African Americans focused on the viability and linguistic integrity of the nonstandard English forms used by African Americans. Research has also focused on ways to accommodate dialectal differences in speech for analysis and assessment to differentiate the language skills of children who are typically developing and those with language disorders.

Studies focusing on speech and language acquisition and development in African Americans have historically targeted the urban, working class. Several studies have been published that provide language comparisons of low-income African American children with those of middle class counterparts. Thankfully, such studies are seldom seen within the linguistic literature today, although the benchmark for typical development continues to be based on norms previously established using the middle class majority culture children. Other studies that have included African American children in the subject pool have included them in numbers that are barely detectable for evaluating significance in performance.

African American children's language skills are frequently assessed using instruments that are more applicable to other groups of children and to other styles of acquisition. Most standardized language tests actually examine the amount of standard language a child has acquired rather than how much of the child's target language he or she has acquired. Because of the misconceptions regarding the language skills of working class African American children in the research literature, there is a need for more culturally sensitive information about the linguistic abilities exhibited by these children. Ethnographic and empirical research methodologies are needed to provide important information about the speech and language skills of working class African Americans and other groups of children from backgrounds other than white middle class.

ᗡ

CURRENT SPEECH AND LANGUAGE ACQUISITION RESEARCH

Despite the existing limitations in language acquisition research that focuses on African American speakers of AAE, some compelling and informative research designs have recently been completed. Let us examine the current research on these children's speech and language acquisition skills. From this we see that most of the current research on African American children has examined the surface structure of the language, such as phonology. An investigation using Bloom and Lahey's (1978) form, content, and use will assist us in targeting what research is needed for these particular children. It is, however, equally important that research be conducted for children from other culturally and linguistically diverse groups. Comparisons in performance will assist us in understanding the similarities and differences that may exist in the language development skills of children from cultural backgrounds different from the dominant culture. This information is important to issues of assessment and intervention and is discussed further at the conclusion of this chapter.

⊐

BLOOM AND LAHEY'S (1978)
CONTENT, FORM, AND USE

LANGUAGE CONTENT

Language content is the meaning represented in language that is shared through common human experiences (Lahey, 1988). It is defined by what people talk about. What people talk about depends on their experiences. The language content categories include objects (specific objects and classes of objects), relations between objects (similarities, differences, and relationships), and relations between events (or within a single event). For language content to be expressed, however, it must have language form. Language content is most commonly referred to as semantics.

Research into the semantic language development of African American children has increased in recent years due greatly to the work of Stockman and Vaughn-Cooke (1986). In a landmark study, these authors questioned whether working class African American children exhibited the same developmental proficiencies in acquiring semantic categories as other groups of working class and middle class American children. The authors examined the stages of acquisition, ages of the children at these acquisition points, and order of semantic category acquisition. They further examined whether the types of words acquired and the order of acquisition were comparable to those of children in other linguistic communities. The results indicated that typically developing nonstandard speakers of English "build their surface linguistic forms on the same kind of semantic base that standard speakers do" (p. 22). In fact, Stockman and Vaughn-Cooke (1986) confirmed that semantic categories such as action, state, location, and possession appeared to be universally acquired in early language.

Craig and Washington (1995) investigated the potential relationship between AAE and semantic complexity. They found that a group of urban, low-income African American preschool-aged children exhibited a statistically significant positive relationship between degree of AAE form use and relational semantic complexity (prepositional meaning). The authors also noted that there were no significant relationships between simpler prepositional meanings and AAE form use.

In the area of vocabulary assessment, Pena and Quinn (1997) examined the vocabulary test performance of working class African American and Puerto Rican preschool-aged children. The researchers were specifically interested in these children's performance on two language tests with varying task demands, one that matched skills trained at home and one that did not. In addition, the researchers were interested in which of the two tests most accurately differentiated children who were typically developing and those with low-language ability. They found that the children in this particular study performed better on a descriptive subtest of the *Stanford-Binet Intelligence Scale* that required description than on the *Expressive One-Word Picture Vocabulary Test* (EOWPVT), a test that requires labeling. Also, the *Standford-Binet* subtest appeared to better differentiate typical development from low-language ability. Overall, the researchers believed that to assess the true language ability of children from diverse cultures, tasks should be matched to sociocultural familiarity. Tasks that match the linguistic demands found within a child's home appeared to better indicate linguistic ability than tasks that do not.

Clarke (1997) assessed differences in 4-year-old African American girls' ability to rapidly grasp the meanings of novel object, action, attribute, and affective state words after testing each child's cognitive style of learning. The results of the receptive and expressive vocabulary tasks revealed that, although the girls exhibited similar receptive vocabulary responses, significant differences were noted in expressive action word responses. Clarke suggested that the girls who were field-dependent had an affinity toward relational meanings that allowed them to perform significantly different from the girls who were field independent on the action word "mapping" task.

These studies seem to suggest that, although African American children share a similar semantic base with other groups of children, their use and expression of the language may differ. In fact, sociocultural experience appears to greatly influence how language is expressed.

LANGUAGE FORM

Lahey (1988) described language form as "the shape or contour of the surface features of what is actually said." The underlying rule system for language form includes syntax, morphology and phonology.

SYNTAX

Language syntax is expressed through rule-governed word order in an effort to express a thought. The rules for syntax assist in expressing an intended meaning (language content).

Craig and Washington (1994) investigated the complex syntax usage of urban, low-income African American preschool-aged children. Analyses of spontaneous language samples indicated that the amounts of complex syntax usage varied across subjects from 0 to 25%. The authors found that the number of different types of complex syntax positively correlated with the percentage of utterances containing complex syntax. Some types of complex syntax were widely used by the children, including: (1) two of the three types of infinitives that were marked with *to,* (2) the conjunction *and* to link two independent clauses, (3) noninfinitive *wh*-clauses, (4) noun-phrase complements, and (5) let's/lemme. The play schemes that the children were exposed to, although spontaneous in nature, may have facilitated use of some forms over others. Children develop their play schemes in the home and broader environment and call on those schemes to assist them in novel play activities. Again, we see that a child's experiences influence current and future activity.

MORPHOLOGY

A morpheme has been described as the smallest unit of speech that carries meaning (Lahey, 1988). These units make up the function words and inflections found in the language. Inflections are bound to parts of speech and mark differences in meaning. The relationship between parts of speech and the inflections are formalized by the syntax of a sentence.

African American English affects morphosyntax in primary ways (Craig, 1996). The mean length of utterance (MLU) is a measure that is widely used to analyze the verbal expressive output of young children. In AAE, several morphological forms differ from SAE. An African American child's MLU can easily be misrepresented regardless of the focus of the MLU analysis, whether for morphemes or for words. Very little difference in morphosyntactic development between speakers of AAE and SAE can be noted before age 3 years. However, between 3 and 5 years of age, when social class differences appear to have the greatest influence on language, the influences of AAE become more pronounced in a young child's speech.

PHONOLOGY

The early phonemic development of speakers of AAE and SAE are quite similar (Battle, 1997). Differences in features are usually not apparent until sometime after age 5 years. Protocols utilized to assess the articulation skills exhibited by African American children, especially speakers of AAE, have come under severe scrutiny in recent years. Cole and Taylor (1990) questioned the extent to which phonological performance varied as a function of test-client incongruence on three different tests of articulation among African American AAE speakers and the extent to which the children's performance on these tests lead to misdiagnosis of pathology when dialect considerations were not recognized.

Ten low-income African American children were individually assessed using the picture test of the *Templin–Darley Test of Articulation* (2nd edition), the *Arizona Articulation Proficiency Scale: Revised,* and the *Photo Articulation Test.* Each response received two scores. One score was given according to the criteria set for each test. A second score was based on the phonological rules of AAE.

Results of testing indicated that the African American children performed differently on the tests as a function of the linguistic norms used to score test items. The results also indicated that when dialectal variation is not taken into consideration, there is an increased likelihood that AAE speakers will be misdiagnosed as having articulation disorders. However, adjusting test scores in consideration of dialectal differences would not necessarily solve the problem (Cole & Taylor, 1990). An integrative approach to evaluation would assist in increasing the validity of testing procedures and results.

Moran (1993) examined the speech of 10 African American children to determine if African American children delete final consonants in a particular manner that may have been previously overlooked. He argued that most assessments of phonology were based on perceptual judgments. These judgments could lead to incorrect assumptions of a child's phonological knowledge.

In the first of two experiments, each child was asked to identify 40 pictures given a carrier phrase. The 40 pictures comprised 20 minimal pairs. Tape recorded speech samples were obtained and were analyzed for evidence of final consonant deletions. A second analysis included examining the vowel length in words from which the final consonant was deleted. Vowel length was determined by sonograph. Experiment 2 involved training the listeners in narrow phonetic transcription prior to analyzing words for final consonant deletions.

The results of the two experiments indicated that African American children possess phonological knowledge of the final consonants that were perceived to be deleted by the trained listeners. The authors suggested that the children may have been using vowel length as a contrastive feature, a point previously noted by other authors. Alternately, the authors pointed out that the children may have been making the articulatory gesture toward the final consonant, but fell short of a complete production.

Of the data-based research that focused on the phonological and articulation skills of African Americans, most have assessed these children's performance based on the performance of children from other groups (normative samples). Typically these other groups have consisted of children whose cultural and linguistic background were different from the children in question. The normative data have provided information about children who are members of that group, but are inappropriately used as a point of comparison against the speech performance of African American speakers of AAE (Bleile & Wallach, 1992).

Few studies have considered cultural attitudes toward speech performance. Bleile and Wallach (1992) embarked on a preliminary investigation to gain insight into how people belonging to the African American community judge the speech of preschoolers from that community. This study focused on African American Head Start teachers who lived and worked in the children's communities. The teachers were asked to identify children in their classes "who understood pretty well, but had trouble speaking." The children who were identified by the teachers were tested using the *Photo Articulation Test*. Results indicated that teachers successfully identified children within their classrooms who exhibited difficulty in articulation. The authors then suggested that community views about who is considered to have disordered speech are as important as "traditional metrics." They added, however, that selecting a group to serve as a judge of behavior within a community must be accomplished carefully and results should be interpreted with caution.

It is important to consider that members of like communities may more accurately identify instances of linguistic incongruence. These individuals have the benefit of cultural experience and can assist speech-language pathologists in achieving diagnostic precision.

LANGUAGE USE

Lahey (1988) outlined three major aspects of language use: (1) the use of language for different goals, (2) the use of contextual information to guide what we say to meet linguistic goals, and (3) the use of the interaction between individuals to initiate, maintain, and terminate conversations.

Language use is called pragmatics. Recent research has little to add about the pragmatic language skills of African American AAE-speaking children. One of the only studies available was a dissertation by Saferstein (1991).

PRAGMATICS

Saferstein (1991) examined the pragmatic language attributes of 8-year-old African American and White American children with disabilities. Utterances obtained from the children were categorized according to the *Advanced Pragmatic Checklist* (APC). Results revealed no statistically significant differences between the two groups on the pragmatic language categories of interaction and intention. Statistically significant differences were noted in appropriate responses, sequencing information in order of time and importance, and identification and possession of events categories. In these categories, African Americans scored significantly higher than their counterparts. White Americans scored significantly higher in establishing a topic and compliance responses.

Battle (1997) pointed out that, young children who are culturally and linguistically diverse, will imitate, ask questions, express their needs verbally and nonverbally, answer questions, and be interested in stories and tales. These children may also respond differently to questions. In certain African American groups, the way that stories and tales are told may differ qualitatively from storytelling of other groups. Due to differences in communicative style and/or a lack of resources (storybooks), the oral tradition may be used to facilitate topic maintenance and conversational turn-taking skills, hence the preference for a topic-associated narrative style within the African American culture. The development of this style could then be related to the ability to sequence information in order of time and importance. If stories are relayed to AAE-speaking children differently then they are relayed to SAE-speaking children, differences in narrative style would be expected.

⊏⊐

CONCLUSION

This chapter examined sociocultural factors that influence and contribute to the acquisition of AAE in young speakers. We have also explored existing research to help determine areas of research need.

Note that the acquisition of AAE includes more than the acquisition of a rule system for syntax, morphology, semantics, phonology, and pragmatics, but is also influenced by the speaker's orientation and experiences within his or her environment. Children learning language acquire more than just the static components needed to communicate. They also learn those elements of the language that facilitate communicative competence. Children who are native speakers of AAE and have developed communicative competence within their cultural group may have a difficult transition to a novel language system such as SAE. After all, to fully acquire a second system, an individual must also acquire the unspoken components of that system. In addition, the age of acquisition and the level of importance the new system has within the child's culture influences the level of proficiency in acquisition and use.

Research investigating the language acquisition skills of African Americans has varied in the manner of data collection, age, class, and method of study (Battle, 1997). In general, data-based research in speech and language development is needed for all children, regardless of their cultural or linguistic origin. To date, however, a vast amount of the completed research has focused on a monolithic group of children. Results and implications from these research paradigms are frequently embraced and have been used to generalize behavioral patterns to other groups.

Using Bloom and Lahey's (1978) form, content, and use paradigm as a guide, it is obvious that not enough is known about African American AAE-speaking children's language skills. Yet, these children are frequently thought to require therapeutic intervention and specialized educational services. Most working class African American children who enter the special education system remain there throughout their school career. This means that a path to failure in adulthood has been established from as young as preschool-age. We can, however, start with what we know about African American children and their path to language acquisition and development to establish a foundation for future studies.

Several conclusions about the acquisition of language in African American children as posed by Stockman (1986) and van Keulen, Weddington, and DeBose (1998) can be drawn:

■ Language is acquired within a particular time frame. Children acquire semantic categories in a developmental sequence and the ability to do so increases with age. Stockman and Vaughn-Cooke (1986) indicated that African American children acquired semantic categories in ways comparable to other groups of children.

■ Locke (1994) posited that children should accumulate a minimal storage of lexical items to facilitate the triggering of the grammatical analysis mechanism. African American children could be included in this group; however, further study is warranted.

■ African American children tend to exhibit topic associating conversational/storytelling styles, comment on the environment, and utilize verbal persuasion.

■ Just as in other groups, African American children's mean length of utterance (MLU) increases with age. However, a clinician should be aware that AAE-speaker MLUs computed in morphemes may differ from SAE speakers, but this may not indicate delayed skills.

■ Children increasingly acquire AAE forms as they develop and have increased experiences around AAE users.

The definition of typical linguistic behavior can be difficult to determine when assessing children from diverse backgrounds. A few suggestions have been offered to remedy this problem:

■ Researchers should continue to provide developmental data (using different research paradigms) on the speech and language skills of African American children, in general, and AAE speakers, in particular;

■ Investigators should not hesitate to investigate the speech and language skills of African American children just because they, themselves, are not members of that group;

■ Before engaging in research to study the speech and language skills of African American children, investigators should first examine their level of cultural sensitivity and, if necessary, seek assistance from others who have more experience with the population in question;

■ Investigators should make special efforts to include low-income African American children in their methodologies (where appropriate) and should also include children from (various) other cultural and linguistic backgrounds to provide information about similarities and differences in performance;

■ Training is paramount. Investigators should train students in the allied health professions to consider sociocultural factors that influence speech and language development in all children;

- Investigators should (whenever possible) consider the attitudes and perceptions of the culture of which an individual is a member to determine normalcy or deficiency of linguistic behavior for that group; and
- Both ethnographic and empirical methodologies are warranted in the study of the speech and language skills of African American AAE users.

⊔

REFERENCES

Battle, Delores, E. (1997). Language and communication disorders in culturally and linguistically diverse children. In D. K. Bernstein & E. Tiegerman-Farber (Eds.), *Language and communication disorders in children.* Needham Heights, MA: Allyn and Bacon.

Bleile, K. N., & Wallach, H. (1992). A sociolinguistic investigation of the speech of African American preschoolers. *American Journal of Speech-Language Pathology, 1,* 54–62.

Bloom, L. & Lahey, M. (1978). *Language development and language disorders.* New York: John Wiley.

Clarke, M. G. (1997). *A study of cognitive style and fast mapping skill exhibited by middle class, Black American four-year-old girls.* Unpublished doctoral dissertation, Howard University, Washington, DC.

Cole, P. A., & Taylor, O. L. (1990). Performance of working class African American children on three tests of articulation. *Language, Speech, and Hearing Services in Schools, 21,* 171–176.

Craig, H. K. (1996). The challenges of conducting language research with African American children. In A. G. Kamhi, K. E. Pollock, & J. L. Harris (Eds.), *Communication development and disorders in African American children: Research, assessment, and intervention* (pp.1–17). Baltimore: P. H. Brookes Publishing Co.

Craig, H. K., & Washington, J. A. (1994). The complex syntax skills of poor, urban, African American preschoolers at school entry. *Language, Speech and Hearing Services in Schools, 25,* 181–190.

Craig, H. K., & Washington, J. A. (1995). African American English and linguistic complexity in preschool discourse: A second look. *Language, Speech, and Hearing Services in Schools, 26,* 87–93.

Creason, P. (1992). *Changing demographics and the importance of culture in student learning styles.* Unpublished paper.

Garcia, G. E. (1992). Ethnography and classroom communication: Taking an "emic" perspective. *Topics in Language Disorders, 12,* 54–66.

Goodenough, D. R., & Witkin, H. A. (1977). Origins of the field-dependent and field-independent cognitive styles. *Educational Testing Service.* Princeton, New Jersey. Unpublished paper.

Hale, J. E. (1994). *Unbank the fire: Visions for the education of African American children.* Baltimore: Johns Hopkins University Press.

Hansen, J. & Stansfield, C. (1980). *The relationship of field-dependent-independent cognitive styles to foreign language achievement.* Unpublished paper.

Hunt, S. (1993, November). *Cultural perspectives and thinking: The African American thinker in the classroom.* Paper presented at the annual meeting of the Speech Communication Association, Miami Beach, FL.

Hymes, D. (1966). *On communicative competence.* Paper presented at the Research Planning Conference on Language Development Among Disadvantaged Children, Yeshiva University, NY.

Lahey, M. (1988). *Language disorders and language development.* New York: Mac-Millan Publishing Co.

Lee, D. L. (1987). *The effects of object-oriented and socially-oriented pictures upon elicited language of children with differing visual perceptual cognitive styles.* Unpublished doctoral dissertation, Howard University, Washington, DC.

Locke, J. L. (1994). Gradual emergence of developmental language disorders. *Journal of Speech and Hearing Research, 37,* 608–616.

Massey, A. (1996). Cultural influences on language assessment and intervention. In A. G. Kamhi, K. E. Pollock, & J. L. Harris (Eds.), *Communication development and disorders in African American children: Research, assessment, and intervention* (pp. 285–306). Baltimore: P. H. Brookes Publishing Co.

Moran, M. J. (1993). Final consonant deletion in African American children speaking Black English: A closer look. *Language, Speech, and Hearing Services in Schools, 24,* 161–166.

Nichols, E. (1987). *The philosophical aspects of cultural difference.* Unpublished outline.

Pena, E., & Quinn, R. (1997). Task familiarity: Effects on the test performance of Puerto Rican and African American children. *Language, Speech, and Hearing Services in Schools, 28,* 323–332.

Saferstein, S. A. (1991). *A comparative analysis of discourse in African American and White learning disabled children.* Unpublished doctoral dissertation, Howard University, Washington, DC.

Stockman, I. J. (1986). Language acquisition in culturally diverse populations: The Black child as a case study. In O. L. Taylor (Ed.), *Nature of communication disorders in culturally and linguistically diverse populations* (pp. 117–155). Austin: PRO-ED.

Stockman, I. J., & Vaughn-Cooke, F. B. (1986). Implications of semantic category research for the language assessment of nonstandard speakers. *Topics in Language Disorders, 6,* 15–25.

Taylor, O. L., & Clarke, M. G. (1994). Communication disorders and cultural diversity: A theoretical framework. *Seminars in Speech and Language, 15,* 103–113.

Taylor, O. L., & Payne, K. T. (1994). Language and communication differences. In G. H. Shames, E. H. Wiig, & W. A. Secord (Eds.), *Human communication disorders: An introduction* (4th ed, pp. 118–143). New York: Merrill: Maxwell Macmillan International.

Terrell, S. L., & Terrell, F. (1993). African American cultures. In D. E. Battle (Ed.), *Communication disorders in multicultural populations* (pp. 3–37). Boston: Andover Medical Publishers.

U.S. Bureau of the Census (1994). Populations of the United States, trends and prospects. In *Current Population Reports*. Washington, DC: U.S. Government Printing Office.

van Keulen, J. E., Weddington, G. T., & DeBose, C. E. (1998). *Speech, language, learning and the African American child* (pp. 81–110). Boston: Allyn and Bacon.

Witkin, H. A., Oltman, P. K., Raskin, E., & Karp, S. A. (1971). *A manual for the Embedded Figures Tests*. Palo Alto, CA: Consulting Psychologists Press.

MICHELE CLARKE WALKER, PH.D.

Michele Clarke Walker, Ph.D., currently serves as a lecturer in the Department of Hearing and Speech Sciences at the University of Maryland—College Park and as an Adjunct Assistant Professor in the Department of Communication Sciences and Disorders at Howard University, where she also received her doctorate. Dr. Walker is a Fellow of the Maternal and Child Health Bureau. Her research interests and publications have focused on typical language development in preschool-age children from culturally and linguistically diverse populations and on language acquisition in children with neurodevelopmental impairments.

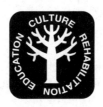

CHAPTER 4

SEMANTIC DEVELOPMENT OF AFRICAN AMERICAN CHILDREN

IDA J. STOCKMAN, Ph.D.

Semantics is concerned broadly with the study of linguistic meaning (O'Grady, Dobrovolsky, & Aronoff, 1989). Meaning is a critical aspect of language as a tool of social communication. At its root, communication is the shared interpretation of messages (Robinson, 1988). It is successful when the semantic value of words creates the same sense of reality in both the speaker and listener. To acquire semantic competence, children rely on their stored knowledge about the world to figure out what words mean in a language (Crais, 1990).

Semantic mapping ought to challenge the child because there is not an inherent relationship between words and the meanings they represent. Moreover, the semantic boundaries of words are not fixed (Labov, 1973). Whereas word forms conform to finite patterns of morphosyntactic regularity in the surface structure of a language, given the natural constraints on perceiving and producing speech sounds, their meanings are neither finite nor overt. Meanings must be constructed from personal experience, which necessarily occurs in a cultural context among other types of contexts (K. Nelson, 1985). Consequently, the meanings of words are portable and variable across individuals within and across cultures to the extent that the contexts of real experiences differ. The word, *house*, can bring to mind an adobe hut for one individual or a mansion for another. It is this individual variability of experience that requires meaning to be negotiated even among competent speakers of the same language, if communication is to be truly a "meeting of the minds."

Semantic competence means that a child has learned how words map onto their shared conventional meanings as understood by other speakers in the linguistic community. However, conventional meaning is not universal. Languages are selective about which aspects of experiences are coded and how they are coded. For example, languages differ in which aspects of experience are lexicalized and therefore efficiently coded. Apparently, the language-specific organization of a lexicon can bias early lexical development enough to question the dominant appeal of a universal cognitive explanation for semantic learning (Bowerman, 1989). For example, when learning to talk about spatial relations, English speakers first use words to code containment (*in*) and support (*on*). Korean children's earliest words refer to looseness and tightness of fit for objects in contact (Choi & Bowerman, 1991). Language-specific lexical biases in early development continue to show up as this kind of crosslinguistic inquiry has been extended to other groups, namely Dutch and Tzeltal Mayan (Bowerman, 1995).

Studies of European languages have led to the conclusion that topological relations among objects such as containment, support, and proximity emerge before projective relations or spatial coordinates of a landscape. But in some cultures (e.g., Mayan Tzeltal in Southern Mexico and Balinese in Southeast Asia), children talk about projective before proximal space (cf. P. Brown & Levinson, 1995; Dasen & Wassmann, 1995). The findings in the Balinese culture were attributed to its religious practices. It is important in the culture to determine direction, which is sacred. The temples of worship are always located north and uphill from the sea. Thus, cultural practices may force children to pay attention to projective spatial notions at earlier ages in some cultures than in others.

This focus on meaning as the product of culture and language-specific differences counters the usual emphasis on meaning as the product of universal human experience. There is, of course, reason to believe that languages do code common meanings despite their different symbolic forms. Otherwise, it would not be possible to translate from one language to another, as we know persons who are bilingual can do. Dialects of the same language are expected to have even greater semantic congruence than different languages, especially if they share a common lexicon, geographical location, and national history. Consequently, it is not surprising that crosslinguistic studies seldom consider dialect difference in efforts to sort out what is universal and particular about semantic knowledge. Yet semantic differences do exist even among different dialects of the same language. The same word can have a broader range of semantic distinctions in one regional dialect than another (Wolfram, 1991). It ought not be surprising to observe more extreme differences among social dialects, particularly when the speakers of one dialect have been culturally isolated from those of another dialect, and therefore, bring different life experiences to the language learning task.

A case in point is the social dialect spoken by many African Americans in the United States. Their U.S. slave history and forced social segregation until the latter half of the 20th century created a unique and separate indigenous cultural experience relative to other citizens even in the same geographical regions. This cultural history has had strong linguistic consequences. It has affected the semantic distinctions as much as it has affected the grammatical rules of the English dialect variously labeled as Ebonics, Black English (BE), or African American Vernacular English (AAVE). The latter term (AAVE) is used in this chapter.

Research on the semantic development of African American children is worthy for both theoretical and practical reasons. It can shed further light on if and how the universal assumptions about language acquisition might be tempered by specific linguistic-cultural experience. At the same time, there has been an urgent need to gather normative data on African American children to improve the adequacy of clinical and educational service delivery.

This chapter aims to take stock of what seems to be known about the acquisition of meaning by African American children who acquire AAVE. Specifically, its goals are to:

1. Describe the ways in which the semantic distinctions of AAVE can be expected to differ from Standard English (SE) dialects.
2. Summarize and evaluate the research on the semantic development of African American children.
3. Identify crosscultural issues that affect the assessment of semantic knowledge for clinical and research purposes.

First, it is necessary to specify the sense in which meaning is viewed in this chapter.

⊔

DELINEATING THE SCOPE
OF MEANING

Meaning is complex, because it can be described on multiple levels that cross domains of inquiry (cf. linguistics, philosophy, and cognitive and social psychology) (N. Nelson, 1986). This chapter focuses on word meaning in native spoken languages as used for social communication. Meaning is the referential content of words and constitutes the semantic structure of a language (O'Grady et al., 1989).

Semantics specifies the relationship of words and sentences to the external reality of objects and events as actually experienced or conceptually known (reference).[1] At the lexical level, for example, semantic knowledge enables children to know that the word **chair** refers to the perceived reality of a particular object (e.g., a rocking chair). It also enables a child to know that the same word **chair** codes a conceptual category that includes rocking chairs never before experienced plus chairs that are not rockers, such as sofa chairs, high chairs, and so on.

Semantics also specifies how the meanings of words relate to one another in the lexicon (sense). For example, it enables a child to know that the meaning of the word **chair** is included in the meaning of other words that have either a subordinate or superordinate referential relationship to the word (hyponomy). For example, **chair** is subordinate to **furniture** (chair is a type of furniture) but superordinate to words that code different types of chairs. Its referents include rocking chair, high chair, and sofa chair, all of which are related to a common sitting function. The word **sit** is the opposite in meaning to the word **stand** (antonymy) and the words **sit, dwell,** and **occupy** all have similar meanings (synonymy). Further, the word **chair** can have multiple meanings (polysemy). For example, **chair** refers not only to an inanimate piece of

---

[1] Reference is conflated here to include the relationship between words and events actually experienced and the relationship of words to a conceptual category, although the latter is often treated separately as **denotation** in some formal linguistic frameworks (e.g., Lyons, 1977).

furniture, but also to a person who leads a meeting, committee, or board, as in *chairs a meeting.*

At the sentence level, semantic knowledge enables children to know the relationship between word combinations and a range of relationships that can hold between objects in the real world. For example, one object can act on another to change its location, physical appearance, or ownership. It also enables children to distinguish sentences that do not express true propositions or reflections of reality from those that do when both include identical words and morphosyntactic structure, as in the following examples:

(1) Chairs eat termites.
(2) Termites eat chairs.

The first sentence is anomalous, except in an appropriate figurative context. The coded relationship between chair and termite does not respect the animate/inanimate semantic distinction in English. Chairs are designated as inanimate and cannot literally eat things, whereas termites are animate and can do so.

Linguistic meaning as reference and sense of a shared conventional code clearly differs from other ways to describe meaning that are not part of this chapter. The focus on linguistic meaning is set apart from meaning in the broader sense of what is involved in the nonverbal mental representation of experience. The focus on the conventional meaning of words obviously differs from their private, idiosyncratic meaning. Bloom (1994) distinguished private and public meanings and argued that children are driven to learn a conventional language to share their private meanings, to get work done in the world, and to be socially and affectively connected to it.

Linguistic meaning as reference and sense also differs from the social or pragmatic meaning of language. Social meaning respects that we usually want people to act or do something in response to the word/referent relations expressed. In generating a sentence such as "Termites eat chairs," we might wish to get listeners to understand a point, carry out an action, laugh, or cry. Although the function of expression may motivate the choice of word/referent relationships coded, behavioral descriptions of pragmatics do not focus on the objects and events that are coded by words. Instead, pragmatics is concerned with how word/referent relationships are used to achieve social interactive goals.

⊔

FORM/MEANING RELATIONSHIPS BETWEEN AAVE AND SE

Acquiring semantic competence is the process of discovering how the rules of a target language or dialect map onto experiences with objects and events. The arbitrariness of form/meaning relations in languages allows many pairing options that may or may not match those expressed even in different dialects of the same language.

Four types of form/meaning relationships can exist between two languages or dialects:

1. They can have identical forms and referents, in which case there are no differences.
2. They can have different forms and different referents.
3. They can have different forms for the same referents.
4. They can have different referents for the same forms.

These four patterns exemplify the relationship between AAVE, the minority dialect acquired by many African American children, and standard English (SE), the dialect of wider communication.

CROSS-DIALECT SIMILARITY

AAVE requires children to learn many words whose form and meaning are identical to the words in SE dialects. These include many commonly and frequently used words for coding objects (car, baby, house, doll), actions (eat, drink, cry), attributes (red, hot), locations (in, on, under), and so on. If dialects of the same language are more similar than different, then we can expect the largest number of words learned by AAVE speakers to be identical to those in SE. But apparently, the differences that do show up are pervasive enough to stress crosscultural communication between AAVE and SE speakers.

CROSS-DIALECT DIFFERENCES

Smitherman (1994) identified more than 1,000 words and phrases with unique Afrocentric meaning. Among them were words like *boojee, bo-*

gue, kwanza, sadiddy, doofus, gumby, hoodoo, ankh, and *wigga,* which are not commonly found in SE speech or print (see also Dillard [1977] and Molefi [1990]). These different dialect forms are the products of innovations, a source of language difference and change. Innovations reflect speakers' creative efforts to make a language fit their particular needs and they exist in every language. Speakers of all languages create words by using such strategies as lexical compounding, blending, clipping, borrowing, and so on (Sornig, 1981; Wolfram, 1991). AAVE speakers have derived new words using the same strategies, as can be seen in Table 4–1. However, such innovations in all dialects are usually treated first as colloquial or vulgar uses of language and often referred to as slang (Andersson & Trudgill, 1990). But clearly some of these uses do become legitimized after a time. Such words as *honeysuckle, bewitched, smog, radar, gas,* and so on are now so commonly accepted in print and speech that it is hard to remember that they were not always regarded as standard usage. Also see examples of Africanisms in English and American culture (Dalgish, 1982; Holloway, 1990; Molefi, 1990).

Given a generally negative view of innovative language use, coupled with the low social status of African American speakers, it is not surprising that innovative words unique to AAVE are slow to be recognized as legitimate forms. The group's unique language forms are treated simply as slang. Yet speakers from nonmainstream cultures and languages may be prone to linguistic innovations to provide meaning to a shared minority group experience and culture that is not coded by a mainstream language or dialect. Although slang has evaded rigorous scholarly definition, scholars agree that its shared use solidifies group identity (Andersson & Trudgill, 1990). According to Smitherman (1994), African Americans deliberately created an in-group code for self-protection during slavery. Obviously, the innovative uses of the language lead to AAVE and SE differences in the form/content relations expressed.

NONOVERLAPPING RELATIONSHIPS: DIFFERENT FORMS AND DIFFERENT REFERENTS

Innovations can lead to unfamiliar forms that also have unfamiliar meaning in two languages or dialects. This maximum difference between two languages requires both a form and a content shift in cross-cultural communication. This difference is probably most common to different languages spoken in separate geographical locations and cultures. It is likely to account for only a small amount of the difference

TABLE 4-1

Examples of innovation in standard English and African-American vernacular English.

Process	Definition	Examples	Examples from AAVE
compounding	two or more existing words are combined to form a new word	ingroup, honeysuckle, badmouth	hotcomb, basehead littlebug, banjyboy
derivation	affixes are added to create new forms or change the part of speech	forestry, badness, bewitched	airish – putting on white ways homey – person from hometown
borrowing	words from other languages are incorporated into the language or dialect	moccasin (American Indian) delicatessen (German) arroyo (Spanish)	hip (Wolof), bogue (Hausa), Kwanza (Swahili)
blending	parts of two words are combined to form a new word	smog (smoke/fog) brunch (breakfast/lunch) sitcom (situation/comedy)	wigga (white nigger) wannabe (want to be white)
acronyms	new words are formed by taking the initial sounds or letters from existing words	radar (radio detecting and range) WASP (white Anglo Saxon Protestant) UN (United Nations)	OG (original gangster) HNIC (head nigger in charge) PP (personal problems)
clipping	words are formed by shortening an existing word	gas (gasoline) dorm (dormitory) perm (permanent)	hood (neighborhood), cuz (cousin) tude (attitude), ig (ignore)
conversion	words are shifted from one part of speech to another without any change in their form	run (as a noun in "They scored a run.") bottle (as a verb in "She bottled the water.") tree (as a verb in "They treed a cat.")	dog – (as a verb in "to dog someone out") humpin (as an adjective in "he's humpin" to mean "very good looking") jet (as a verb in "he gotta jet now" to mean "run fast") book (as a verb in "he's gotta book" to mean "to leave")

Source: Adapted with permission from *Dialects and American English*, by W. Wolfrom, 1991, p. 39. Englewood Cliffs, NJ: Prentice Hall.

68

between two dialects with a common lexicon such as AAVE and SE. Exceptions are the clearly borrowed words from other languages that refer to ethnic customs (e.g., special celebrations, foods, dress, and so on), which have no parallels in mainstream life. For example the word Kwanzaa was recently created (Karenga, 1985). The word, borrowed from Swahili (kwanzee for first fruit) refers to a special African American celebration in winter. Words also are created to refer to ethnic dress and hair style (e.g., hotcomb, cornrows, ankh). However, nonoverlapping form/meaning relationships between AAVE and SE dialects are far less common than are the overlapping ones.

OVERLAPPING RELATIONSHIPS: DIFFERENT FORMS/SAME MEANING

Two languages or dialects can use different words to mark the same semantic distinctions. The same semantic distinctions in SE can be marked by different AAVE lexical and grammatical forms. AAVE has a range of unique lexical forms such as *boojee* (high class as in bourgeois), *bogue* (deceitful), *sadiddy* (snooty), *doofus* (disorganized), *gumby* (awkward), and so on. Although frequently regarded as slang, Smitherman (1994) reported that many of the words are commonly used across the various social strata of African American speakers. Some words have been created using the innovations shown in Table 4–1. Others just sound different from SE, because of phonological rule differences. Some AAVE phonological rules create lexical forms that are homonymous with SE words that code a different meaning. For example, the word *bust* /bʌst/ is pronounced as *bus* /bʌs/ by AAVE speakers who reduce final clusters under certain conditions. Thus the word **bust**, which refers to an action, as in the utterance, *"Bus you upside of your head,"* is homonymous with the word **bus,** which refers to a motorized vehicle.

AAVE speakers also use different grammatical constructions to code the same semantic distinctions in SE. For example, **stress *been*** as in "He **been** married" is a remote time marker. It means that the man was married a long time ago (and could still be married). SE speakers, who ignore the phonological stress intensifier, interpret this form to mean that the man was married sometime in the past. SE does not code remote "**BE**" with the same efficiency as AAVE. One must construct a sentence such as the following: "The man was married a long time ago" (Baugh, 1983).

Perfective *done*, which is used to code completed action in the past (e.g., "He **done** broke his toy") is another example of a different morphosyntactic AAVE form used to code the same semantic distinction in

SE (e.g., "He had broken his toy") (Baugh, 1983; Molefi, 1990). The "be done" form also is used to mark actions to be completed in the future (cf., "We **be done** cooked by the time he gets here" [AAVE] and "We will **have cooked** by the time he gets here" [SE]).

OVERLAPPING RELATIONSHIPS: SAME FORMS/DIFFERENT MEANING

When two dialects of a language share the same lexicon, it is probably most common for them to use the same stock of words to mark different meanings. Intuitively, this kind of difference also is likely to create the most cognitive dissonance, because speakers/listeners expect identical linguistic forms in two dialects to mark the same semantic distinctions. Crosscultural communication becomes more difficult when one dialect has a broader range of meanings attached to the same word than does another. In AAVE, a given word may have a culture-specific meaning and a meaning that fits with the dialect of wider communication. A well known example is the use of the word **bad.** Although typically used to mark a negative condition, or state in SE, the word **bad** refers to both a negative and a positive condition or state in AAVE. Children may acquire the special cultural meaning of a form before they acquire the meaning assigned to the form in the dialect of wider communication.

Using the same words to code different meaning can be viewed as double talk, or camouflage form use. A camouflage form is identical in SE and AAVE, but carries a different meaning in each. This tendency shows up in both lexical and grammatical uses. Lexical uses, often viewed as slang, extend the meaning of a word in ways that are not covered by conventional use. Examples include such commonly used words as **bad** (good), **bag** (person's trade or interest), **apple** (wide brimmed man's hat), **bite** (exaggerated praise), **clean** (stylish dress or to quantify a state as total or complete, e.g., "I clean forgot"), **crib** (home or house), and **drop** (to inform), and so on.

Camouflage grammatical forms in AAVE often lead to the wrong semantic interpretation in SE (Baugh, 1983). Examples include the frequently used habitual be (e.g., *They be working down there*), which codes a past event that continues to occur on a regular basis. The durative, habitual aspect is missing in an SE interpretation. It can be incorrectly assumed by SE speakers that such an utterance refers to an event that is occurring at the present time (i.e., "They are working down there right now"). However, the correct SE translation is "They usually work down there." In AAVE, an event that happens at the present time is coded without copula, for example, "They working down there."

Other examples of camouflage forms in AAVE include the grammatical uses of **steady** and **come** as modal verbs. These express particular meanings more efficiently than does SE. The use of **steady** in AAVE refers to the manner of activity as intense, consistent, and continuous. Baugh (1983) traced its origin to Bantu languages. It can be used with or without habitual be. For example, compare "They steady working down there" and "They be steady working down there." The word **steady** also may be stressed. The SE approximation (e.g., "They are steadily working down there") does not capture the intensity of the activity.

Spears (1982) described the semantic use of **come** as a modal verb in AAVE. It refers to the mood or attitude of a speaker toward an event as one of indignation (e.g., "He come telling me to go"). Its meaning is not simple reference to the act of coming. **Come** can co-occur as a modal and a primary verb in the same sentence (e.g.,"He **come** *coming* to my house"). In SE, such expressions could be grammatically framed as "He had the nerve to tell me to go" or "He had the nerve or gall to come to my house."

RESEARCH ON THE SEMANTIC KNOWLEDGE OF AFRICAN AMERICAN CHILDREN

Only a few studies have focused on the semantic knowledge of African American children who acquire AAVE. However, in all populations of speakers, semantic development has been less often targeted for study than the grammatical and pragmatic aspects of language. This bias is because meaning is difficult to study. It is not directly accessible to observation. Therefore, taxonomies for describing meaning objectively and reliably are difficult to create. As individual words are easy to identify, count, and test in a standardized way, it is not surprising that vocabulary, or lexical, meaning has been the predominant focus of the research on semantic development.

For the most part, descriptions of vocabulary, or lexical, meaning have been isolated from the modest attempts to describe the meaning of children's word combinations or sentences. Descriptions of relational meaning have been based on the semantic/syntactic relationships expressed in early grammars using the method of rich interpretations introduced by Bloom and her colleagues in the 1970s (Bloom & Lahey, 1978; Bloom, Lightbown, & Hood, 1975). With older children, the study of relational meaning has been narrowly confined to the understanding and use of figurative meaning, such as proverbs and other idioms (see Nippold, 1988; Nippold, Uhden, & Schwarz, 1997).

The types of studies on the semantic knowledge of AAVE speakers reflect these two research orientations to developmental semantics. That is, some studies have focused on vocabulary, or lexical, meaning with others focusing on relational, or syntactic, meaning. The following literature survey is organized to reflect this trend. Studies were included in the review, if they focused specifically on African American children's semantic knowledge. Thus, observations of vocabulary knowledge that are embedded in studies of academic achievement and performance on intelligence tests were excluded.

The general questions about the acquisition of meaning by African American children have been no different than those for studying the rest of language. Investigators have wanted to know what meanings children express, in which order, at what age, and why. The next section considers how far we have come in answering these questions about AAVE speakers.

LEXICAL OR VOCABULARY DEVELOPMENT

The study of vocabulary growth focuses on the meaning of individual words in the lexicon. Vocabulary encompasses both the breadth and depth of word knowledge (Mount-Weitz, 1996; Nagy & Herman, 1987). Breadth can be estimated by the number of different words that are understood and used. Depth can be estimated by the variety of meanings understood and used for one word. Lexical competency also includes the knowledge of the semantic relationships among words in the lexicon, such as their similarity (synonymy) and contrasts (antonymy) in meaning, and so on. Given the range of semantic aspects that can be studied, it is clear that the vocabulary research on African American children is very limited in scope. The following studies, with one exception, have focused on the number of words that the children know, as evidenced by standardized vocabulary tests and spontaneous speech use.

STANDARDIZED VOCABULARY TESTS

The *Peabody Picture Vocabulary Test* (PPVT) (Dunn, 1959; Dunn & Dunn, 1981) has been used to study African American children's vocabulary. This widely used test of receptive vocabulary requires children to point to the picture that best corresponds with the word given by the examiner.

Kresheck and Nicolosi (1973) studied 50 Black and 50 white children from low-middle class families who were matched for age and grade level. The subjects were presumed to be normal language learners and ranged from 5;6 to 6;6 years of age. The children were given the A form of PPVT (Dunn, 1959). For the Black children, the scores ranged from 33 to 68 with a mean of 48. For white children, scores ranged from 42 to 76 with a mean of 59. A statistically significant difference was observed between the mean scores of the two groups. Some items were missed by a larger percentage of the Black than white children. For example, the word *caboose* was missed by more the 80% of Black children. The authors did note that Black children may have used a different name for *caboose*. Ten other words that were missed by 10% to 50% of the Black children included *building, badge, coach, freckle, dial, yawning, tumble, submarine, thermos,* and *counter.* The response pattern did not reveal a reason for the missed items. In a few instances, the visual similarity between the pictures for the correct and erred responses suggested lack of familiarity with decontextualized picture representation. For example, some children pointed to the picture of a dial in response to the word *spider web.* Kresheck and Nicolosi's (1973) results were not surprising, given that the PPVT was not originally standardized on African American children.

However, African American children also obtained lower than average scores on the revised PPVT-R (Dunn & Dunn, 1981), which did include the population in the standardization sample. This was essentially the point that Washington and Craig (1992) made in a later study. They observed 105 low-income African American children in the Detroit metropolitan area. Their subjects' responses to the PPVT-R were scored using both the established scoring criteria and an adjusted score designed to take dialect differences into account. The two groups of preschool and kindergarten children spanned the ages of 4;5 to 6;3. The mean standard score equivalent obtained for the whole group averaged 79.7% and corresponded to the 10th percentile rank of the standardization sample. The mean for the African Americans was more than one standard deviation below the mean for the standardization sample as a whole and these findings did not vary according to age or grade grouping. When scores were modified to take dialect variants into account, the adjusted mean scores were higher than the unadjusted ones, but these gains did not make a clinical difference for the sample as a whole. As many as 11 items were failed by at least 50% of the children. The failed items did not form a particular response pattern. The response choices seemed random rather than deliberate. Washington and Craig (1992) concluded that the PPVT-R was not a representative measure of the vocabulary of low-income African American children, despite the inclusion of African American children in the standardization sample.

SPONTANEOUS SPEECH

Standardized tests are generally criticized for not being representative of word use in ordinary contexts. Children may actually use words that they fail to identify on a standardized test. Ideally then, research should focus on word use in spontaneous habitual speech, as Hart and Risley (1995) set out to do. Unlike the studies of standardized test responses, their longitudinal study aimed at documenting vocabulary growth. The 42 children studied were stratified by social class and ethnicity. The subjects included 17 African Americans. Vocabulary was compared among children from professional families and those from working class and welfare families in Kansas. Within the working class group, Hart and Risley made ethnic group comparisons. An ethnic analysis was not possible for the professional group, which included just one African American child nor the welfare group, which was exclusively African American. The number of new words used in home speech samples during habitual activities was tracked once every month for 2½ years. Each audiovisual recorded sample lasted an hour. Observations of the children began around the first birthday soon after they had said their first words.

The results revealed that all the children had an increased number of new words used spontaneously as age increased, but there were pronounced social class differences. Children from the professional class showed the most rapid and largest vocabulary growth. Those from the working class had larger vocabularies than those from welfare families. Thus, the higher the social class, the larger and more precipitously was the word gain across time. Social class accounted for 42% of the variance in vocabulary growth. In the working class group, for which ethnic comparisons could be made, the vocabulary gains for African American and white children were comparable.

The differences in vocabulary growth were significantly correlated with several variables related to language input, as indexed by the following caregiver interactive characteristics: (1) talking or listening to children beyond what is required to manage their care, (2) being nice as they correct errors, (3) asking before demanding compliance for more mature behavior, (4) providing basic education or elaborating answers more than necessary to answer a question. In sum, the quality of parenting amounted to responsiveness, prompting, gentle guidance, and feedback. Parents from welfare families talked the least to their children and their talk was more frequently geared to parent-initiated topics, imperatives, and prohibitions. Hart and Risley (1995) stated that:

> the magnitude of children's accomplishments depends less on the material and educational advantages available in the home and more on the amount of experience children accumulate with parenting that provides language diversity, emphasis, gentle guidance, responsiveness and affirmative feedback. (p. 211)

They concluded that intervention before age 3;0 is critical to the vocabulary growth trajectory. It was recommended that social policy be geared to parental intervention for welfare families. The goal of such intervention would be to educate parents to interact with their children in ways that stimulate language use.

Whereas Hart and Risley focused on the number of words used in spontaneous speech over time, Davis, Williams, Vaughn-Cooke, and Wright-Harp (1993) described the **types** of words used across time. In a longitudinal study, they tracked the lexical development of two African American boys across a 6-month period between 18 to 23 months of age. One child was developing normally,while the other one was not. The data were taken from the CAL (Center for Applied Linguistics) archives (Stockman & Vaughn-Cooke, 1982a,1989). The database consisted of audiovisual records of spontaneous speech samples collected in low structured natural situations in children's homes. The subjects were monolingual English speakers living in families and communities of Washington DC where AAVE was commonly spoken. Annual incomes qualified the families for participation in Head Start programs. The database included language samples from children who were developing normally and from one child who subsequently turned out to have a moderate delay in language development. He was enrolled in special education programs after entering school.

Davis et al. (1993) sampled the words used in 1-hour samples of spontaneous speech. Benedict's (1979) taxonomy was used to classify the words as nominals, actions, modifiers (e.g., attributes, states, locatives, possessives) and personal-social words. All four categories of words were observed in both subjects' repertoires. Nominals and actions comprised the largest categories of use across time. The number of words used increased with age for both the child deemed normal and the child with language delay, but clearly more slowly for the child who had delay. The typical child used twice as many words as the child with language delay and the gap became larger with age. The typical child also differed in the distribution of word types over time. Nominal words were more frequent than action words at just the earliest age (18 months). At older ages, action words were used just as often as nominals. In contrast, nominals dominated the repertoire of the child with language delay at every age sampled and this gap was significant at 23 months, the latest age sampled. The results suggested that reduced vocabulary is associated with language delay in low-income African American children.

RELATIONAL MEANING

The study of relational meaning was an important expansion of semantic acquisition research. Words are not typically experienced as isolated linguistic forms. More often than not, words occur in syntactic context in which they take on new meaning in relationship to other words. For example, in the sentence, "**Dog** bites the boy," the word *dog* refers to more than an animate object with certain physical and functional characteristics. It also refers to the agent of the action that affects the boy. Case grammar (Fillmore, 1968) predicts that the same object word can take on varying semantic roles depending on its grammatical position and role in sentences. In the sentence, "The bug was on the **dog**"; the word **dog** refers to a location. It refers to the recipient of an action (dative case) in "Give the meat to the **dog**," and to the possessor of an object in "It is the **dog**'s meat." A small set of such semantic/syntactic relations appear to be coded in every language and therefore are assumed to be universal (R. Brown, 1973).

A few studies (Blake, 1984; McWhirter, 1988; Stockman, 1991, 1992; Stockman & Vaughn-Cooke, 1982b, 1984, 1986, 1992) have examined the relational meaning expressed in the early grammars of African American children. They have done so in the tradition of rich interpretative analysis introduced by Lois Bloom and her colleagues (Bloom & Lahey, 1978; Bloom et al., 1975). In all these studies, investigators have focused on children's spontaneous speech in typical caregiver interactions. Data analyses have been framed around some version of the semantic/syntactic categories described in Bloom et al. (1975), and elaborated in Bloom and Lahey (1978). The original taxonomy was based on white middle class children. Utterances are first categorized in terms of the major verb relations expressed, (existence, action, locative action, state, locative state, notice, and so on), and then in terms of minor or coordinated categories that include Wh-question, instrumental, action plus place, inverted question, place, notice plus place, quantity, recurrence, and so on. Children are judged to productively code a semantic category if it occurs in three to five or more different spontaneous utterances. Using this approach, studies have sought evidence for semantic relational meaning coded by African American children.

GLOBAL SEMANTIC/SYNTACTIC CATEGORIES

Stockman and Vaughn-Cooke (1982b) used a taxonomy adapted from Bloom et al. (1975) to describe the semantic relations expressed in the spontaneous speech of 12 African American children (6 males, 6 females) at three age cross-sections: 18 months, 36 months and 42 months. The data were taken from the CAL archives. Analyses were based on single 2-hour language samples that had been recorded from each child during low structured activities in the home. Altogether, the data analysis was based on about 5,367 utterances across the 12 children, and ranged from 87 to 1,034 per child. A category was judged to be productive in a child's repertoire, if it was produced in four different utterances.

Stockman and Vaughn-Cooke (1982b) showed that the children in their Washington, D.C. sample were combining words at 18 months of age and learning to code a variety of semantic relationships. The earliest categories at 18 months commonly included existence, action, and locative action. The number of categories increased from 3 to 5 for every child at 18 months to a range of 13 to 15 at 36 months and 15 to 17 at 42 months. Naturally, there was individual variability in the frequency with which individual semantic categories were expressed, given the different types of speaking contexts. Stockman and Vaughn-Cooke (1982b) concluded that the children's speech expressed the same types of semantic distinctions expressed by white children, as described by Bloom et al. (1975).

Blake (1984) corroborated these findings in a longitudinal study of three African American children (2 males and 1 female) in New York City. The semantic-syntactic category analysis was part of a comprehensive study of form, content, and use interactions. Blake described how the children's acquisition of semantic and pragmatic categories shifted in relation to mean length of utterance. The children were from working class backgrounds and maternal speech patterns exhibited characteristic features of AAVE. Using the taxonomy employed by Bloom et al. (1975), their semantic development was tracked at 4-week intervals between 18 and 27 months of age. Spontaneous speech samples were videotaped during low-structured interactive play with their mothers in the playroom at Columbia University. At least one sample was taken in the home. Each sample lasted for an hour. Blake (1984) reported that only 1% of the 2,228 complete, spontaneous utterances could not be categorized according to the original taxonomy developed by Bloom et al. (1975).

A criterion of three different utterances was used to judge the productivity of a category in the repertoire. The action, locative action, and state categories were productive in the first session for all three children. Action was more often coded than was state. The number of semantic/syntactic categories used in spontaneous speech increased across time. Major semantic relations accounted for a larger proportion of the utterances than did the minor ones. Further, Blake (1984) reported tradeoffs in language form (measured by mean length of utterance), content (measured by semantic/syntactic categories) and pragmatics (measured by functional taxonomy of social language use) during the acquisition process. In the time period of the greatest shift in the number of semantic and pragmatic categories used, there was not a corresponding increase in sentence length. Blake (1984), like Stockman and Vaughn-Cooke (1982b), concluded that her African American subjects were acquiring the same categories as those that had been documented in the language of white middle class speakers of SE in a comparable age range.

Stockman and Vaughn-Cooke (1986) systematically compared the findings from the above two studies on African American children with those obtained for working class white children (Miller, 1982) and for middle class white children (Bloom et al., 1975). The meta-analysis, based on 22 children, included four studies that had used a similar semantic relational taxonomy. Criteria were devised for comparing the number and types of semantic/syntactic categories represented in comparable MLU-related stages of development, according to R. Brown (1973). All 11 major categories and 5 of the minor (Wh-question, place, action + place, dative, instrument) semantic categories were defined in comparable ways across studies. Figure 4–1 presents a summary of the findings.

The analysis revealed that every comparable category coded by white middle class and white working class children was also coded by one or more African American children at some age. This observation suggested that all the children coded the same types of semantic notions regardless of social class or ethnic group membership. The number of categories expressed increased across age for all groups, although individual differences in the number and types of categories used at a given stage were apparent in every study.

EARLY STAGE I — MLU = 1.01-1.30, Age = 18-21 months

SUBJECTS / SEMANTIC CATEGORIES	(RJ	AG	MW	CH)[3]	(Peter	Eric	Gia)[1]
MAJOR CATEGORIES							
Existence	●	●	●	●		X	X
Action	●	●	●	●	X	X[L]	X
Locative Action			●	●			X
State							
Locative State							
Negation	●	●		●		X[L]	
Possession	●						
Attribution			●				
Notice							
Intention							
Recurrence							X
MINOR CATEGORIES							
Wh Question							
Place							
Action + Place							
Dative							
Instrument							
Quantity							
Time[a]							
Mood							
Coordination							
Causality							
Epistemic							
Antithesis							

MID STAGE I — MLU = 1.31-1.55, Age = 19-23 months

SUBJECTS / SEMANTIC CATEGORIES	(Amy)[2]	(Ben	Martin	Jane)[4]	(Peter	Eric	Gia	Kathryn)[1]
MAJOR CATEGORIES								
Existence	○	●	●	●	X	X	X	X
Action	○	●	●	●	X	X	X	X
Locative Action	○	●	●	●	X	X	X	X
State	○[L]	●	●	●		X		X
Locative State	○[L]		●[L]					X
Negation	○		●[L]	●	X	X	X	X
Possession	○		●[L]		X	X	X	X
Attribution		●	●[L]	●	X	X	X	X
Notice	○[L]	●		●		X	X	X
Intention		●	●	●				X
Recurrence			●[L]		X	X	X	X
MINOR CATEGORIES								
Wh Question			●[L]	●				
Place	○		●[L]	●	X			
Action + Place	NC[b]						X	
Dative	NC		●[L]					
Instrument	NC		●[L]					
Quantity	NC		●[L]		NC	NC	NC	NC
Time[a]								
Mood								
Coordination								
Causality								
Epistemic								
Antithesis								

LATE STAGE I — MLU = 1.56-2.0, Age = 22-25 months

SUBJECTS / SEMANTIC CATEGORIES	(Amy	Wendy)[2]	(Ben	Martin)[4]	(Peter	Eric	Gia	Kathryn)[1]
MAJOR CATEGORIES								
Existence	○	○	●	●	X	X	X	X
Action	○	○	●	●	X	X	X	X
Locative Action	○	○	●	●	X	X	X	X
State	○	○[L]	●	●	X	X	X	X
Locative State	○	○	●	●	X	X	X	X
Negation	○	○		●	X	X	X	X
Possession	○	○		●	X	X	X	X
Attribution	○	○	●	●	X	X	X	X
Notice	○	○	●	●	X	X	X	X
Intention	○	○	●	●	X		X	X
Recurrence				●	X	X	X	X
MINOR CATEGORIES								
Wh Question	○	○	●	●	X		X[L]	X
Place	○	○	●	●	X	X	X[L]	X
Action + Place	NC	NC				X	X	X
Dative	NC	NC		●		X	X[L]	X
Instrument	NC	NC		●				
Quantity	NC	NC		●	NC	NC	NC	NC
Time[a]								
Mood								
Coordination								
Causality								
Epistemic								
Antithesis								

STAGE II — MLU = 2.01-3.0, Age = 21-28 months

SUBJECTS / SEMANTIC CATEGORIES	(Amy Wendy Beth)[2]	(Ben	Jane	Martin)[4]	(Peter Eric Kathryn	Gia)[1]
MAJOR CATEGORIES						
Existence	○	●	●	●	X	X
Action	○	●	●	●	X	X
Locative Action	○	●	●	●	X	X
State	○	●	●	●	X	X
Locative State	○	●	●	●	X	X
Negation	○	●	●	●	X	X
Possession	○	●	●	●	X	X
Attribution	○	●	●	●	X	X
Notice	○	●	●	●	X	X
Intention	○	●	●	●	X	X
Recurrence	○	●	●	●	X	X
MINOR CATEGORIES						
Wh Question	○	●	●	●	X	X
Place	○	●	●	●	X	X
Action + Place	NC		●		X	X
Dative	NC	●	●	●	X	X
Instrument	NC			●		X
Quantity	NC		●	●	NC	NC
Time[a]						
Mood						
Coordination						
Causality						
Epistemic						
Antithesis						

POST STAGE II — MLU > 3.0, Age = 32-35 months; MLU > 4.0, Age = 53-54 months

SUBJECTS / SEMANTIC CATEGORIES	(LA DD KM	CW)[3]	(EC	DW MN	ST)[3]
MAJOR CATEGORIES					
Existence	●	●	●	●	●
Action	●	●	●	●	●
Locative Action	●	●	●	●	●
State	●	●	●	●	●
Locative State	●	●	●	●	●
Negation	●	●	●	●	●
Possession	●	●	●	●	●
Attribution	●	●	●	●	●
Notice	NC	NC	NC	NC	NC
Intention	NC	NC	NC	NC	NC
Recurrence	●	●	●	●	●
MINOR CATEGORIES					
Wh Question	●	●	●	●	●
Place	●	●	●	●	●
Action + Place	●	●	●	●	●
Dative	●	●	●	●	●
Instrument	NC	NC	NC	NC	NC
Quantity	●	●	●	●	●
Time[a]	●	●	●	●	●
Mood	●	●	●	●	●
Coordination		●	●	●	●
Causality		●	●	●	●
Epistemic				●	●
Antithesis					●

Footnotes: [a] Time, Mood, Coordination, Causality, Epistemic and Antithesis were included only in Stockman and Vaughn-Cooke's study as separate categories.

[b] NC - Refers to noncomparable categories for the study specified.

References:
1. Bloom, Lightbown & Hood (1975)
2. Miller (1982)
3. Stockman & Vaughn-Cooke (1982)
4. Blake (1984)

FIGURE 4–1

The sematic categories that reached criterion of productive usage for working class Black children (●), working class white children (○), and middle class white children (x) in four studies. (Reprinted with permission from "Implications of Semantic Category Research for the Language Assessment of Nonstandard Speakers," by I. Stockman and F. Vaughn-Cooke, 1986, p. 19. *Topics in Language and Language Disorders, 6,* 15–25.)

The analysis permitted direct comparison of African American and white children in just the first four of the five MLU-derived developmental stages shown before 30 months of age. At each stage, no semantic category was coded by all the middle and/or working class white children and by none of the African American children. Conversely, there was no category coded by all African American children and by none of the white children. This observation suggests that all the children were acquiring a common core of semantic relational knowledge within the same developmental time frame, regardless of social class or ethnicity. The data provided further support for the universal nature of the semantic categories studied.

BRIDGING THE GAP—COMBINING LEXICAL AND RELATIONAL MEANING

Later studies of semantic relational knowledge were motivated by the global nature of the semantic relational categories originally described by Bloom et al. (1975). Once a semantic category such as action or locative action emerges early on, the descriptive framework does not provide a way to document its continuing development. Earlier studies (Coggins, 1979; Leonard, Bolders, & Milller, 1976), which had employed a global category taxonomy, revealed little or no qualitative difference between children with normal and delayed language. A fine grained analysis of a global semantic category is needed to develop assessment protocols that can identify language delay beyond the earliest ages.

Several semantic relational studies responded to this issue by examining the types of words used within a global semantic category, such as action, locative action, locative state, and so on. This strategy was well motivated because vocabulary is expected to increase with age. Moreover, words are seldom experienced in isolation of syntactic frames, although lexical and syntactic meaning are typically studied as separate semantic systems. When words are embedded in phrases and sentences, meaning is extended beyond their respective lexical definitions. Meaning reflects the word's syntactic relationship to other words in sentences. Stockman and Vaughn-Cooke (1984, 1992) hypothesized that the type of semantic-syntactic context in which words occur influences their developmental order in expressive speech. They studied the emergent use of spatial locative words (particles, prepositions, adverbs) used by African American children to code **locative action.** This global semantic category refers to a change of location or the movement of an object from one place to another. It is expressed by the co-occurrence of a movement action verb (e.g., go, come, walk, take) with a locative preposition or adverb in such sentences as the following:

Source	**Path**	**Goal**	**Combined**
Go out ____	Go up ____	Go in ____	Go out in ____
Go off ____	Go over ____	Go on ____	Go over on ____

The resulting semantic fields respect the reality of any locative displacement event—namely, that it necessarily involves a source location, movement path, and a goal location. Languages differ on if and how each aspect is coded (Talmy, 1985). The English lexicon marks each aspect separately as shown in the columns.

Stockman and Vaughn-Cooke (1984, 1992) longitudinally tracked the emergent use of spatial locative words in the **locative action** sentences used by four African American children who were developing typically between 18 and 36 months. The number of different locative words used in these sentences increased significantly across age for every child. This increase was not random. Source/path words (e.g., *away, off, out, up, down*) emerged and proliferated in frequency of use earlier than did goal words (e.g., *in, on, under, beside*), although the combinatorial use of locative words in the same sentence (e.g., *out in, down in, over in*) emerged latest of all.

Stockman and Vaughn-Cooke appealed to both linguistic and cognitive factors in accounting for their observed developmental trends. It was speculated that source/path words (e.g., *off, out, away, up*) appeared earliest because they are salient in the language input. They frequently appear as adverbial particles at the ends of sentences (e.g., *Go away, Go up*). In contrast, words used to mark goal of movement (e.g., *in, on, under*) are often embedded in prepositional phrases (e.g., "Go in the room"; "Put it on/under the bed."), although they, too, can appear as adverbial particles (e.g., "Put it on" or "Put it in").

At the same time, appropriate use of source/path words requires a child to pay attention to just one locative reference point. Source/path words can code an object's relocation relative to the place of origin without regard to its new resting place or destination. Utterances such as "Go out" and "Go up" entail knowing that the object moves **from** some place but not the place to which it moves. In contrast, reference to the goal or destination of the movement entails coordination of two locative reference points: (1) the existing site or point of origin and (2) the relocated or goal site. For example, expressions such as "Put the ball in" or "Put the ball in the box" require a child to regard both the ball's existing and future locations. As the ball cannot occupy both sites at the same time, only one location is observable while the other one must be mentally inferred. Therefore, it was speculated that a more stringent cognitive requirement had to be met to understand and use goal rather than source/path words in sentences coding locative action.

This "cognitive constraint" interpretation of the data appeared justified by the observations of locative word use in sentences that code **locative state** (Stockman, 1991). In locative state sentences, the order of emergent use was reversed for source/path and goal words. Locative state is an object's place or spatial position in terms of its proximal relation to another object without reference to the action that led to the location. It is expressed by the co-occurrence of a nonmovement verb with a locative adverb or preposition as realized in sentences such as:

Source/Path	**Goal**	**Combined**
It's out ___	It's in ___	It's out in ___
It's up ___		

Although source/path words such as *out, off, away, up* also appear as sentence final particles or adverbs in locative state sentences, their use in this context emerged later and was less frequent than was goal word use (*in, on, under*). Thus the developmental trend for using locative words in locative action sentences was reversed in locative state sentences, even though the linguistic characteristics remained the same. These developmental differences reflected constraints on learning the varying semantic properties of words in the two types of semantic/syntactic contexts. It was speculated that source/path words emerged later than goal words in locative state sentences, because two locative reference points must be coordinated instead of one, as is the case of locative action sentences. For example, the utterance, "It is out of/from here," requires one to consider the object's locative relation to a former place and an unspecified new place. That is, the child must understand that the object is located at a different place than where it used to be. Conversely, the utterance, "It's in the box," requires one to view the object's location in relation to one proximal site instead of the two required to understand locative action sentences, as in "Go in here."

When using locative word combinations in the same sentence such as "It's out by the closet," the children clearly coded both aspects. Stockman (1991) concluded that the development of lexical meaning involved more than learning the meaning of individual words. The differential order in which locative words first emerged in locative action and locative state sentences suggested that development was influenced by the semantic role of locative words in sentences.

Although the source/path/goal/combinatorial categories of word use in locative action sentences are still rather coarse, Stockman (1992) showed that they could differentiate normal and slow language learning after productive use of a global semantic relational category was evident. This longitudinal study of four children between 18 to 36 months of age was based on videotaped samples of oral speech in the CAL archives (Stockman & Vaughn-Cooke, 1982a, 1989). Three of the children were typical (two females and one male) and one was subsequently identified as having language delay and received speech-language therapy. The sentences that just coded locative action were reliably identified. The number and types of locative source/path/goal words and their combinations were tracked before and after the children achieved a productivity criterion of four different semantic/syntactic constructions that included at least two different verbs.

The child with language delay reached the criterion of productive use at a later age (2;2 years) than did each of the normal children (1;6 to 1;11 years). Once his locative action utterances were productive, he added fewer locative words to his vocabulary over time than did the other children, and used each one less frequently. Further, at every stage of comparison, he was at least one step behind his typical age peers in the categories of locative words used. When typical children were using mainly source/path markers at the earliest stage of their development, the child with language delay did not productively use locative action utterances. By the time locative action was productive for the child with language delay, the children, who were typical, had shifted to using predominantly goal expressions, whereas the child with language delay was using mainly source/path words. As the typical children began combining locative terms, the child who had delay, proliferated in the use of goal expressions. He also began to combine locative words much later than did his typical age-matched peers and few locative combinations were observed.

McWhirter (1988) focused on lexical subcategories within the global semantic/syntactic category of **action.** The lexical verb in sentences codes action. Bloom and colleagues defined action as a semantic category of movement that does not change the object's location and it is differentiated from the category of state (Bloom et al., 1975). However, McWhirter's taxonomy encompassed the entire verb system. Action was defined broadly as reference to a happening or event. The question, "What is/was X doing," can be answered with a sentence such as "He's holding the ball." Therefore, the verb, **holding,** was classified as a type of action, although it may be treated as a state in other taxonomies. Verb categories or semantic fields were identified by their reference to two aspects: movement versus nonmovement and change versus no external change in the object affected by the action. Subfields were differentiated further by their reference to change or no change of an affected object's locative, physical, or possessive attributes. For example, verbs were distinguished by their reference to movements such as *throw, cut,* and *give,* which code a **change** of an object's locative, physical, or possessive state, respectively, and movements that do not change the **external** state of the affected object, at least in a predictable or obligatory way (e.g., **look** – *look at the ball;* **rub** – *rub the ball.*). Movement verbs differed from nonmovement ones. The latter verb types included *wait, think,* and *keep,* which do not change the affected object's locative, attributive, or possessive state, respectively, along with nonmovement action verbs such as *sleep,* which do code an observable change of state, but the change is not implicit in the type of action coded by the verb.

One goal of McWhirter's (1988) study was to determine whether one action verb category occurred more frequently in the spontaneous speech of typically developing African American children than did others. Another goal was to determine if these categories could differentiate between children with normal and delayed language. To answer the first question, the frequency of each of the action verb categories in the spontaneous speech of African American preschoolers was tabulated. The data were taken from the CAL archives. The first hour of a 2-hour language sample was taken from 8 children (4 boys and 4 girls) between 4;3 to 4;6 years of age. The home samples had been obtained in low-structured play situations. The number of utterances and contexts of language use differed across the children, but their coding of action subcategories reflected diverse verb use . The number of different verbs used varied from 109 to 274 across children. Movement/change verbs were uniformly the most frequent—accounting for 60% to 72% of all verb uses. Movement (change plus nonchange) verbs altogether accounted for 88% to 97% of the verbs used. The categories were ranked in the order of most to least frequent as movement/change followed by movement/nonchange, nonmovement/change, and nonmovement/nonchange.

The next goal was to determine if the action subcategories derived from African American children could distinguish between normal and slow language learners. A pilot study of four white male children (3;11 to 4;5 years of age) was done. They were selected from public schools in Michigan. The children formed two subject pairs, each comparable age pair consisting of a child who was typical and one atypical child with language delay. The typical children in each pair scored at age-appropriate levels on the receptive and expressive portions of the *Northwestern Syntax Screening Test* (Lee, 1971). Both atypical children were judged to be about 9 to 12 months delayed in expressive language based on standardized test scores and they were receiving therapy at the time of the study. Audiovisual recordings were made of the 50- to 60-minute spontaneous speech samples elicited. The samples were elicited using a standard set of toys in a laboratory playroom environment. McWhirter applied the same criteria for identifying action subcategories as had been used to classify the verbs used by the African American children.

For the older subject pair, age 4;5, the typical child used significantly more action verbs than did the child with language delay. The verbs represented the same categories observed in African American children and the rank order distribution of verbs for both boys was the same as well. For the younger subject pair at age 3;11, the child with language delay used more verbs than did the typical child, who was shy and reticent during the language sample. Nevertheless, the same action subcategories and their rank order distribution for both boys were the same as that observed in the typical African American children. These results suggested that for white children, regardless of normal or delayed status, frequency of verb use also was significantly affected by reference to movement and change, as had been observed among African American children. However, as all the action subcategories were represented in the speech of children who were normal and delayed in the 4- to 5-year-old age range studied, they may still be too coarse to differentiate between older children with normal and delayed language.

SUMMARY AND EVALUATION OF SEMANTIC DEVELOPMENT RESEARCH ON AFRICAN AMERICAN CHILDREN

The semantic knowledge of African American children appears to have been investigated in just a small number of studies. Fortunately, they have spanned both lexical and relational meaning and have included both elicited and self-generated speech. However, the studies have not been uniformly motivated by the basic goal of describing semantic development. Most vocabulary studies, in particular, have been driven by issues of negative test bias and social welfare policy. In three of the four studies reviewed, the underlying goal was to determine how well African American children performed relative to white children or on a vocabulary test normed on mostly white children.

In contrast, studies of semantic relational knowledge abandoned the methodology of racial group comparisons and included just African American subjects. But these studies did not escape the influence of the deficit hypothesis that was inspired by the outcomes of racial group comparisons. Investigators were drawn to a descriptive framework that assumed early semantic knowledge to be universal across languages because this orientation allowed the deficit hypothesis to be countered by revealing similarities rather than differences between African American and white children. The point is that the deficit hypothesis has historically had the effect of diverting scholarly attention away from basic research on African American children.

Nonetheless, all the semantic studies taken together have revealed useful outcomes. They have shown that African American children learn words and sentences to express a variety of meanings and that their semantic knowledge increases with age. Their words and sentences code the same kind of meanings expressed by children who learn SE and other languages. They talk about action, location, time, possession, causality, and so on, but they seem to know fewer words than SE speakers. They score lower on standardized vocabulary tests and add fewer words to their vocabularies over time. However, vocabulary knowledge appears to be related less to their African American ethnicity than to their social class. Children from low income families (those on welfare, specifically) learn fewer words than those from working class and professional families. African American and white children from comparable social classes do not differ in their vocabulary size, although the evidence is available now for just those children from working class families. We can expect both lexical and relational semantic knowledge to differentiate children who have normal and delayed language among young African Americans.

Still, so much is unknown about the semantic knowledge of a group claimed to have so many linguistic and cognitive deficits. The scope of semantic research has been limited on many fronts. Vocabulary studies have emphasized the breadth of word knowledge. Virtually nothing is known about the depth of vocabulary knowledge. African American children's understanding of multiple word meanings, word relationships (e.g., synonymy, hyponymy), and figurative meaning has not been investigated.

The study of multiple word meanings ought to be especially important, because speakers of nonstandard social dialects may use the same word to code a meaning that is specific to the local culture in addition to the meaning coded in a standard dialect. When such extended semantic reference exists, young children are likely to encounter the word first as it is used in the local community culture. So far, though, semantic studies have emphasized what African American children know about word meanings that match those in the dialect of wider communication. Consequently, little is known about the dialect-specific aspects of meaning that do not. For example, nothing seems to be known about the development of AAVE grammatical features that have idiomatic meaning to its speakers (e.g., **habitual be, steady, come**).

Inadequate knowledge about the acquisition of dialect-specific meaning may be because semantic studies have focused on young preschool children. Grammatical studies (Cole, 1980; Stockman, 1986a, 1986b) suggest that AAVE features are not evident at the early developmental stages, but become prominent as age increases after 3 years or so. Normative descriptions of preschoolers well serve the goal of early identification of language delay. However, a comprehensive normative description of African American children's language ought to also include the later learned dialect-specific features.

Research on African American children with language delay is even scarcer than that on typical speakers. In the two studies of language delay reviewed, just one child with language impairment was described and both studies focused on the same subject in the CAL archives. The literature surveyed support the following conclusions, which can serve as working hypotheses for future research:

1. African American preschoolers learn the same kind of lexical and relational meanings as those expressed by SE speakers at comparable ages.
2. The number and types of words used in self-generated speech increase with age.
3. Vocabulary growth is tempered by social class, such that African American children from low-income families comprehend and use fewer words than those from higher social classes.
4. Typical and delayed language among African American children can be distinguished by the number and type of lexical and relational semantic distinctions expressed.

CROSSCULTURAL CHALLENGES
TO SEMANTIC ASSESSMENT

Assessment is an important activity for researchers and clinicians alike. Clinicians must first assess language to determine if a problem exists. Researchers must assess language to know whether learners who are normal or impaired are selected as subjects. Both researcher and clinician often rely on the same methods to identify whether a language problem exists.

A long-standing concern has been the over- and underidentification of minority language speakers in clinical populations. Although norm-referenced standardized tests are typically used for this purpose, it has become clear that they are limited in ways that challenge fair crosscultural assessment. The challenge for semantic assessment is no different than that which applies to the rest of language. The basic issue is how to document competence accurately and efficiently. However, if meaning is inherently difficult to observe, then a semantic assessment could pose an even bigger problem to achieving fair crosscultural assessment than do other aspects of language. This is particularly true for assessing vocabulary knowledge. Ironically, a vocabulary index is the most popular and efficient way to assess semantic knowledge; yet it is likely to be the most vulnerable to bias when assessing speakers from varying languages and cultures. One person does not learn all the words of a language and the ones that happen to be known surely result from personal experience as shaped by the functional practices of a culture. So there is bound to be a lot of variability in the words children learn, especially in the case of open class words such as nouns, verbs, adjectives as opposed to the finite closed class words such as determiners, prepositions, or grammatical operators that occur in many sentences. Given the expected variability in word knowledge, test makers are faced with several types of problems in trying to create an unbiased standardized test that requires all children to know the same words.

SEMANTIC ASSESSMENT USING
EXISTING PROCEDURES

ASSESSING LEXICAL MEANING (VOCABULARY)

CHOICE OF WORDS ASSESSED.   There is no agreed upon way to select the initial pool of words to be included in a test. In some cases, the words are chosen from dictionaries (e.g., *Peabody Picture Vocabulary Test-Revised* (PPVT-R) (Dunn & Dunn, 1981). In other cases, parents and teachers are polled (e.g., *Receptive One Word Picture Vocabulary Test* (ROWPVT) (Gardner, 1985). It is not surprising that tests can end up with entirely different words, as is the case for the PPVT-R and the ROWPVT. Such differences could differentially affect performance if the words on one test happen to be more familiar to a group of children than those on another. It is noteworthy that standardized vocabulary tests can yield different outcomes for the same general population of children, even though the testing procedures and stimulus characteristics are virtually identical. Flipsen (1998) concluded that the ROWPVT is less suitable than is the PPVT-R for screening the kindergarten children in a small western Canadian community. His conclusion was based on two screening studies. Each study included 70 or more kindergarten children. The scores were distributed such that too few were more than one standard deviation below the mean relative to the expected normal distribution on the ROWPVT (Flipsen, 1993). Consequently, Flipsen speculated that the ROWPVT would not identify enough children as having language delay. The PPVT-R, on the other hand, did yield a normal distribution with the expected percentage of scores at the low end of the distribution (Flipsen, 1998). Although the test differences were attributed to the sizes of the standardization samples, the inventory of words was a confounding factor.

SCOPE OF WORD MEANING ASSESSED. Once words are chosen for a test, another issue that challenges crosscultural assessment is the aspect of meaning targeted. A given word can have more than one meaning and it can be known and used in more than one context, particularly by speakers of minority languages or dialects. Children in different communities may code the same concept with different synonyms; compare *boat, ship, sailboat, canoe*. Most vocabulary tests do allow for some lexical variation. However, they are not likely to allow for the full range of variants that can occur across different groups. In the case of AAVE, innovative variants that fall outside of standard usage are either unknown or not allowed. Yet children may hear and use the nonstandard variant earlier or more often than the standard one. Likewise, second language speakers may learn and use a word in one language and not another. Patterson (1996) concluded that children who are Spanish/English bilingual are not delayed in lexical acquisition relative to monolingual English speakers when the vocabularies of both languages are combined.

ELICITATION CONTEXT. Even if there is agreement on the set of words that children typically ought to know at a given age, there remains the problem of how to determine that knowledge in a standardized way. It is now well known that test bias does not arise simply from the choice of linguistic stimuli presented. It also stems from the material or stimuli used to elicit responses. Pictures are often used and they often dictate the kind of words tested. It is possible for a wrong response to reflect poor interpretation of pictures rather than lack of word knowledge. Test makers undoubtedly try to create the most neutral or generic stimuli possible by using black and white line drawings. Otherwise, the features would have to be related to a particular object or event that could favor some experiences over others. A neutral black and white line drawing of a dog ought to elicit images of a collie, dalmatian, greyhound, and so on. At the same time, generic representations decontextualize the elicitation task so much that some children can be penalized if they are not accustomed to print media. Advocates of dynamic assessment point out that typically developing children from minority languages may perform poorly on standardized tests, because they lack experience with using language in a testing context. Snow (1990) concluded that even word definition skill requires experience with the linguistic form for giving definitions. Consequently, typically developing children are likely to fare better on formal testing after they have been oriented to the test-taking task.

Test makers must be as savvy about the alternative pictures chosen as the incorrect response as they are about the target response. Washington (1996) reported that in response to the word **uniform** on the PPVT-R, some African American children in their sample pointed to the picture of a man behind prison bars (an incorrect response by test definition) and not to the policeman in uniform (the correct answer). As prisoners also wear uniforms, this response choice for the word, **uniform,** is appropriate in the experience of some African American children.

ASSESSING RELATIONAL MEANING

Taxonomies for describing semantic/syntactic relations add a rich new dimension to linguistic description. Words are seldom learned, understood, or used in isolation of other words. It has helped matters that the larger event relations expressed by language have been observed cross-linguistically and seem to be universal. The implication is that a child is likely to be at-risk for language impairment, if action relations are not coded by a certain age regardless of cultural or linguistic background. Conceivably then, a semantic relational analysis, which does not require children to know the same exact words, ought to be less vulnerable to crosslinguistic bias than are the measures of vocabulary knowledge.

Nonetheless, there are at least two problems that prevent semantic/syntactic analyses from being fully exploited in assessment procedures aimed at identifying a language problem. The first is that the clinical taxonomies used so far yield a rather coarse analysis of the meaning relations expressed. This analysis is so coarse that most children, including those who acquire AAVE, acquire productive use of the major semantic categories at an early age. After 3 years or so, there is not a metric for assessing normal language.

A second problem relates to the implementation of the semantic relational analysis. Even a coarse analysis cannot be done too quickly or in the standardized manner required to identify language delay. This is because the analysis is typically based on an oral speech sample. Thus the assessment procedure inherits all the problems that are related to using this kind of assessment procedure. See Stockman (1996) for a discussion of some of these problems. Just getting an adequate sample is a crosscultural challenge when the clinician does not represent the child's linguistic or ethnic group, as is often the case for African American children. The children may not talk, particularly if they feel that their speech patterns are inadequate and subject to negative judgments by people outside of the linguistic community.

ALTERNATIVE SOLUTIONS TO SEMANTIC ASSESSMENT

The challenges to semantic assessment that are created by linguistic and cultural differences cannot be met simply by creating a separate test for each minority language group. There are too many groups and this solution also ignores the within-group variability that is likely to still render a common standard as ineffective. The dependency of test performance on language-specific experience makes crosscultural identification of language delay a formidable, if not impossible, problem to optimally solve by using any kind of broad standardized measure.

One solution is to dispense with the idea that a general unbiased test of vocabulary can be developed with the implicit assumption that all children at a given age ought to know the same set of words. There are many words to be known in a language and speakers typically acquire just a subset of them, anyway. Thus alternative assessment strategies that allow inferences to be made about semantic knowledge are desirable. Three such strategies are considered here.

STANDARDIZED LANGUAGE PROCESSING TESTS

One alternative is to foreground on-line language processing ability rather than the child's stored knowledge of words. Campbell, Dollaghan, Needleman, and Janosky (1997), pointed out that performance on vocabulary tests are particularly vulnerable to the kind of words that children have experienced and, therefore, are prone to the risk of confusing a language difference with a disorder. They studied 156 males (average age of 12;6 years), who included white, African American, Asian, and Native Americans. Campbell et al. (1997) showed that minority children did not differ from white children on language processing tests involving nonword repetition, working memory for competing stimuli, and auditory processing of linguistic commands using a closed set of words. But significant differences between white and minority subjects were observed on the Oral Language Scale from the *Woodcock Proficiency Battery-Revised*, which relies heavily on vocabulary knowledge.

The use of on-line processing tasks to identify language delay is a promising strategy to pursue provided that (1) the tasks can be done by children at much earlier ages than the 11- to 12-year-old children studied by Campbell et al. (1997) and (2) the tasks yield performances that are highly correlated with "real" estimates of semantic knowledge.

FAST-MAPPING:
DYNAMIC ASSESSMENT STRATEGY

Using an on-line processing task to identify at-risk children would not eliminate the need to assess semantic knowledge directly. After identifying a problem (however that is done), clinicians determine a baseline of functioning to justify, plan, and evaluate therapy. Semantic knowledge is evaluated along with other aspects of language.

Even so, therapy is not expected to teach all the words that a child will need to learn. Relative to phonologic and morphosyntactic rules, semantic knowledge is not finite. Vocabulary continues to expand across the life span (Obler, 1997, p. 450). Thus, it may be more clinically useful to know how well one can acquire new words (i.e., extract the features of unknown words and use them in grammatical context) than it is to estimate vocabulary that has already been acquired.

It is possible to get more direct information about word learning by creating a standard word learning task that requires on-line processing of novel words. This strategy places assessment of word meaning into a "dynamic" assessment context. Broadly speaking, dynamic assessment stresses one's potential to learn (Lidz, 1991; Pena, 1996). A dynamic assessment procedure can exploit the evidence that children with either typical or delayed language are capable of "fast word mapping." That is, they can learn new words incidentally after brief exposure to them in semantic/syntactic context (e.g., Dickinson, 1984; Dollaghan, 1987). Such learning reflects the ability to bootstrap one's own word acquisition by combining existing linguistic knowledge with the ability to process novel words in an actual situation. For example, hearing a sentence such as "John wugged the ice," a child is likely to conclude that the strange unfamiliar word "wugged" refers to an action, given its position in the verb slot of the sentence. It ought to be possible to standardize novel word learning tasks that can discriminate between normal and slow word learners, as has been done. Rice, Buhr, and Nemeth (1990) created 6-minute animated video narratives in which different classes of new words were presented a certain number of times. Children's comprehension of new words was assessed before and after the media viewing. The researchers observed that children with language impairment mapped fewer words than did their age- and language-matched peers.

TARGETING SEMANTIC FIELDS

When assessment and therapeutic goals target specific words in the vocabulary, it might be better to focus on a semantic field of related words rather than isolated words. A semantic field is a category of words that shares a common meaning. This strategy is helpful to cross-cultural assessment, because it allows variable word use within a range of possible words whose shared semantic features are critical to functional language use. For example, speakers of all English dialects and other languages can profit from having words to talk about space, action, possession, time, and so on. But different groups need not use the same vocabulary terms to do so. Specifying semantic fields for relational words in terms of their semantic/syntactic relationships in sentences may be useful for four reasons. First, the strategy links lexical and relational meaning, as is done in real language learning. Second, AAVE and SE may differ less in the meaning of relational words (e.g., spatial and temporal prepositions) than on the open class words, such as the nouns, which are so often targeted in standard vocabulary tests.

Third, relational words are likely to be the most problematic for children with language delay. Fourth, semantic fields provide boundaries within which to focus vocabulary intervention in principled ways related to sentence use.

Studies of African American children's use of locative words in locative action and state sentences suggest that development is patterned by semantic fields, as defined by the semantic relationship of verbs and other words in sentences. This means that therapy could target words belonging to the same semantic/syntactic subclass, with the expectation that their shared semantic/syntactic patterns will facilitate more rapid learning of new words belonging to the same field. Studies of locative development (Stockman, 1991; Stockman & Vaughn-Cooke, 1992) suggest that one should pay attention to whether locative prepositions co-occur with movement action or nonmovement action verbs. Within each semantic/syntactic context, source, path, and goal words may be targeted as separate groups.

⊥⊤

FUTURE RESEARCH DIRECTIONS

Research goals should continue to provide the most comprehensive view of developing semantic knowledge in AAVE as is possible. This requires focusing on the semantic features that are both similar to and different from those of other English dialects.

INVESTIGATING NORMAL SEMANTIC ACQUISITION

FOCUSING ON AAVE AND SE SIMILARITIES

So far, studies of African American children's semantic knowledge have foregrounded what they know about the meanings of words and sentences that are shared by SE speakers. Continuing this focus is defensible for three reasons.

First, AAVE and SE dialects share a common lexicon. A comprehensive description of AAVE speakers must include the words whose meanings are similar to SE and those that are not. In the absence of empirical documentation, even the assumptions about which features are shared must remain tentative.

Second, studying similar features is necessary because African Americans have, for the most part, been excluded from research studies designed to establish norms. Generalizing existing developmental findings to them based on other groups is often tempered by continuing suspicion that they either do not develop as much language as other groups, or do so at a slower rate. Only empirical observations can determine whether this view is myth or reality.

Finally, if the cultural context and language socialization experiences of African Americans are different as argued (e.g. Hart & Risley, 1995; Heath, 1983; van Kleeck, 1994), then a different developmental schedule may well show up even for the semantic features that presumably are identical. But to the extent that development is the same for children across cultures, there is further evidence for linguistic universals and a biological substrate for language learning. Universal aspects of language are helpful to clinicians practicing in culturally diverse settings. They can use the same guidelines to evaluate speakers from varying backgrounds including those who acquire SE.

In focusing on African American children's semantic features that are like those in SE, we need to move beyond the goal of documenting the number of words known. What we need are richer descriptions of language that focus on the depth of semantic knowledge, including the acquisition of multiple meanings, sense, and organization of the semantic space as well as literal and figurative meaning.

Studies of semantic acquisition are no exception to the predominant current focus of research on finding solutions to the practical problems of social welfare and clinical service delivery. Therefore, it is not surprising that basic theoretical issues have gone unexplored. There is little in the research done so far that contributes to theoretical issues on the structure of semantic memory from either a normal (e.g., see Markman, 1994; K. Nelson, 1985) or clinical (e.g., Kail & Leonard, 1986) perspective. This trend needs to be reversed in future research.

FOCUSING ON AAVE AND SE DIFFERENCES

There is equally good reason to investigate the acquisition of dialect-specific meaning. A comprehensive description of AAVE acquisition demands it. The semantic characteristics of some AAVE forms have not been fully described, even for its adult speakers. The "go copula" is a case in point. It is expressed in utterances such as "There go the ball," or "Here go the ball," or "There/Here go the ball right here." Such utterances have the earmarks of camouflage forms. Their surface structure conforms to SE, but their meaning appears superficially to be quite the opposite, given preliminary observations of the contexts of use. The "go copula" does not occur in the context of dynamic movement events, as is expected in SE when the "go" verb is used in many linguistic contexts. It is used in the context of static events to refer to an object in the perceptual field. In SE, such events are coded by existential locative expressions such as "There's the ball" or "Here's the ball."

The "go copula" has been documented in the speech of African American children in different geographical regions. It has been observed in a Chicago, IL sample (Cole, 1980), a Washington, DC sample (Stockman & Vaughn-Cooke, 1984), and a Hartford, CT sample (Wyatt, 1991, 1996). A careful study of the "go copula" in adult and child AAVE speech is needed.

Even among the dialect-specific semantic features that have been described in adult AAVE, little is known about children's usage of them except in an incidental way. One or both of the following AAVE forms with well-described idiomatic AAVE meaning appeared in studies by Cole (1980), Wyatt (1991; 1996), and Washington and Craig (1994):

1. Stress **been** used to mark remote past.
2. **BE** copula used to mark habitual action.

Although these studies were concerned with AAVE morphosyntacic forms instead of meaning, their outcomes suggest that three factors should be considered in future research aimed at tracking the semantic development of dialect-specific forms.

AGE AS A VARIABLE IN AAVE USE. Cole's (1980) study showed that age is a factor in children's use of AAVE features. Both **remote past been** and **habitual be** (in addition to "go copula") were elicited as early as 3 years of age in response to photographs and verbal prompts. There was a modest increase in the number of children using **go copula** and **habitual be** as age increased from 3 to 5 years but not for **remote past been.** The number of children using the latter feature actually declined with age—a trend contrary to the expectation that dialect-specific features become more prominent with age. More robust data are needed to show if and how the use of AAVE forms change with age. The assumption that AAVE and SE speakers do not differ much until after 3 years of age (Stockman, 1986a,1986b) is challenged by Hart and Risley's (1995) study of early vocabulary growth. The question for future research is whether the age-graded hypothesis applies equally across all domains of language, including the semantic representation of AAVE forms.

INDIVIDUAL VARIABILITY IN AAVE FORM USE. Studies (Washington & Craig, 1994; Wyatt, 1991) suggest that some African American children use more AAVE features than do others. In Washington and Craig's sample of 61 low-income children (4 and 5 years old) in Detroit, **remote been** was never observed. They elicited responses to a picture elicitation task and recorded 15-minute speech samples. **Habitual be** was used by 40% of their high-frequency AAVE users, 17% of the moderate users, and none of the low-frequency users.

Wyatt (1991) observed just two instances of **habitual be** in 50 transcripts of oral language taken from ten 3- to 5-year old children in Hartford, CT. This number amounted to less than 1% of an entire corpus of declarative sentences. None of the high frequency users of the dialect exhibited this feature. The "go copula" was more frequent, although it is not known from the aggregate data if every child used it.

These are interesting outcomes, because it has been generally assumed that children from a low-income or low-social class are most prone to use AAVE forms (see recent study by Washington & Craig, 1998). Although such observations may be accurate, what the above cited studies show is that even low-income African American preschoolers are not uniform in their use of AAVE forms. It is not known from the aggregate group data reported on the "go copula" if the same small percentage of children accounted for all the AAVE forms used, or if every child studied used the AAVE form some of the time. Within-group variability must be taken into account in efforts to build suitable assessment procedures.

More careful study of the social class variable is needed as well. It could be that low income is such a global measure of social class that it does not adequately reflect the cultural patterns that are most likely to correlate with language. It is generally expected that low income also means low levels of education, a variable correlated with language use; but it is not a perfect correlation. People have low incomes for reasons unrelated to educational achievement. Some African American parents may be better educated than their low-income status reflects. Research is needed that documents the boundaries of the relationship between AAVE use and social class. Little is known still about if and how low and middle class African American children differ, although preliminary observations point to social class differences (Hart & Risley, 1995; Washington & Craig, 1998).

CONTEXT VARIABILITY AS A CONDITION FOR AAVE USE. It may well be that **remote past been** and **habitual be** were not elicited more often in the cited studies because the elicitation tasks did not target the contexts in which they are most likely to be used. In spontaneous speech samples, there is little control over what children will say. More information is needed about the pragmatic contexts that are likely to prompt the expression of meaning specific to AAVE.

At the same time, more needs to be known about how meaning may influence the variable rules governing the phonologic and morphosyntactic forms of AAVE. The frequently investigated morphological inflections immediately come to mind. AAVE forms are characterized by inflectional morpheme absence. But inflections are not invariably absent in AAVE speech (Wolfram, 1991). Variable use is rule governed even in children's speech (Wyatt, 1991, 1996). For example, inflections that occur in word final position may be influenced by a final consonant deletion rule. A final consonant is more likely to be deleted when it is followed by another consonant than by a vowel, as in the following two morphophonemic contexts: stepp<u>ed </u>back and stepp<u>ed i</u>n, respectively. However, final consonants that mark semantic contrasts, as in the case of the **-ed** (stepp<u>ed </u>back) may be less vulnerable to deletion than are final noninflected consonants that do not mark semantic contrasts (e.g., ba<u>d b</u>ack).

This kind of exploration, which is aimed at identifying the variable rules governing inflectional use, could be relevant to explanations of specific language impairment (SLI) that are framed in terms of a universal grammar. This notion rests on the argument that decreolized languages such as AAVE have evolved toward a standard parent language (e.g., English) in accord with natural or biological constraints on learning language forms (Bickerton, 1984). For example, retaining the final consonant before the vowel instead of the consonant favors the universal preference for CV syllable structure. Children with SLI are prone to delete inflectional morphemes across languages (Leonard, 1992). Still, research is revealing that slow language learners do use them (Lahey, Chesnick, Menyuk, & Adams, 1992) and more frequently in some contexts than others (Rice & Oetting, 1993). Their variable use of morphological inflections may be constrained by the same natural learning factors that govern AAVE usage. In fact, some patterns of morphological deletion in children with SLI parallel AAVE rules. Like AAVE adult speakers, children with SLI are prone to delete the /s/ plural in words preceded by a quantifier (cf., two shoe and two shoes) (Rice & Oetting, 1993). This pattern has the effect of simplifying the lexical patterns by eliminating redundant features. In the case of "**two** shoes," quantity is coded by both the adjective modifier, "**two**," and the inflectional "s" morpheme in "shoes." AAVE variable rules could provide clues to the variable constraints on SLI morphology.

OTHER ISSUES. The nature of the AAVE dialect and its social history ought to provide a unique opportunity to reveal some interesting features of human learning. There may be consequences for speaking an oral language or dialect that provide insight into the nature of human learning and adaptation in a way that languages with parallel written systems cannot do. For example, Craig (1992) noted that all nonstandard languages (Creoles included) have in common a tradition of oral language use that does not require written or highly formal communication. He speculated that there are probably consequences for the kind of verbal communication system that evolves. The size of the vocabulary or lexicon could be one consequence, given that the vocabulary of a Creole is limited. Predominant reliance on face-to-face communication means that the same words can have a greater variety of meanings, because the discourse context can be used to eliminate semantic ambiguity. The implication is that speakers can get by with fewer words, yet communicate a wide range of semantic distinctions.

Such speculation encourages study of the interface between semantic knowledge and the nonverbal context of verbal discourse, including its paralinguistic and other features. It also raises the question about whether speakers of oral languages acquire semantic depth in word meaning at earlier ages than speakers of languages with a parallel written code. Intuitively, it seems that if the same words are used to convey many meanings with help from the nonverbal context, then this semantic workload ought to show up in the number of different meanings attached to them. Children with an oral language as L1 may have early access to the variety of meanings to the extent that learners can more easily decode the nonverbal than the verbal contexts for using words appropriately in different ways.

No research appears to have been done on the nonverbal communication patterns of AAVE speakers or the relationship between discourse genre and vocabulary use. This is a worthy issue to pursue, because reduced vocabulary among African American children is usually interpreted as reduced potential to mark semantic distinctions. Reduced verbal input to children by caregivers also is now taken as evidence of no communicative interaction at all. These assumptions would be challenged by evidence of rich nonverbal interactions within which semantic distinctions are marked, and by evidence of unspoken communication between caregivers and their children.

A decreolizing social dialect such as AAVE offers a unique opportunity to study lexical innovation in a language that is not written. Innovation may be more pervasive for an oral dialect whose speakers have low social status. Terrell and Terrell (1993) reported that African American speakers use more slang terms than other groups, although empirical evidence for this claim was not offered. Innovations, which include slang, have not been respected phenomena to study in their own right. However, they clearly reflect the creative power of speakers. As transient language forms, the study of slang also provides a medium for exploring the factors underlying language change.

CLINICAL RESEARCH NEEDS

Obviously research needs to focus on clinical issues related to the assessment and treatment of semantic problems. Crosscultural language assessment is less formidable when impairment co-exists with clear physical, sensory, or cognitive deficits that are known to affect language development. In contrast, assessment is challenged by the largest group of children that is likely to be served—namely, those with specific language impairment (SLI) whose delay cannot be attributed to obvious causes. In such cases, a language difference and a disorder are more likely to be confounded. Semantic knowledge may prove to be a better metric for exposing such within-group differences than are the grammatical forms that variably apply.

Research aimed at determining the effectiveness of alternative approaches to semantic assessment is likely to be fruitful. Studies designed to determine the usefulness of existing criterion-referenced procedures also are likely to be helpful, particularly those procedures that assess vocabulary in ways that do not require children to know the same words, and make use of parental input in judging what words a child understands and uses. For example, Rescorla (1989, 1991) has developed a lexical criterion based on caregiver report that claims to identify lexical delays as early as 24 months of age. It predicts that normal learners will have at least 50 different words in their vocabularies by age 2;0. In a recent study (Watkins, Kelly, Harbers, & Hollis, 1995), it was reported that the total number of different words used in a speech sample may be an even better index of vocabulary size than is the traditionally used type token ratio. Future research can determine whether these two quantitative procedures are useful for revealing differences between African American children with, and those without language delay.

⌐

CHAPTER SUMMARY

In this chapter, it was pointed out that semantic competence in the language is more dependent on culture/language specific patterns than we might like to imagine—even for dialects of the same language. Some ways that AAVE differs from SE varieties were pointed out. Then the small set of studies on African American children's vocabulary and relational meaning were reviewed and critiqued. The chapter also called attention to the difficulty of studying meaning and the challenges that meaning poses for crosscultural language assessment that serves clinical and research goals. Alternative assessment approaches were identified and encouraged as a fruitful venue for future research. Finally, some ways to extend the research agenda on the normal semantic development of AAVE speakers were identified.

⌐

REFERENCES

Andersson, L., & Trudgill, P. (1990). *Bad language.* Cambridge, MA: Basil Blackwell, Ltd.

Baugh, J. (1983). *Black street speech.* Austin: University of Texas Press.

Benedict, H. (1979). Early lexical development: Comprehension and production. *Journal of Child Language, 6,* 183–200.

Bickerton, D. (1984). The language bioprogram hypothesis. *Behavioral and Brain Sciences, 7,* 172–221.

Blake, I. (1984). *Language development in working class black children: An examination of form, content, and use.* Unpublished doctoral dissertation, Columbia University, New York.

Bloom, L. (1994). Meaning and expression. In W. Overton & D. Palermo (Eds.), *The nature and ontogenesis of meaning* (pp. 215–235). Hillsdale, NJ: Erlbaum.

Bloom, L., & Lahey, M. (1978). *Language development and language disorders.* New York: John Wiley.

Bloom, L., Lightbown, P., & Hood, L. (1975). Structure and variation in child language. *Monographs of the Society for Research in Child Development, 40*(Serial No. 160). Chicago: University of Chicago Press.

Bowerman, M. (1989). Learning a semantic system: What role do cognitive predisposition's play? In M. L. Rice & R. L. Schiefelbusch (Eds.), *The teachability of language* (pp. 133–169). Baltimore: Brookes.

Bowerman, M. (1995, September). Learning to talk about space: A crosslinguistic perspective. Symposium on Cognitive Anthropology and Human Development. The Centennial Jean Piaget conference, *The growing mind.* Geneva, Switzerland.

Brown, P., & Levinson, S. C. (1995, September). Frames of spatial reference and their acquisition in Tenejapan Tzeltal. Symposium on Cognitive Anthropology and Human Development. The Centennial Jean Piaget conference, *The growing mind.* Geneva, Switzerland.

Brown, R. (1973). *A first language: The early stages.* Cambridge, MA: Harvard University Press.

Campbell, T., Dollaghan, C., Needleman, H., & Janosky, J. (1997). Reducing bias in language assessment: Process dependent measures. *Journal of Speech, Language and Hearing Research, 40*(3), 519–525.

Choi, S., & Bowerman, M. (1991). Learning to express motion events in English and Korean: The influence of language-specific lexicalization patterns. *Cognition, 41,* 83–121.

Coggins, T. (1979). Relational meaning encoded in the two-word utterances of Stage 1 Down's syndrome children. *Journal of Speech and Hearing Research, 22,* 166–178.

Cole, L. (1980). *A developmental analysis of social dialect features in the spontaneous language of preschool Black children.* Unpublished doctoral dissertation, Northwestern University, Evanston, IL.

Craig, D. (1992). Communication differences between standard and nonstandard speakers. In M. Cummings, L. Niles, & O. Taylor (Eds.), *Handbook on communications and development in Africa and the African diaspora* (pp. 140–153). Needham, MA: Ginn Press.

Crais, E. (1990) World knowledge to word knowledge. *Topics in Language Disorders, 10*(3), 45–62.

Dalgish, G. M. (1982). *A dictionary of Africanisms: Contributions of Sub-Saharan Africa to English language.* Westport, CT: Greenwood Press.

Dasen, P., & Wassmann, J. (1995, September). Absolute and spatial orientation in Bali: A reversal in Piagetian stages? Symposium on Cognitive Anthropology and Human Development. The Centennial Jean Piaget conference, *The growing mind.* Geneva, Switzerland.

Davis, P., Williams, J., Vaughn-Cooke, A. F., & Wright-Harp, W. (1993). A comparison of lexical development in a child with normal language development and in a child with language delay. *National Student Speech Language Hearing Association Journal, 20,* 73–77.

Dickinson, D. K. (1984). First impressions: Children's knowledge of words gained from a single experience. *Applied Psycholinguistics, 5,* 359–374.

Dillard, J. L. (1977). *Lexicon of Black English.* New York: Seabury Press.

Dollaghan, C. A. (1985). Child meets word: "Fast mapping" in preschool children. *Journal of Speech and Hearing Research, 28,* 449–454.

Dollaghan, C. A. (1987). Fast mapping in normal and language-impaired children. *Journal of Speech and Hearing Disorders, 52,* 218–222.

Dunn, L. M. (1959). *Peabody Picture Vocabulary Test-Revised.* Circle Pines, MN: American Guidance Service.

Dunn, L. M., & Dunn, L. M. (1981). *Peabody Picture Vocabulary Test-Revised.* Circle Pines, MN: American Guidance Service.

Fillmore, C. (1968). A case for case. In E. Bach & R. Harms (Eds.), *Universals in linguistic theory* (pp. 1–88). New York: Holt, Rinehart & Winston.

Flipsen, P. (1993). Use of ROWPVT with small-town Canadian kindergarten children. *Journal of Speech-Language Pathology and Audiology, 17,* 145–148.

Flipsen, P. (1998). Assessing receptive vocabulary in small-town kindergarten children: Findings for the PPVT-R. *Journal of Speech-Language Pathology and Audiology, 22,* 88–93.

Gardner, M. F. (1985). *Receptive One-Word Picture Vocabulary Test.* Austin, TX: PRO-ED.

Hart, B., & Risley, T. (1995). *Meaningful differences in the everyday experience of young American children.* Baltimore: Brookes Publishing Co.

Heath, S. B. (1983). *Ways with words.* Cambridge: Cambridge University Press.

Holloway, J. E. (1990). *Africanisms in American culture.* Bloomington: Indiana University Press.

Kail, R., & Leonard, L. B. (1986). Word-finding abilities in language-impaired children. *ASHA monographs 25.* Rockville, MD: American Speech-Language-Hearing Association.

Karenga, M. (1985). *The African American holiday of Kwanzaa.* Los Angeles: University of Sankore Press.

Kresheck, J. D., & Nicolosi, L. (1973). A comparison of black and white children's scores on the PPVT. *Language, Speech, Hearing Services in Schools, 4,* 37–40.

Labov, W. (1973). The boundaries of words and their meanings. In C. J. Bailey & R. Shuy (Eds.), *New ways of analyzing variation in English* (pp. 340–373). Washington, DC: Georgetown University Press.

Lahey, M., Chesnick, M., Menyuk, P., & Adams, J. (1992). Variability in children's use of grammatical morphemes. *Applied Psycholinguistics, 13,* 373–398.

Lee, L. (1971). *Northwestern Screening Syntax Test.* Evanston, IL: Northwestern University Press.

Leonard, L. (1992). The use of morphology by children with specific language impairment: Evidence from three languages. In R. Chapman (Ed.), *Processes in language acquisition and disorders* (pp. 186–201). St. Louis: Mosby Year Book.

Leonard, L., Bolders, J., & Miller, J. (1976). An examination of the semantic relations reflected in the language usage of normal and language disordered children. *Journal of Speech and Hearing Research, 19,* 371–392.

Lidz, C. S. (1991). *A practitioner's guide to dynamic assessment.* New York: Guilford Press.

Lyons, J. (1977). *Semantics* (Vol. 1). Cambridge, UK: Cambridge University Press.

Markman, E. M. (1994). Constraints on word meaning in early language acquisition. In L. Gleitman & B. Landau (Eds.), *The acquisition of the lexicon* (pp. 199–227). Cambridge: MIT Press.

McWhirter, S. (1988). *Subcategories of action verbs in children's language.* Unpublished master's thesis, Michigan State University, E. Lansing, MI.

Miller, P. (1982). *Amy, Wendy and Beth.* Austin, TX: University of Texas Press.

Molefi, A. (1990). African elements in African American English. In J. Holloway (Ed.), *Africanisms in American culture* (pp. 19–33). Bloomington: Indiana University Press.

Mount-Weitz, J. (1996). Vocabulary development and disorders in African American children. In A. Kamhi, K. Pollock, & J. Harris (Eds.), *Communication development and disorders in African American children: Research, assessment and intervention* (pp. 189–226). Baltimore: Brookes Publishing Co.

Nagy, W. E., & Herman, P. A. (1987). Breadth and depth of vocabulary knowledge: Implications for acquisition and instruction. In M. G. McKeown & M. E. Curtis (Eds.), *The nature of vocabulary acquisition* (pp. 19–35). Hillsdale, NJ: Lawrence Erlbaum.

Nelson, K. (1985). *Making sense: The acquisition of shared meaning.* Orlando, FL: Academic Press.

Nelson, N. (1986). What is meant by meaning and how can it be taught. Semantic factors in language development and disorders. *Topics in Language Disorders, 6*(4), 1–14.

Nippold, M. (1988). Figurative language. In M. Nippold (Ed.), *Later language development: Ages 9 through 19* (pp. 179–210). Austin, TX: PRO-ED.

Nippold, M. A., Uhden, L. D., & Schwarz, I. E. (1997). Proverb explanation through the lifespan: A developmental study of adolescents and adults. *Journal of Speech, Language and Hearing Research, 40,* 245–253.

Obler, L. K. (1997). Development and loss: Changes in the adult years. In J. B. Gleason (Ed.), *The development of language* (pp. 440–472). Needham Heights, MA: Allyn & Bacon.

O'Grady, W. O., Dobrovolsky, M., & Aronoff, M. (1989). *Contemporary linguistics: An introduction.* New York: St. Martin's Press.

Patterson, J. (1996, November). *Expressive vocabulary development of Spanish-English bilingual toddlers.* Paper presented at the annual convention of the American Speech-Language-Hearing Association, Seattle, WA.

Pena, E. (1996). Dynamic assessment: The model and its language application. In K. N. Cole, P. S. Dale, & D. J. Tahal (Eds.), *Assessment of communication and language* (pp. 281–307). Baltimore: Brookes Publishing Co.

Rescorla, L. (1989). The language development survey: A screening tool for delayed language in toddlers. *Journal of Speech and Hearing Disorders, 54,* 587–599.

Rescorla, L. (1991). Identifying expressive language delay at age two. *Topics in Language Disorders, 11,* 14–20.

Rice, M. L., Buhr, J. C., & Nemeth, M. (1990). Fast mapping word-learning abilities of language-delayed preschoolers. *Journal of Speech and Hearing Disorders, 55,* 33–42.

Rice, M. L., & Oetting, J. B. (1993). Morphological deficits of children with SLI: Evaluation of number marking and agreement. *Journal of Speech and Hearing Research, 36,* 1249–1257.

Robinson, J. A. (1988). "What we've got here is a failure to communicate": The cultural context of meaning. In J. Valsiner (Ed.), *Child development within culturally structured environments* (Vol. 2, pp. 137–198). Norwood, NJ: Ablex Corporation.

Smitherman, G. (1994). *Black talk: Words and phrases from the hood to the amen corner.* Boston: Houghton-Mifflin.

Snow, C. (1990). The development of definitional skill. *Journal of Child Language, 17,* 697–710.

Sornig, K. (1981). *Lexical innovation.* Amsterdam: John Benjamins.

Spears, A. (1982). The Black English semi-auxiliary *come. Language, 58,* 850–872.

Stockman, I. (1986a). The development of linguistic norms for nonmainstream populations. *Asha Reports, 16,* 101–110.

Stockman, I. (1986b). Language acquisition in culturally diverse populations. In O. Taylor (Ed.), *Nature of communication disorders in culturally and linguistically diverse populations* (pp. 117–155). San Diego: College Hill Press.

Stockman, I. (1991, October). *Lexical biases in dynamic and static locative expressions.* Paper presented at the Boston University Conference on Language Development, Boston, MA.

Stockman, I. (1992). Another look at semantic relational categories and language impairment. *Journal of communication disorders, 25,* 175–199.

Stockman, I. (1996). The promises and pitfalls of language sample analysis as an assessment tool for linguistic minority children. *Language, Speech and Hearing Services in Schools, 27,* 355–366.

Stockman, I., & Vaughn-Cooke, F. (1982a). Re-examination of research on the language of working class Black children: The need for a new framework. *Journal of Education, 164,* 157–172.

Stockman, I., & Vaughn-Cooke, F. (1982b). Semantic categories in the language of working class Black children. In C. Johnson & C. Thew (Eds.), *The proceedings of the Second International Congress for the Study of Child Language* (pp. 312–327). Washington, DC: University Press of America.

Stockman, I., & Vaughn-Cooke, F. (1984, July). *A closer look at the dynamic and static distinctions.* Paper presented at the Third International Congress on Child Language, University of Texas, Austin.

Stockman, I., & Vaughn-Cooke, F. (1986). Implications of semantic category research for the language assessment of nonstandard speakers. *Topics in Language and Language Disorders, 6,* 15–25.

Stockman, I., & Vaughn-Cooke, F. (1989). Addressing new questions about Black children's language. In R. Fasold & D. Schriffrin (Eds.), *Language change and variation* (pp. 275–300). Amsterdam: John Benjamins.

Stockman, I., & Vaughn-Cooke, F. (1992). Lexical elaboration in children's locative action constructions. *Child Development, 63,* 1104–1125.

Talmy, L. (1985). Lexicalization patterns: Semantic structure in lexical form. In T. Shopen (Ed.), *Language typology and syntactic description: Vol. 3. Grammatical categories and the lexicon* (pp. 49–57). Cambridge, UK: Cambridge University Press.

Terrell, S. L., & Terrell, F. (1993). African-American cultures. In D. Battle (Ed.), *Communication disorders in multicultural populations* (pp. 3–37). Boston: Andover Medical Publishers.

van Kleeck, A. (1994). Potential cultural bias in training parents as conversational partners with their young children who have delays in language. *American Journal of Speech-Language Pathology, 3,* 67–78.

Washington, J. (1996, March). African American English. Lecture presented at Michigan State University, E. Lansing, MI.

Washington, J., & Craig, H. K. (1992). Performances of low-income, African American preschool and kindergarten children on the Peabody Picture Vocabulary Test. *Language, Speech and Hearing Services in Schools, 23,* 329–333.

Washington, J. & Craig, H. K. (1994). Dialectal forms during discourse of urban, African-American preschoolers living in poverty. *Journal of Speech and Hearing Research, 37,* 816–823.

Washington, J., & Craig, H. K. (1998). Socioeconomic status and gender influences on children's dialectal variations. *Journal of Speech, Language, and Hearing Research, 41,* 618–626.

Watkins, R.V., Kelly, D. J., Harbers, H. M., & Hollis, W. (1995). Measuring children's lexical diversity: Differentiating typical and impaired language learners. *Journal of Speech and Hearing Research, 38,* 1349–1355.

Wolfram, W. (1991). *Dialects and American English.* Englewood Cliffs, NJ: Prentice-Hall.

Wyatt, T. (1991). *Linguistic constraints on copula production in Black English child speech.* Unpublished doctoral dissertation, University of Massachusetts, Amherst.

Wyatt, T. (1996). Acquisition of the African American English copula. In A. Kamhi, K. Pollock, & J. Harris (Eds.), *Communication development and disorders in African American children: Research, assessment and intervention* (pp. 95–116). Baltimore: Brookes Publishing Co.

IDA J. STOCKMAN, PH.D.

Ida J. Stockman, Ph.D., is Professor of Speech-Language Pathology in the Department of Audiology and Speech Sciences at Michigan State University. Dr. Stockman's research on the spoken language of African American children has emphasized semantic and phonological development and the use of such data for improving diagnostic assessment of minority language speakers.

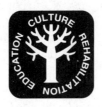

CHAPTER 5

GRAMMATICAL ACQUISITION OF AFRICAN AMERICAN ENGLISH

HARRY N. SEYMOUR, PH.D.
THOMAS ROEPER, PH.D.

In this chapter we attempt to describe the acquisition of syntax by children who speak African American English (AAE). This description is guided by (1) descriptive accounts of adult AAE, (2) prevailing theories of language acquisition, and (3) a limited descriptive profile of child AAE. Our approach is unique in that it integrates theoretical principles of acquisitional syntax with sociolinguistic accounts of AAE. We address the challenge of describing how and when a child learns the AAE dialect when surrounded by both AAE and standard American English (SAE). This challenge is reflected in Example 1:

(1) "I ain't got none cause he be eatin it. He don't share stuff. He bad."

This remark (Example 1) was made by a 3-year-old African American boy who speaks African American English (AAE). It includes features that are commonly found in AAE. These include multiple negation involving "ain't" and "none," the use of aspectual "be" as a part of the main verb, third person singular substitution of "don't" for "doesn't," and absence of copula "is." Were this child 5 or more years of age there would be little doubt that he is simply producing features of the adult AAE linguistic system. However, assume that a 3-year old produces "He don't share stuff. He bad." Here, there are other possible explanations for this child's "nonstandard" productions. It is quite possible that these features are simply immature products of an emerging language system as they also may be observed in developmental speech patterns of young children who speak other dialects of English such as SAE. Every language or dialect is a mixture of elementary structures, those that children grasp quickly and those that demand much more exposure. We return to the features of AAE that are particularly sophisticated below.

Let us assume the child is indeed a speaker of AAE. Support for this claim would be in expressions of the form "he be eatin," which show an awareness of a habitual meaning that cannot be grammatically expressed in SAE, except through an adverb like "habitually." We return to this intriguing feature of AAE below. On the other hand, the expression "he bad" is typical not only of adult AAE, but also of child grammar in both AAE and SAE. Such forms make it difficult to determine, at the outset, whether "he bad" is like adult AAE or a sign that a child was still in an early stage of grammar.

A further diagnostic would be required. In this instance, it refers to time. The early emerging grammars appear to allow expressions like "he bad" to refer both to "he is bad" and " he was bad," while AAE restricts the expression to present "he is bad." There is a large difference between a child who does not recognize tense and therefore can use "he bad" for present or past and the child or AAE speaker who limits the noun–adjective construction to a here and now interpretation. This subtle distinction is difficult to recognize in naturalistic data and therefore calls for the use of more sophisticated means of elicitation. Well targeted and subtle linguistic experiments can accomplish this task. Their development is an important current task for the field of communication disorders.

Linguistic progress works on two fronts. We have descriptive accounts of when new forms typically appear in the growth of SAE. And we have theoretical studies that identify the presence of basic principles of grammar. Both are of value in descriptions of an emerging grammar such as AAE. The descriptive sequence is a useful benchmark and the theoretical models promise more precise definitions of various abilities.

The effort to examine AAE development promises to shed light on AAE itself, on the acquisition process in which a dialect is present, and on the interesting microscopic features of acquisition.

Recent theoretical work (Green (1993) has advanced both the insight we have into grammar and the range of descriptive observations about AAE. Some of her important data can serve as indicators of grammar growth, even when their theoretical analysis continues to undergo evolution. Ultimately, when "explanatory adequacy" is achieved, we will have an account of Universal Grammar (UG) within which we can locate every special feature of every grammar. Until that time, many important and useable insights are available.

As in medical research, it is imperative to use what one knows, even when knowledge is imperfect. In describing our notion of crucial facts of language acquisition, we take a particular position about UG that is widely shared within linguistics, but not necessarily in the more applied disciplines. It is an exciting and enriching prospect to integrate dialect issues in speech pathology and education with linguistic theory and ongoing research. We begin this process by briefly reviewing how the syntax in adult AAE is typically described.

꒒

DESCRIPTION OF ADULT AAE

Unlike child AAE, there is substantial literature describing linguistic features of adult AAE, which focus primarily on syntax and phonology. However, for our purposes, we provide an overview description of only the syntactic profile. In doing so, it is important to point out certain inherent problems with such descriptions. In each instance of linguistic description of AAE form, we have a description, but not necessarily a full understanding of how a speaker represents the rule causing the form. Moreover, because most AAE descriptions are from a standard English perspective of how AAE diverges from SAE, these descriptions can be misleading in several respects. First, it does not reveal that a particular difference may have several origins. For instance, past tense -*ed* may be absent for phonological, syntactic, or semantic reasons. Second, it does not reveal that fundamental differences in grammar organization may be involved. For instance, languages of the world differ in whether they emphasize tense distinctions (past or present) or aspectual distinctions (progressive, resultant). AAE has properties of aspectual languages, although SAE is primarily tense-oriented. Third, it does not reveal where interpretive variation absent in SAE is present in AAE, such as the aspectual "be." In later sections of this chapter we discuss how current work has begun to recast our representation of AAE.

Notwithstanding the above limitations associated with the following overview, an adult AAE profile is nevertheless important as a maturational benchmark for interpreting and describing child AAE. Hence, the following adult AAE features are prominent in the literature.

Absence of -ed suffix: Some examples are:

A. past: He polished the table → He polish the table.
B. participle: He has polished the table → He has polish the table.
C. adjective: She is a blue eyed girl → She is a blue eye girl.

Representation of this phenomenon is partly phonological in that certain consonant clusters reduce *test* → *tes;* and when -ed is added to a verb such as miss, the outcome is likely *missed* → *miss.* Also, the -ed representation is partly grammatical: when past tense is invisible (as in *hit*), or in AAE, present *rub* → rub[+past]. added to a word, rubbed → rub.

The regularization of irregular verbs: Some verbs that have irregular past tense forms may be produced by adding *-ed* to the present tense form: He drank water → He drinked water. Universal Grammar (UG) represents external affixes (such as -ed) more easily than internal ones (drank). Therefore, overgeneralization is always towards external affixes (drinked).

Absence of forms of have: The contracted forms 've and 's for the auxiliary have in the present tense forms may be absent. Examples include: He's gone home → He gone home. I've two books → I two books. UG allows possession to be expressed without verbs, as in John's hat. Therefore, it is not surprising that an implied form of possession occurs in the verbal domain.

Absence of s-suffix: Third person singular subject verb agreement is not obligatory in AAE. Examples would be:

A. He runs home → He run home.
B. *Have* and *do* = / → has and does
[He have an apple; He do tricks.]

As we discuss below, it may be that AAE speakers associate different semantics with + or − s.

Absence of s-suffix plural marker: A plural quantifier (e.g., five) substitutes for inflectional plural (-s): I have five cent.

Absence of s-suffix possessive marker: The possessive marker is indicated by the order of the words and not by the present of 's. For example, John's cousin → John cousin.

Forms of gonna vary: Gonna may be expressed in the following ways: I am going home:

→ I gonna go home
→ I'mana go home
→ I'mon go home
→ I'ma go home.

It is not obvious that each of these forms have the same meaning. One hypothesis is that "I'mana" has an extended future reading.

Absence of contracted form of will: The future indicator will may be deleted when contracted and particularly so when followed by a labial consonant, that is, He'll marry her → He'uh marry her; He gon' marry her.

Invariant form of the verb to be: The form *be* may be used as a main verb (he be angry) or an auxiliary verb: *He be eating.* This form refers to a habitual or intermittent action as opposed to a single event.

Absence of contracted is and are: When is and are can be contracted in standard English they can be deleted in AAE. Examples are: He's strong → He strong; They're strong → They strong.

The features offer a descriptive outline of often cited aspects of AAE and provide a backdrop for our discussion of acquisiton.

⊔

CRUCIAL FACTS ABOUT
LANGUAGE ACQUISITION

UNIVERSAL GRAMMAR

Our description about AAE acquisition must at the same time encompass and capture the essence of the acquisition of all languages and the specifics of the English language. There are important properties of English that bind its various dialects together, as there are properties that connect English to other languages of the world. The theory of commonalties is called Universal Grammar, which is the basis of most current linguistic theory. From the opposite perspective, AAE illustrates some properties found in quite different language families, for instance, those where "aspect" is grammatically marked.

To ignore these properties would be to present a distorted and incomplete picture of any child's language. Thus, our description, in addition to describing how AAE acquisition may differ from other dialects of English, addresses language properties that are common to all languages, as well as to all dialects of English. We take this position not simply because we lack developmental milestone data on AAE, but because we believe the most important aspects of language acquisition are universal.

All children begin with a minimal form of UG that is represented in their minds as a system of principles and parametric choices. Principles are universal and apply equally to English, French, Arabic, and so on. They capture fundamental features of all grammars: the presence of words, phrases, and displaced elements. Phrases are the larger units present in all languages. Displacement occurs (what did John say) when something appears in one position but functions in another (say what). Words have discrete labels, phrases represented in the concept of a tree hierarchy, and "displacement" is captured by the concept of a transformation (which we illustrate below). The evidence for these principles is interconnected, but it lies in everyday observations about language. Thus, if we say:

(2) "The strange man saw the large hat"

And we transform it by passive into:

(3) "The large hat was seen by the strange man"

We have moved an entire object (so the subject is displaced from its object function) to a new position. Taking a whole phrase is defined by the combination of a transformation operating on a higher node (NP):

(4) NP1-V-NP2 → NP2 was V-d by NP1

It is commonsense that we cannot move half the phrase:

(5) *The large* was seen *hat* by the strange man

So there is a sense that the NP in the tree reflects a real unit—a moveable unit. A random part of that unit is not eligible for movement, as our intuitions tell us in judging Example 5 to be ungrammatical. Principles capture much that is commonsense and it is for this reason that it took an act of imagination by Chomsky (1957) to realize that these principles must be stated to represent universal language abilities. Once stated formally, they allow us to make other generalizations. The formal generalizations are themselves fundamental claims about how the mind is organized. Such principles may or may not extend to other realms of mind.

PARAMETERS

Parameters offer a universal set of choices, but each language takes a different choice path. Parameters involve many of the subtle details of language and therefore are under a great deal of discussion. One important parameter is word order: some languages are subject-object-verb, with others being subject-verb-object. This can be described as a simple choice, but it can feel to the learner of a second language like the whole grammar is backwards. Nonetheless, interestingly, a German child will decide that German is object-verb while at the two-word stage and feel that it is perfectly natural. This fact about early grammar suggests that it is indeed a simple choice which—if the mind is aimed at the right point—a child can make easily. What is the "right point"? Presumably it is a trigger in the biological sense—something that the organism is programmed to recognize although it is not logically necessary. Thus, a child might look automatically to intonation as the source of sentence force (question, declarative, imperative), although this is not a logical necessity.

Acquisition data from the two-word stage that shows that object-verb or verb-object order has been selected as a strong form of support for the parameter + triggers approach. It leads us to imagine that there must always be a simple trigger that gives the child crucial information, although the language the child hears is full of confusing examples, like the passive of Example 3, where (if one ignores "was"), it seems that the object precedes the verb. It may be that the simple word-order trigger lies in imperatives in German and English: "wash your hands" or "Hände waschen" (hands wash) in German.

INNATE LANGUAGE FACULTY

Because principles of language are universal they are therefore biological, in that infants all over the world are born with some innate capacity for language. They have what Chomsky (1972) refers to as a *language faculty,* which permits all children to acquire the language to which they are exposed with relative ease. This *language faculty* makes up what Chomsky has labeled the linguistic acquisition device (LAD).

This LAD is a biological endowment providing all children with the internal mental structure for language. All that is required for this language capacity to be realized is exposure to a language—any language. A combination of universal principles, setting of parameters, a vocabulary knowledge, and peripheral knowledge makes it possible to speak English, French, Arabic, Russian, or whatever human language to which a child is exposed. This exposure creates triggers that actualize what may be thought of as dormant knowledge about language. Once actualized, language unfolds and progresses without adult coaching in a manner almost impervious to disruption.

TRIGGERING EXPERIENCE

An essential dimension of LAD is what Chomsky refers to as the "triggering experience." His choice of terms merits attention. He does *not* say: invoke structure, or context, or meaning. The word "experience" refers to the combination of those factors. Let us imagine a case. How does a child learn that a passive must have been applied:

(6)　the milk was drunk

Let us equip the child with three levels of representation each of which must be compatible with the other to trigger passive voice:

Context: someone drinks a glass of milk
Meaning assumption: milk can be object, not subject
Structural observation: object (milk) is in subject position

Is there an operation that will make each observation above compatible? If the acquisition device satisfies these levels of analysis in a given situation, then it can project an autonomous syntax by the addition of a specific operation, a passive transformation:

Move the object to the subject position
(someone) drink milk → milk was drunk

This syntactic projection, in concert with pragmatics and meaning, triggers passive voice.

Once triggered, the environmental factors disappear. Context is not required for the interpretation of a sentence, just as it is not required in reading the example sentences in this essay. That is: we can understand passive sentences of the following form with no context:

(7) a. the hamburger ate the policeman
    b. the policeman was eaten by the hamburger

For us to recognize these sentences as grammatical nonsense, which violates pragmatics and natural meanings, we have to attribute independence from context to a grammar user. It is a correct understanding of Example 7a, which is the test of grammar acquisition.

The intricate interaction of nonlinguistic meaning apprehension and an autonomous grammar can be seen in these examples. By hypothesis the child will fix meaning inside grammar construction by construction. Therefore we predict correctly that a child will use grammar to recognize Example 7a as nonsense first, at a point where if given Example 7b, the child will have the policeman eat the hamburger, using context or common sense alone. What shows that a child is using common sense? Evidence suggests that children will treat Examples 8a and 8b differently:

(8) a. The policeman was eaten by the hamburger
    b. The milk was drunk by the child

A child will interpret Example 8b correctly apparently because it is implausible to have milk drink a child. However failure to see that Example 8a is nonsense means that the child has not fully acquired the passive transformation but has, instead, chosen to ignore passive markers and reduce it to a plausible sentence (the policeman ate the hamburger). It is important to realize that the true acquisition of grammar requires that we determine fundamental features of meaning without contextual support.

In other contexts, contextual support is required by the grammar itself in highly circumscribed ways. For instance, the following sentence is uninterpretable without context:

(9) I want that.

We must have context to interpret the deictic pronoun. Nonetheless we must be careful not to confuse this grammar-controlled use of context with the use of context in the process of "triggering experience."

POVERTY OF STIMULUS ARGUMENT

Cook (1987) discussed Chomsky's response to the "Plato Problem," as it relates to language. This problem poses the question: "How do we come to have such rich and specific knowledge, or such intricate systems of belief and understanding, when the evidence available to us is so meager?" (p. 55)

Chomsky's response was to put forth the "poverty of stimulus argument," which asserts that the available data to which young children are exposed is too impoverished to account for the scope and depth of knowledge they have when they acquire language. Thus, he concluded that the knowledge associated with language must derive from another source, which he attributed to properties of the mind, that is, the LAD.

This poverty of stimulus position has particular implications for AAE, because it reduces the importance of the quality of language exposure in determining whether a child will acquire appropriate and functional language. In fact, Chomsky (1972) has gone so far as to suggest that children could acquire language from the "scraps of the table." If Chomsky's claim is correct—albeit there are dissenters—children will acquire functional and competent language despite adverse environmental circumstances such as poverty, limited education on the part of parents or guardians, and noisy and even chaotic home settings, and so on.

Clearly, there must be a certain quality of exposure to language. But, the point is that this exposure can be very different among language learners and may not require motherese and it may be from rather disjointed sources including people, songs, stories. Yet, for much of its history, AAE has been viewed as a corrupt and cognitively deficient form of English whose origin is rooted in cultural disadvantage. This perception persists in the public at large, despite strong opposing arguments by linguists and other educators.

The simple claim that language will be acquired regardless of the cultural and language background, socioeconomic level, and educational environments of infants places all children on equal footing regardless of their language, culture, and educational background. This includes African-American children who speak AAE as their first language. Barring severe physical abnormality and extremely harsh environmental deprivation, African American children will acquire language in the same manner and to the same degree as anyone else. Although this position should be obvious and should not need saying, one must recognize that in many areas and segments of our society, the language development of African American children has been viewed from a deficit perspective.

POSITIVE VERSUS NEGATIVE EVIDENCE

The actual language evidence to which children are exposed is primarily positive. By positive evidence we mean that they only hear linguistic forms and structures that should be spoken in their language. For the most part, they don't get error messages to allow self-correction, or have a model of incorrect production against which to calibrate their own productions. Moreover, they cannot observe the impossible in their language, and there is much about their language they never observe directly at all, because some aspects occur so rarely. Yet, these rare forms are learned and used without ever hearing them produced by others. So, how do children learn their grammar from only positive evidence or no evidence at all. One answer to this question is that they cannot do so from what they hear alone (positive evidence), and, thus, there must be some internal and intuitive mechanism guiding them.

Of course there is some external feedback received by children as they monitor their own language use, the response from others, and as they do some internal comparisons against what they hear. But by and large, language cannot be acquired in this monitoring and feedback fashion. Contrary to a commonly held view, rarely are children corrected for their own error patterns and given the correct forms to say. When this kind of correction does occur it is a form of "negative evidence."

Negative evidence in child language acquisition can be indirect or direct. An indirect form may occur when a child never hears a subject-less sentence and sets a parameter that there must be a subject at the head of a declarative sentence. Brown and Hanlon (1970) suggested a number of possible indirect sources of negative evidence, but concluded that none were sensitive to grammatical ill-formedness and, thus, did not constitute evidence that a child was provided with indirect evidence. Although claims in more recent studies suggest a contingency relationship between mother's language behavior on children's grammatical ill-formedness (Demetras, Post, & Snow, 1986; Penner, 1987), the prevailing conclusion, nevertheless, remains that children do not receive systematic input about ill-formed sentences (Atkinson, 1992; Pinker, 1989).

Indeed, the more commonly described example of negative evidence is the direct, in which a parent corrects something a child has said. This direct appeal from parents is rarely successful (Pinker, 1984), and it is not clear that children even understand the concept of grammar correction, as opposed to content correction. An often cited example of negative evidence was reported by McNeill (1966):

Child: Nobody don't like me.

Mother: No, say "Nobody likes me."

Child: Nobody don't like me.

(dialogue repeated eight times)

Mother: Now listen carefully, say "Nobody likes me."

Child: Oh! Nobody don't likes me. (p. 13)

Adults, as well, resist correction. This is obvious when one tries to force a foreigner to pronounce something without an accent. They may succeed in direct imitation, but then quickly revert to pronunciation with a foreign accent.

There is little evidence that negative evidence as a corrective model is effective or that it is widely used in child-rearing practices. Even in the domain of clinical treatment of children and adults with language disorder, there is debate over the efficacy of correction models versus more naturalistic and whole language treatment strategies (Lahey, 1988; Lund & Duchan, 1993). Indeed, parents correct their children, but the practice seems more directed at semantic and content areas and not specific linguistic syntactic structures (McNeill, 1970). The informed view is that negative evidence has little to do with the acquisition of language among children whose language is developing normally.

Yet, it appears that only in the case of AAE that there has been major programs developed to provide a heavy dosage of negative evidence as a corrective model for normal children (Bereiter & Engelmann, 1966). These programs were unsuccessfully administered by professionals who were working under the assumption that large numbers of African American children were linguistically deprived as a result of being exposed to an "aberrant" model of English. Thus, not only was the input from community language provided to many young African American children viewed to be impoverished, it was also considered a corrupt form of English. The perceived consequence of children exposed to this "aberrant" language input, were children viewed to be linguistically and cognitively deprived, as evidenced by the following quote:

The speech of the severely deprived children seems to consist not of distinct words, as does the speech of middle-class children of the same age, but rather of whole phrases or sentences that function like giant words. That is to say, these "giant word" units cannot be taken apart by the child and re-combined; they cannot be transformed from statements to questions, from imperatives to declaratives, and so on. Instead of saying "He's a big dog," the deprived child says "He bih daw." Instead of saying "I ain't got no juice," he says "Uai-ga-na-ju." Instead of saying "That is a red truck," he says "Da-re-truh." Once the listener has become accustomed to this style of speech, he may begin to hear it as if all the sounds were there, and may get the impression that he is hearing articles when in fact there is only a pause where the article should be. He may believe that the child is using words like it, is, and in, when in fact he is using the same sound for all of the—something on the order of "ih." (This becomes apparent if the child is asked to repeat the statement "It is in the box." After a few attempts in which he becomes confused as to the number of "ih's" to insert, the child is likely to be reduced to a stammer.) (Bereiter & Engelmann, 1966, p. 34).

To consider a whole community of speakers to be aberrant, as suggested in the above quote, is absurd. Indeed, there is ample evidence of language impairment among individuals, but never an entire dialect. For similar reasons, it is equally absurd to claim that the offspring of AAE speakers will have a deprived or deficient language because AAE is their model of exposure. Of course an important basis for these claims is the contrast between young AAE and SAE speakers in their development and use of language. Most notably, there are far more morphemic inflections and verb forms absent in child AAE than in child SAE. However, in an important sense, AAE clearly represents the direction of language change. Modern SAE lacks most of the inflections that Middle English exhibited, or that children speaking Germanic languages exhibit.

These absent AAE forms are typical in adult AAE, as well, and therefore one should not be surprised at their absence in child AAE. In fact, so-called forms "absent" in child AAE are evidence of the character and power of the community language in shaping one's language structure. For unlike the SAE-speaking child, the AAE speaker is exposed to both the AAE and SAE dialect forms. In many respects these two dialects would provide contradictory evidence to the child. However, despite this dual exposure, the child acquires the adult AAE system. In effect, the child must keep each grammar separate in order to not regard the input as unresolveably incoherent. In fact, an argument can be made that all speakers learn more than one dialect inside the same language.

The evidence which the AAE child draws for his or her language is no greater or less than that of other children of different language backgrounds. The youngster is only exposed to positive evidence. Moreover, there are no sideline coaches signaling when an utterance is nonstandard, contrasts with SAE, or in any other way is deviant. As discussed, when such efforts are made, they are unsuccessful. As with all children, African American children simply acquire that to which they are exposed, which is as rich and as fully developed a language system as any other.

⊔

ACQUISITION VERSUS DEVELOPMENT

How exactly the journey occurs from innate capacity of infants to the actual production of a full-fledged adult language is not altogether clear. This is a nativistic question to which psycholinguists devote much of their effort trying to figure out. Explanations of first language acquisition in children has from the very beginning been a debate centering on the nature versus nurture issue. Undoubtedly, children's language is shaped by both internal biological factors and external social experiences. Clearly, AAE's development is a product of both. Thus, our account draws theoretical frameworks that are both nativistic and social. As such, we integrate current theories in psycholinguistics and sociolinguistics in describing what AAE speaking children know about language and how they appear to use their language.

One possible way of reconciling somewhat incompatible theories from psycholinguistics and sociolinguistics is to consider a distinction, sometimes made by psycholinguists, between acquisition and development (Cook, 1987). Acquisition of language refers to an idealized model of principles that appear to be innate and that make up LAD. Development, on the other hand, may be those aspects of language associated with parameter setting and are influenced by an interaction with other faculties of the mind such as cognitive factors, as well as external factors associated with environment. Cook (1987) made the point that acquisition is concerned with evidence about what children know and development with evidence from what children say. The former requires no direct observation of children, whereas the latter does.

If we were to apply this acquisition versus development distinction to AAE child language, the description of acquisition should be identical to other dialects of English and, for that matter, to other languages as well. On the other hand, the development of AAE will show both differences and similarities as a child progresses through various stages. We discuss this acquisition/development distinction in terms of both psycholinguistic and sociolinguistic perspectives.

PSYCHOLINGUISTIC PERSPECTIVE

What language factor does a child have when first born? The infant certainly has a range of grammar-specific analytic powers. Concepts such as words, hierarchy, and transformation are available as soon as triggering environments allow them to be used. The acquisition of AAE presents no unique problems, but it does belong to a family of language phenomena that are just now receiving theoretical attention: bilingualism and second language acquisition.

How does a child cope when confronted with incompatible grammars? One approach to this question is to argue that a child just keeps two languages phonologically distinct and therefore acquires two grammars with no overlap. Here we have an easy answer to the question of dialect variations. But suppose there is no reliably distinctive phonology.

Then we might take another approach and argue that all speakers have several dialects. This means that the AAE/SAE speaker is identical in all respects to the so-called SAE speaker because, though unacknowledged, pockets of dialects exist for everyone. Consider the dialect speaker who says either "he here" or "he is here." Now consider the speaker of SAE who allows inversion with quotation but not with normal transitive sentences:

(10) a. "Nothing" said Bill
     b. *ball threw John

If we have object-verb-subject in Example 10a, then why not in Example 10b? In fact, the Examples 10a,b combination is equivalent to German. Can the presence of both Examples 10a and b be described as properties of the same grammar? In a strict sense, they cannot. Either one moves main verbs to the second position or one does not. If one divides the vocabulary so that quotation verbs are distinct from nonquotation verbs, then one can say that different sections of vocabulary undergo different rules (although in German both undergo the same rule). In effect, we argue that one section of the vocabulary (quotation verbs all allow this operation: "So what," murmured John) is Germanic and one is not. This claim, of course, fits the history of the language, as it originally had a verb-raising structure.

When do SAE speakers exhibit knowledge of a subpart of the grammar that undergoes different rules? In fact, the verb-second operation affects more than quotation environments. It also affects *have* and *be*. It is well known that we are still shifting from a grammar in which *have* can be fronted to one where we must insert a dummy element *do*:

(11) a. Has he any money
     b. Does he have any money

Older speakers allow Example 11a more readily. Perhaps the language is moving toward the requirement that we insert *do* everywhere, although historical change is a complex phenomenon. The same evolution occurs with *be*:

(11) c. Is he here
     d. Does he be here/do he be here

The case of Example 11d reflects AAE and a more consistent approach to verb-fronting in which no main verb can front. Note that in imperatives we have already made the shift: "don't be late." One would expect, ultimately, a parallel shift in quotation:

(11) e. "Nothing" did he say

This evolution may yet occur. Until it occurs, SAE is in an intermediate dialect, with AAE having progressed somewhat further toward regularization, as has British English, which allows both "Do be nice," as well as "Be nice."

The conclusion of this discussion is that there is nothing inherently unusual in being surrounded by a language environment in which partly incompatible grammars with the same phonology are at work.

Our social perceptions, of course, like fashion, generally, are linked to strong feelings unjustified by the facts. We easily perceive "have you any money" as stilted and "he don't be happy" as uneducated. In reality both forms are participating in the same language change in different ways. However social perceptions are a reality as well. Whether and how we choose to honor them, reflects how far we care to make language prejudice legitimate.

Nonetheless, two general descriptive questions arise about the development of AAE: (1) how far does it parallel Standard English and the development of any language, (2) how and when does it diverge? There is a theoretical answer to each of these questions. In principle, invariant universal features of grammar should exhibit the same growth pattern for all grammars. And language-particular features should produce a distinctive acquisition schedule at the moment they become relevant. These ideas become more accessible in the following examples.

SEMANTICS

First, we indicate where principles suggest a common developmental sequence. Semantic distinctions are often universal. For instance, the definite and the indefinite article involve an automatic capacity to distinguish between set-reference and individual reference. Maratsos (1974) showed that such capacities were available as soon as experimentation could be done. Experimenters made up a word that could either be a common noun or a proper noun: Dax. Children under 2 years were then shown two identical dolls. And to one doll they pointed and said: "Here's Dax." to the other they said: "Here's a dax." Then they asked the children to point to "a dax" or "Dax." Only in the former case did the children sometimes point to the identical doll instead of the original doll. This indicated that they understood that "a Dax" meant any member of a set of items of the same kind. No one instructs a child about such things. There is no reason to expect a dialect difference in the semantics (although "definiteness" may be represented differently in languages without articles).

SYNTAX

Syntax shows substantial variation, but little variation between SAE and AAE. There is no distinction between the categories noun and verb when we look across languages. Therefore "see" and "dog" should be equally accessible in any language (assuming that the phonology is clear). The next step after nouns have been identified is to identify noun phrases. This requires a child to recognize articles. Here languages differ syntactically (but not semantically as we have just shown), though AAE and SAE do not. In some languages, like German, the article can be a pronoun. This never occurs, even erroneously, in English because no child has ever been reported as saying: *"I want the," although this is quite possible in German ("Ich möchte den"). How does a child know that the article cannot stand alone in English. Although it is true that the German article carries more information (gender), it does not follow from this that it should be able to stand alone. Therefore, that children never make this mistake suggests a universal acquisition principle that is not evident in the surface of the language: An article can operate as a pronoun only if it carries more information. Does the incorporated article in English change the acquisition schedule? It is not clear. If having a separable article makes it clearer, then German should allow the identification of articles first. If having no ambiguity between article and pronominal use is an advantage, then English should be first. It is an empirical matter.

French has articles that are cliticized. They seem to be part of the noun. This is actually true in part for English because the article changes its phonology: For many speakers "thuh hat, but thE apple." The /e/ is long before a vowel which means it is being treated as part of the word. This means that, in effect, the child hears two forms of the same word and must somehow be sure that it is not two words. These features again do not distinguish SAE and AAE (although in some dialects of English there is no lengthening, just /thuh apple/). Finally in some languages, like Faroese, the article appears in the middle of the word: "app-the-le." This means that the English-speaking child must be ready to hear German, Faroese, French, or English. These phonological features could complicate recognition. However we have no major SAE/AAE contrast, so our expectations for acquisition should be the same for the acquisition of articles, and the descriptive literature reports no problems with articles.

WORD ORDER AND AGREEMENT PARAMETERS

It is not yet clear how many parametric decisions a child must make. However, the concept is inherently simplifying, because it allows a whole set of decisions to be made at once. For instance, in most cases verbs and prepositions are parallel. If it is object-verb, then it will be object-preposition. So if one decides the order of verb-object, one may know automatically that it is preposition-verb as well. However, life is not always so easy, as some languages appear to be mixed (like German) and there are lexical exceptions in English (where from/ what with/where to). The child must not be led astray by these lexical items and suddenly think that they represent an object-verb or object-preposition language. Enabling a child to discriminate between exceptions and rules is a major challenge to the child and to acquisition theory. It is complicated in a dialect situation. How does a child keep two dialects apart? In fact, there are points where we can identify code switching and points where the existence of one or two grammars may be very obscure. We can illustrate this with the phenomenon of agreement.

We know that the AAE dialect allows invisible agreement or nonagreement in third person. How do we determine the difference between invisible agreement and nonagreement? This is a deep question that is currently debated in linguistic theory. One possible piece of evidence for invisible agreement lies in the obligatory subject/verb connection in ellipsis. If I say "Who has a hat," we can answer "me" or "him" (which never show agreement (*him does and seems to be a default form) or "I do" but never *I or *he alone. Why does it not appear alone? It is not a pure phonological clitic because one can have an intervening adverb (I never do). Therefore one can argue that there is an invisible agreement between subject and verb that demands that both be present even when the agreement marker is invisible. This means that at the earliest stages, the so called optional infinitive stage (Rice & Wexler, 1996; Wexler, 1994), where children say "she go" but never "she" alone, an invisible agreement marker must be present. In effect, then, more than an infinitive is present because an invisible agreement node is operative. In German or Arabic, the default is the nominative "I" and it occurs freely by itself (Abdulkarim & Roeper, 1996).

Now that there is an "optional" agreement in AAE that is often reported, is open to several interpretations. First it may indeed be optional. If it were really optional, then we would expect AAE speakers to be able to say "I" by itself. This is not reported and therefore it seems that some agreement is present at an abstract level.

Second -s might mark a different distinction, such as emphasis. Thus we find speakers who say "I says" and "you says" where the -s clearly cannot carry third person agreement at all, but must have some other function. Third, the child may be bidialectal. When the -s is present on third person, then it is SAE, and when it is absent, then it is AAE and is present invisibly. So at a very subtle level, code switching rather than optionality would be present. It is evident that dialect choice is linked to subtle social factors (Wyatt & Seymour, 1990). In one situation, one dialect may be chosen, although, again, "situation" may be very subtle. Suppose I were to say "It isn't so, I mean it just ain't so," I may have shifted to an informal mode within a single sentence. Dialects are extremely subtle and linguistic analysis has not yet identified all of the relevant social factors.

SUBJECTLESS SENTENCES

Let us consider one final example. Subjectless sentences are found in Italian as a rule, but they are found in English as a reflection of an informal social register. That is, we allow ourselves to say:

(12) Seems like a nice day

when the grammar as a rule requires the presence of subjects. This informal social register borrows, in effect, from a different language family (much like the quotation examples above). There is no way to make English have a single grammar that both predicts the presence and the absence of subjects. In a reduced form, once again, we have the equivalent of a dialect that obeys different rules. In sum, the patterns of interwoven dialect are, from a theoretical perspective, much like the pattern of varying speech registers to be found in any language.

FUNCTIONAL CATEGORIES

We return now to issues of the acquisition process by focusing on functional categories. Grammars bear a variety of relations to the core principles of UG that may have profound effects on the course of acquisition. There are five categories which we can articulate:

1. Default Values: Direct reflection of core default values in UG. Universal grammar, in its simplest form, defines a set of core relations that all humans can generate. Thus "he big" is found in AAE and in many other grammars of the world, although it is not a direct possibility in SAE. It is an indirect possibility in sentences of the form: "He arrived tired," which involves two forms of predication—He arrived and he tired. Only AAE allows the latter to exist without an overt inflectional morpheme, but the relation exists in both AAE and SAE.

2. Lexical Extensions: Grammars vary in how many lexical items will occupy certain formal roles. Thus AAE uses both "it" and "there" in environments where SAE uses "there" alone, as in "There is nothing going on" → It is nothing going on.

3. Parametric Choices: Here is where languages acquire their distinctive character. Some grammars may not articulate an independent category to represent negation. Negation can be either a modifier or a category of its own. This is like the distinction between contraction (didn't) and a full form (did not). This distinction affects how the negative system will be developed.

4. Invisible Presence: The foremost theoretical possibility is that forms are not absent, but present invisibly. Intuitively, for instance, we sense that in elliptical utterances forms are still present when not pronounced:

(13) John is tall and Bill is too = Bill is tall too.

This may be true of missing tense and copula forms as well, because in AAE the copula is invisible, as in "John big"(instead of "John is big"). This is different from the claim—in some theories—that there is a relation of *predication* that makes the copula unnecessary. For instance, if we say:

(14) I consider John tall

we find no verb. The same kind of predication, or sometimes called "small clause" can be present in AAE forms like:

(15) John tall

Theories depend on descriptions, but we must be careful that our choice of descriptive terminology does not influence our theoretical direction. The term "deletion" can obscure the possibility that invisible forms are present.

   In addition, new hypotheses emerge under these theories. If predication is present automatically in UG, then a child who says "John big" must have it. If there is a deletion or an invisible copula in some languages, then a child with a deficit might have predicational "John big," while a normal AAE child would have "John big" with an invisible copula. The same form would have two different grammars. The invisible copula could become visible under movement for one but not the other (I know how John big → move big left → I know how big John *is*). It is often the case that core data is opaque and only subtle data reveal structure. It is then the subtle structures that must be used for diagnosis.

5. Theoretical Variants: We do not know exactly which of these theoretical representations should be advocated. The accumulated evidence, most recently discussed in Green (1993), suggested that AAE represents a radical departure from SAE in the structural representation of the inflectional and aspectual systems. For instance, the habitual "be" form (see below) allows do-insertion (he be playing baseball, don't he), which suggests that it occupies a unique position in the tree-hierarchy above the verb phrase and below auxiliaries. It moves toward aspect-dominated grammar families. The progressive loss of inflection in SAE historically over the last 300 hundred years suggests that it too will move in that direction.

ACQUISITION IMPLICATIONS

The implications for acquisition are unknown and must simply be studied empirically. One major claim is: Default UG structures may appear with no overt input evidence. There are many forms of default structures in language. In adult language they appear innocuously in many environments: "He likes ice cream more than me/more than **I**." "**Me**" is a default, assigned without appropriate case, but not disturbing to most speakers in this context. The same operation occurs when a child says "me want."

Modal interpretation may also have a default value. For instance, a child may be able to link modality to an abstract morpheme without input of that kind. Thus if a child says: "ride bike" and the parent knows that it means "can I ride a bike" the child is able to represent a meaning that is technically at odds with reality (he or she is not riding a bike) and that reflects a mental attitude (a desire is expressed), and consent is sought (parental approval). It is also possible that the notion of "can" is in the grammar, although the remainder is part of contextual interpretation. The line between what is invisible in the grammar and what is a contextual extension is very difficult to draw.

Second we can expect lexical items to show many kinds of personal and temporal variation. The comprehension of a subject as object is generally linked to particular lexical items. Thus if I say:

(16) that's easy

it means:

(17) that is easy (to do that)

and the "that" is really the object of a hidden verb. But this complex grammatical relation may await the learning of individual adjectives like "easy."

Third we may expect parametric choices to be either early or late depending on how much structure they involve. We have found that children learn the aspectual "be," which has no counterpart in SAE at a very early age. Let us suppose it requires a distinct structural home. One might expect that this would appear late in children's grammars, but as it is prominent in the input and the environment it is quite evident. On the other hand, the negative system of AAE presents unusual challenges and may be learned rather slowly.

DEVELOPMENTAL PERSPECTIVE

The developmental aspect of AAE emergence in children arises from an interaction of internal and external factors. We have discussed the UG principles that make up the language faculty that all children appear to have at birth. This language facility must be accommodated simultaneously by both a biological and social maturation. The brain undergoes considerable and rapid change during the first few years of life, with a corresponding change in language performance. Although the modular view of language faculty would have this module operating independently of other modules of the brain, there must be some coordination and interaction as a child's nervous system matures. It is this interactive property that provides the capacity for setting parameters and for learning the lexicon of one's language and the subtle distinctions of markedness of his or her particular language.

These subtle distinctions have been linked sociolinguistically to social factors of race, socioeconomic class, and culture. This sociolinguistic position is a prominent one and cannot be ignored in our discussion of AAE acquisition. In fact, social variation may be the most challenging aspect of learning a dialect. When is the dialect appropriate and when not? Where children experience only dialect, the social status of the grammar may be quite different from SAE. Thus the social status of AAE may be different in the USA South from the USA North, where SAE is omnipresent. Questions of this kind engage all of our social sophistication and cannot be easy for a child to determine. Therefore we expect children to be uncertain about where informal language is permissible.

To conceptualize the grammar a child must develop to be an AAE speaker, one might envision English that is influenced by the various adult features discussed previously. Although AAE and SAE differ in where they allow complexity, there is no aspect of SAE grammar that cannot be expressed in AAE. Although dialects may exhibit only superficial differences, they may also be profoundly different in some components, as our discussion of aspectual differences illustrates. Still, others make claims for stronger differences rooted in separate and distinct African language origins. We do not address this question of origin in this chapter. However, we take the position that differences manifest in the two adult dialect systems require somewhat different developmental paths.

The question before us is—in what manner do African American children progress from principles of UG to the production of adult AAE? To answer this question, we must untangle the contributions of UG from those of socialization, which, as pointed out earlier, is tantamount to a "nature/nurture" puzzle. It would be easy to solve this puzzle, if we had a complete profile of each minute and detailed accounting of the progressive changes as a child's language unfolds and advances. This profile would also include the environmental events associated with each behavioral change, so that triggers could be identified. Of course, such a description is not possible.

The behavior observed in children's language can be highly variable across children, even for speakers of the same dialect. The source of this variability can be biological in that children arrive at various milestones at different rates. However, a major source of variability is from factors external to a child's grammar, which relate to such things as cognitive maturation, social maturation, environmental influences, learnability among many other possible contributors.

There are many accounts of the development of English in children. Several attempted to describe stages through which all children pass even though they may do so at different rates (Brown, 1973; Miller, 1981; Morehead & Ingram, 1973). Table 5–1 depicts a summary of five major stages reflected in many stage accounts.

Each of the various stage models attempt to link language milestones to a language index, which is either mean length of utterance (MLU), mean length of response (MLR), or an average between the two. MLU is calculated by dividing the number of overall utterances in a child's language corpus by the number of morphemes (free and bound) in that corpus. MLR is similar except its calculation is based only on free morphemes (full word forms). Brown (1973) claimed that language complexity was directly correlated with language length as reflected in MLUs. This claim appears supportable up to about MLU 3.5, at which point complexity of language becomes much more subject to pragmatic factors. Table 5–1 shows a typical kind of profile according to stages of development that are associated with MLU.

The MLU measurement is widely used in child language research to establish and match subjects' language levels. However, it is not a theoretically definable concept and, therefore, it cannot serve as more

TABLE 5–1
Five stages of language development.

Stage	MLU Range	Age Range (months)	Language Description
I	1.0 –2.0	12–26	One Word Stage—Linear semantic rules
II	2.0 –2.5	27–30	Morphological inflection development
III	2.5 –3.0	31–34	Sentence form development
IV	3.0 –3.75	35–40	Embedding of sentence elements
V	3.75–4.5	41–46	Joining of clauses

Source: Adapted from R. E. Owens, 1988. *Language development* (2nd. ed.). Columbus, OH: Merrill.

than a rough guideline. In fact, it may be misleading for the study of SAE in precisely the same way as we argue that it is misleading for AAE. The claim that two children of equivalent MLUs are considered to be functioning at the same language level with very similar language complexity does not hold for AAE. The reason is the many morphemes not realized morphologically, as with a zero morphemes. Consider the following utterances spoken by an SAE child and an AAE child:

(18) a. Two cats are in John's house. (SAE)
 b. Two cat in John house. (AAE)

In Example 18a, there are eight morphemes and in b there are five. These two children may very well be at equivalent syntactic levels, but would have very different MLUs. Because of the many absent morphemic inflections in AAE, no claims can be made about AAE developmental level for particular MLU measurements. Moreover, because these absences are conditioned by variable social and linguistic constraints, claims about language equivalence between two matching MLU levels may be questionable as well.

Despite these problems with applying MLU as an index of language level among AAE child speakers, major stages of development and the sequence in which they occur should not differ for AAE. There are three reasons for this conclusion. First, stages typically are characterized by major milestones that must be acquired by any child learning English. Secondly, the developmental span between stages is so broad that milestones characteristic of each stage are likely to be acquired regardless of within stage variations from dialect differences. And third, the sequence depicts milestone behaviors that progress from simple to complex, which should also occur regardless of dialect variations.

The ways in which AAE differs from SAE and other varieties of English likely will not be evident across the five stages shown in Table 5–1, but instead will be revealed within particular stages. In many cases, these differences may be quite subtle and less apparent in production than comprehension. Because there are serious gaps in knowledge about the specific details of AAE acquisitional milestones, it is impossible to construct a developmental profile that can parallel the stage descriptions found in Table 5–1. Therefore, we avoid such a description. Instead, we discuss what we consider to be important issues necessary for understanding AAE acquisition and for conducting research on this topic . We do this by focusing on dividing the grammatical acquisition into two broad periods: early syntax development and later syntax development.

EARLY SYNTAX

During the one-word stage, there is little evidence that the AAE-speaking child will differ in any substantive way from other children acquiring English. Somewhere around the first year, the AAE child speaker will produce his or her first word. This does not mean that the child knows only one word. During the first year of life, the child has learned much about objects in the world—what they are, how they relate to each other, and to him or her. This knowledge is in the form of comprehension and will rapidly be expressed soon after the first word is uttered.

The early lexicon of children is made up first of nominals and then action words. These words are sometimes referred to as holophrastic, in that they take the form of single words in representing whole phrases. Much of these holophrastic utterances are about "here and now" and about objects that are easily moveable within the child's physical and visual space. Children are less likely to talk about large and immovable objects such as the stove or refrigerator (Lahey, 1988).

Although there is no syntax expressed until the child combines more than one word, there is obviously understanding of adult syntax. The exact nature of this understanding is not clear. It is almost a truism of acquisition work that comprehension precedes production. What is obscure, at times, is whether comprehension is accurate. The field of experimental acquisition work has focused on demonstrating subtle knowledge where inference is not a reliable guide.

In the extreme case, it is not clear that there is any production data at all. For instance, we (Weissenborn, deVilliers, & Roeper, 1996) have undertaken a study of when children comprehend sentences of the form: who bought what. There are no examples in CHILDES (MacWinney, 1991) of these sentences being produced by children. Nevertheless we found that 3-year-old children comprehended the bound variable nature of such sentences. That is, children give a paired list answer to the question "who bought what": John bought potatoes, Bill bought oranges, Fred bought cherries, and so on. Universal grammar must inform the child (a) that a question word is a variable (who or what calls for a list answer) and (b) that when two wh-words are present, the answer is a paired list.

Is there a stage when children do not know that questions involve variables? Sometimes parents will ask a child: "Who was at the birthday party"? and the child answers "Johnny" and then the parent asks, "and who else"? It seems as if the child does not grasp that the question calls for a multiple answer.

Similarly children may not initially know that a question word has a "long-distance" origin. What occurs at early stages when we say to a child:

(19) What did you say you want to eat?

This is a complex sentence that involves moving what over three main verbs (say, want, and eat). Suppose the child says "hot dog." Was it a guess? Did the child understand "what you eat" without the "say" and "want"? It is not clear from ordinary interactions exactly how much grammar is needed to accomplish ordinary understanding.

Within about 6 to 8 months after the first word is produced, children begin to combine words. Often first combinations are simply single-word utterances joined together (Lahey, 1988). These single word utterances are not syntactic as they do not convey a hierarchical structure or combine to form a unified meaning. Also, their prosodic shape is that of two single words. Not until the two words form a unified unit and intonational contour, or a rise or fall is on the second word is there syntax (Cairns, 1996). As we said before, this does not take into account expectation of dialect differences.

In addition to joined single-word utterances there are multiple words that have syntactic shape and will begin to dominate Brown's (1973) Stage 2 as the child progresses. These are words joined together that compose a verb phrase (VP) with either an noun phrase (NP) preceding it ("Mommy bake") or a NP following ("bake cake"). Also, there can be two NPs without the VP as in "Daddy shoe." These phrasal configurations are strong indicators of a rigid compliance with English word order.

In English the basic word order is subject-verb-object. This order is a reflection of UG principles that a child does not have to learn. Crucial features of this system are that one element licenses another: A verb licenses an object and therefore the verb precedes the object. At a subtler level, the modality licenses the verb. Thus we say "can see Bill." Modality includes temporal reference that is sometimes represented in an inflection on a verb. Consistency then demands that we say that it is actually the inflection that licenses the verb, even though it appears after the verb. This consistency is captured by saying that there is an inflectional phrase, carrying time and modality, above the VP. We then, in effect, have this order:

Inflection	Verb	Object
-s	play	ball

Now the order of dominance is at odds with the surface of the language. Therefore, a verb movement operation has been proposed that moves the verb: -s play → play + s. This may seem to be an unmotivated abstraction, but subtle aspects of the grammar show that this movement is real. One such feature is that verbs will not move over negation. Thus when movement fails, *do* is inserted. Now we are able to predict that English has:

(20) a. John does not play ball.
      b. *John plays not ball.

The AAE grammar has generalized the do-insertion operation to include "be" as well as "not" ("John don't be angry").

Moreover, there appears to be no difference between AAE and SAE for this word order parameter and there is no reason to suspect that there would be a difference. Stockman and Vaughn-Cooke (1986) examined the early emergence of semantic categories in AAE-speaking children and found that children's two-word utterances expressed the same semantic categories found in SAE children (Bloom & Lahey, 1978). Also, in examining the language development of toddlers of AAE backgrounds who had been exposed to cocaine in utero, Bland, Seymour, Beaghley, and Frank (1996) observed the same word order composition as described for other English speaking children.

EARLY SUBJECTLESS SENTENCES

In considering the compositions noted above, the VP + NP is far more common than the NP + VP. Cairns (1996) described this difference as a subject-object asymmetry, wherein subjects are omitted much more frequently than are objects. Radford (1990) accounted for this asymmetry with the claim that early two-word phrases lack functional categories like inflectional phrase (IP). The subject occurs as what is called a specifier of IP. He argued that because of the absence of functional categories, subjects in the specifier of the IP are required, compared to no such requirement for subjects in the specifier of VP. Thus, we predict that subjects arise just when modality and tense of the IP are present.

There is evidence that subjectless sentences exist until children acquire auxiliaries and modals (Hyams, 1986). Also, children with specific language impairment (SLI) use subjectless sentences long after that of nonimpaired children and until they consistently use auxiliaries and modals. An intriguing question for AAE is whether this relationship between subjectless sentences and auxiliaries and modals also holds. If this relationship can be established, the occurrence of subjects might indicate knowledge about auxiliaries and modals that may not be evident from productions in which these forms are omitted. The prediction is that subjects should be present when modals are present. However, Ramos and Roeper (1996) found a more complex picture in a case study. While IP does correlate with some nominative uses for one 4-year-old child, expressions like "Her can cook something" are used to the complete exclusion of "she."

Currently, there appears to be no overall data on emergence and mastery of auxiliaries and modals in AAE. We know that Brown's Stage 2 (Brown, 1973) in SAE marks the emergence of morphological inflections, which are not mastered until later stages. Mastery of morphological inflections in SAE is often associated with Brown's 90% criterion, in which children must demonstrate the production of a form 90% of the time when required in an obligatory context. For example, the /s/ plural marker would be obligated whenever a regular noun is pluralized (book → books). In such cases, children who produce this marked form 90% or greater are considered to have mastered it. This 90% criterion has been applied in various examinations when morphological inflections are mastered in English-speaking children.

VARIABILITY

What SLI children acquire has a property of variability that appears to differ dramatically from other dialects of English. For example, the auxiliary form of "is" may be produced by the same AAE speaker within the same conversation as:

(21) a. He runnin
     b. Yes, he is
     c. That man is runnin
     d. What's going on?

At some point along the developmental path, AAE speakers must learn that it is possible to produce certain linguistic constituents in more than one way. In Example 21b the inclusion of auxiliary "is" may be conditioned by syntactic constraints such as whether the NP preceding the auxiliary has a noun (Example 21c), or a pronoun (Example 21a) as its head—or whether there is a phonological representation of a vowel (Example 21b) versus a consonant preceding the copula (Example 21d).

Sociolinguists view this kind of variability as rule governed (Bailey, 1973; Cedergren & Sankoff, 1974; Labov, 1969). They argued for a variability paradigm in which regularities can be discerned for the ways behaviors vary. These regularities may be traced to linguistic and non-linguistic contexts, which function as constraints that operate in conjunction with rules of grammar. Rules of grammar are viewed as operating independently of context and that there can be a predicted relative frequency for the variability observed in language behavior. For example, in Example 21 of auxiliary "is" utterances, Labov (1969) would argue that the variations observed are predictable and conditioned by the linguistic environments surrounding the auxiliary. In effect, then, if they are rule-governed and context-governed, then one may argue that they are not variable but, in fact, obligatory once the conditioning factors are understood.

The variation paradigm can be applied to child language with the understanding that variability may be explained by factors external to language: cognitive and neurological development. Child language acquisition is variable across children, who reach developmental milestones at different rates. However, there are answers to questions about the rate and developmental sequence of specific language features. Indeed, the literature is replete with developmental data on SAE, of which the most notable account was generated over 20 years ago (Brown, 1973). Although the rate and the sequential order in which specific linguistic features are acquired continue to be important areas of interest among researchers in child language, particularly within disciplines such as speech-language pathology, these two sources of variability—the sociolinguistic and the biological—can be difficult to disentangle in child AAE. The absent forms of our 3-year-old African American child discussed at the beginning of this chapter could be the result of a variation rule or a developmental error. How does one determine the difference?

This question need not be asked of child SAE, because there is no variation rule or optionality in simple declarative clauses, although in related structures the same variability arises: "me" or "I do." All speakers can answer the question "Who wants lemonade" either way. Children below 2;6 only say "me" and possibly those with SLI do the same. (See Abdulkarim and Roeper, 1996.)

Either the SAE child produces the adult targets or produces a pattern classifiable as developmental. The problem with child AAE is that one does not know whether many patterns are developmental or adult. This ambiguity can in part be traced to current notions about variable paradigm, as absent constituents are viewed to be optional for both children still within the emerging language period and for those with mature systems. In reality of course, large percentages of white children are also dialect speakers exhibiting precisely the same diagnostic ambiguity. For instance, many dialect forms allow the nonagreeing expression "that don't matter."

One might argue that the ambiguity about so-called variable forms arises from our inability to accurately discern the conditions under which these forms are produced. Once such a discernment is made, there would be no ambiguity and perhaps even no variable rule. The very concept of a variable rule rests on the assumption that a single linguistic constituent can change its shape in accordance with linguistic and nonlinguistic conditions while preserving its meaning. For Example 22, a and b represent variable use of copula with presumably no alteration in meaning:

(22) a. He angry
     b. He is angry

But despite the usual assumption that Examples 22a and b are equivalent, they may have different meanings. This difference may not reside in the lexicon or even the syntax, but in a semantic difference recognizable through context. For instance, Example 22a may invite the view that he is permanently angry (an angry person), while Example 22b may be a temporary state linked to a situation. Such a difference would challenge the notion of a variable rule. This choice would be obligatory: and what appeared to be optional (variable) really is not.

If usage of AAE features are obligatory and not optional, the concept of variable rule would have to be reconsidered. We raise this issue here simply to offer a viewpoint that can place child AAE within the same theoretical place as other children acquiring any language system. This theoretical place is one in which children acquire principles, or rules, for language use. These rules are not variable but obligatory. Otherwise, they could not be regarded as rules.

To extend this position to the problem posed above—to differentiate or disambiguate the developmental errors from adult forms when those adult forms appear to be identical to the developmental patterns—we must do what is done for any other dialect or language. We must determine precisely the rules for adult usage, so that we can be clear about developmental patterns. In SAE, evidence of this descriptive validity derives from a strong descriptive account of the adult system and a rich developmental profile of children as they progress toward adult SAE. When "normal" SAE children produce language behavior deviant from the adult forms, they are in the developmental stages of their language. If we assume that all features of AAE are obligatory as with SAE, why can't the same approach be applied to AAE?

First of all, we don't have the same knowledge base for AAE as compared to SAE for either a complete description of adult AAE or a developmental profile. Therefore, there remains considerable need for more research data on AAE. However, a research agenda based on the assumption that AAE features are obligatory versus one that accepts the variable paradigm could yield very different results. Consider the prevailing views about third person subject-verb agreement, in which sociolinguists have not been able to identify any grammatical or phonological conditioning effects for this form's absence in AAE (Myhill & Harris, 1986). As a result, the conclusion is that the absence of the /s/ marker occurs randomly, much like an "errant vagrant" (Poplack & Tagliamonte, 1989). One could accept this position and the conclusion that the third person /s/ marker is not in the AAE grammar and that its appearance likely is a form of code switching.

CODE SWITCHING

However, it is important to note that code switching is in response to a social perception. Therefore it is equivalent to a changing speech register, and from a theoretical point of view, it is equivalent to bilingualism. How is this difference represented in a system that functions in milliseconds? If it is rapid, then there must be a feature, like any other syntactic feature that is written into the rule system triggering application of the rule. In this respect, we can continue to see code switching as being like any other feature of grammar. It becomes a matter of greater interest when code switching means shifting to a different grammar that is in some sense opposed to the one usually spoken.

Hence, the conclusion that the /s/ marker is random suggests little or no control of this form when switching to SAE, a performance curiously unique to this particular constituent. On the other hand, a position that all AAE features are obligatory would require continued examination with a resolve that the conditioning effects simply have not been identified.

The issue of code switching raises still another problem in developing accurate and completed descriptions of AAE. Clearly, the AAE child is exposed to two dialects—that is, AAE and SAE. This dual exposure produces what may be described as a form of bidialectism. Thus, once again, a child's productions of "He tall" and "He is tall" may represent code switching between two dialects, which further complicates our consideration of the variable rule versus obligatory rule conundrum.

Let us extend an analogy to bilingualism. Assume a bilingual child speaks both language x and y. In language x, there is no article "a," but in language y, the article "a" is obligatory. When the child speaks language x, the article is not used, but when speaking y, it is produced. We would not assign a variable rule status to the child's production of the article "a." This form is simply obligatorily present in one language and obligatorily absent in the other.

To determine the conditions that are requisite for the production of AAE features, we must gain insight into what child AAE speakers know. This internal knowledge pertains to linguistic knowledge (grammar) and to nonlinguistic knowledge (social and environmental factors or triggers). Because AAE and SAE are both dialects of the same language it is reasonable to assume that child AAE and SAE share the most important knowledge about their common parent language. Indeed, there is somewhat of a consensus that the language behavior of AAE speakers differs little from SAE in early language stages and begins to diverge in the later stages. Some have even suggested that below 3 years of age there is little difference between child AAE and SAE (Cole, 1980; Kovac, 1980; Reveron, 1978; Stokes, 1976; Wyatt, 1995).

Although we agree that these two dialects are more alike in the early stages of language production than in the later stages, the extent to which they are alike is unclear. In fact, they may be far more different than we realize from the kinds of descriptive observations that we have been able to make thus far. Most descriptive accounts of early AAE have focused on the particular features that contrast between AAE and SAE in the adult systems. Clearly, until those features are produced in child systems, they are alike simply by virtue of their common absence. However, comprehension of these particular features may differ, as input from the two adult systems are different. Also, even the most casual listening to the one- and two-word utterances of young AAE speakers reveals nuance of meaning that is precursory to highly rhythmical and expressive adult forms. Until we have closely examined and scrutinized these early AAE forms, we should not conclude that they differ little from AAE.

It is clear that in the early stages, particularly Brown's Stages 1 & 2, both child AAE and SAE are marked by a reduced or telegraphic language with many missing production elements. In fact, every theory of early grammar predicts the absence of agreement—each theory employing a different basis. Lebeaux (1988) and Radford (1990) argued that functional categories are absent in general. Wexler (1994) argued that it is tense which is absent. Roeper and Rohrbacher (in press) argued that it is agreement that is absent as this is an option in UG. However, these various theories focus on children's production capacities and thus, show performance limitations without necessarily revealing a child's overall language competence. This is not an easy issue to resolve because one cannot ever directly observe what a child knows. Competence is inferred from evidence observed about a child's performance. However, a major dilemma with any inference about observed behavior is sorting out the myriad of possible factors that may be contributing to that behavior.

This dilemma is particularly acute for child AAE, as we are trying to establish regularities in behavior under circumstances in which the child's language exposure is a bidialectal context. This task then, in a scientific sense, is tantamount to searching for minute clues buried under shifting sand. Typically, in many aspects of child language research, we approach the task of finding out a child's language knowledge of a particular constituent by examining the frequency of that constituent in obligatory contexts and evaluating that frequency within a pragmatic and discourse framework. However, there can be an effective alternative to this tactic. For example, if a question is posed about the acquisition process of the past tense morphological inflection -ed, we might determine how and when children know the difference between:

(23) a. The plant dropped
     b. The dropped plant

In both examples it is possible for an agent to be present . However, in Example 23a "The plant dropped" does not refer to an implicit agent.

But, in Example 23b "The dropped plant" does. There is an invisible reference to an agent—an implicit agent. "The dropped plant" is a passive derivative, as in "The plant was dropped."

How does a child know—and when—that "The dropped plant" and "The plant was dropped" have an agent, but "The plant dropped" may not? Moreover, how do they exclude any interpretation that "The plant dropped" has an agent? See Roeper (1987) for a discussion showing that the distinction is present by 3 years, but not earlier in normal children.

These are important questions for understanding the acquisition of -*ed* suffix. Insight into the acquisition process can come from examining the most obscure, the rare, and the subtlest aspects of linguistic structures. The beauty of such an approach is that invisible information and excluded interpretations cannot be explained by environmental exposure, but only by principles of the grammar.

Thus, knowledge of constituents as reflected in comprehension tasks such as described might confirm competence in AAE speaking children when production comparisons with SAE children suggest otherwise. This is an important issue in light of deficit claims about AAE. Such tasks may also prove valuable as a diagnostic in identifying children whose comprehension knowledge lags behind that of their peers.

LATER SYNTAX

The literature suggests that contrasts between the dialects appear to be most evident above 3 years of age. Kovac (1980) suggested that a shift occurs between developmentally based productions patterns to dialectally based production patterns between 3 and 5 years of age. In support of Kovac's claim, Cole (1980) observed an increase in AAE forms after 3 years of age. Also, studies examining African American children of different socioeconomic status revealed greater use of AAE patterns between 3 and 5 years for working class and lower class children compared to middle class children. And, in the case of zero copula, as children got older there was an increase in use among working class children, but a decrease in this pattern for middle class children (Kovac, 1980).

We recognize and accept claims that AAE and SAE must go through a stage or stages when they appear alike and at some later point in development they diverge. However, the evidence marking this divergence is yet to be identified and the designation of a particular age at which this divergence occurs should be questioned.

In addressing the issue of point of divergence between the two dialects, let us return to the matter of agreement. All children must decide if their language marks agreement. In theory this can be stated as: does the language have an agreement feature. Under Chomsky (1995) agreement is a feature on a tense node, not an independent node. Therefore it is natural in this theory to assume no agreement until there is evidence for it. In that sense, the AAE dialect represents a default dialect and may be evident before the SAE usage of agreement. This has been observed (Weverink (1989)) and it has been called "optional root infinitive" stage (Wexler (1994)). Although at the point where these forms are used, they are optional, and the child presumably passes through a stage silently (at the comprehension level) where no agreement or tense information is represented. Roeper and Rohrbacher (in press) argued that it is agreement and not tense that the child fails to represent (see Schutze & Wexler, 1996), for a further extension of this view).

In general, this means that children begin with more limited structures, which follows from Chomsky's (1995) recent views of "economy" in grammar. However, it also means that SAE in this domain should pass through an AAE stage. There is evidence that this is true and that AAE remains a part of the SAE dialect.

It follows that if the child hears nonagreement sentences from adults, then such forms will remain in the grammar. Therefore the AAE speaker must not simply learn to add overt agreement, but to add agreement in only SAE contexts. Therefore the AAE speaker is learning a more complicated rule: Add X in Y environment. Therefore we can expect that this rule may be delayed.

There are further consequences. Suppose some children fail to make the grammar distinction. They may then use AAE in contexts where SAE is called for. Such contexts include speaking to whites or Blacks in authority positions. Those who have learned the distinction use AAE among themselves but not with adults. This can be a problem when professional speech pathologists attempt to elicit AAE (Seymour & Ralabate, 1985).

The point at which divergence between child AAE and SAE is most evident is when children are producing sentences with all three constituents—subject-verb-object—and several morphologic inflections are expected. However, as pointed out, it would be misleading to suggest that there is a particular age when this occurs. Clearly, by 3 years of age, most children are well beyond Brown's Stage 2. Some are even as far along as Stage 5 and some may still exhibit some Stage 2 behaviors. This variability is precisely the problem with designating an age cutoff such as 3 years for the divergence transition. We suspect that this transition is likely to be highly individualistic and best represented by a language level than by age. Certainly, by Stage 3, the differences between AAE and SAE should be apparent.

DEFAULT STRUCTURES IN UG

We turn now to a discussion of AAE syntax that connects to theoretical research in the acquisition of SAE. Every grammar utilizes some of the default structures available in UG. These default structures tend to be more "economical," which is a technical term for preferring less structure and shorter movement. A default structure that arises in acquisition and also in production is the use of resumptive pronouns. Instead of 20 trucks that I counted, we find:"twenty trucks that I counted them." This occurs because it is easier to link a noun and a pronoun than to move the noun.

The absence of visible agreement in AAE matches default structures and therefore it occurs early and reflects a stage through which all grammars pass. Other features of AAE are far more sophisticated and demand an articulated structure. Therefore they allow us to see more clearly how a child progresses in the acquisition of a dialect. Unfortunately we are at the outset of this form of research. We can however discuss a few results.

NEGATIVE CONCORD

AAE has a particularly intricate form of negation, which involves discontinuous relations. It is commonly assumed that "negative concord" is a random strewing of negative particles across a sentence. This is not true. Negation requires a certain order of constituents and may not cross certain boundaries in both AAE and SAE. When children show mastery of these subtler, nondefault features of grammar, they are using some of the most sophisticated principles of grammar in a unique way.

(24) a. The boy doesn't like any dog
      b. I didn't see the boy that likes any dog

In Example 24a the boy likes no dogs, while in Example 24b the boy likes every dog. The negative element on "didn't" agrees with "any" in Example a but not in b because it does not extend into a relative clause. So "any" in Example 24b refers to any-one-of-the-set of dogs and not none of the dogs. Example 24b reflects a fundamental principle of grammar: almost all invisible connections are limited to a single clause, so negative concord cannot extend into a relative clause. Therefore, negative concord and negative polarity are not the same. Children are born with this principle, but it may apply in different places, as we will show.

SAE children are known to misuse "any" to be negation outside of concord and say:

(24) c. "I want anything" to mean "I want nothing"

In effect they take the neg feature on any to be independent and therefore without a need for a licensing neg. In other words "anything" equals "nothing." Will children interpret Example 24b as if "any" could be equal to "no," as in Example 24d.

(24) d. I didn't see the boy that likes no dog

Here are the predictions: in AAE the children will understand "no" in Example 24a (as in 24e) as negative concord:

(24) e. the boy doesn't like no dog,

but not in Example 24b because "any" is not seen as a negative (although the SAE children do see "any" as a negative). The AAE children should not be subject to this confusion if they always use "no" in the single clause environments (or *nothing* instead of *anything*). They should be able to recognize immediately that "any" in Example 24b is not a negative element, while the SAE children should allow 24b to mean:

(24) f. I didn't see the boy that likes no dog

because they initially allow "any" to mean "no," even if there is no other negation in the clause "I want anything." The child does not violate UG here, but simply substitutes one lexical item (any) for another (no).

We can see that the same principles are at work in SAE and AAE, but the avoidance of negative-"any" in AAE should permit a more rapid comprehension of Example 24b, because it is evident that the clause-barrier effect blocks the negative reading. Therefore, the negative concord system of AAE, although it may lead to apparently odd double-negatives "I don't want none," may facilitate the acquisition of more sophisticated uses of "any."

Is this supposition true? It is part of our ongoing program of research to find out. We believe that AAE children will control this distinction at an early age, because we have evidence that they understand sentence boundaries for construal of wh-expressions (Seymour, Bland, deVilliers, Roeper, & Champion, 1992). For instance, there is a long distance interpretation of "when" into a lower clause in the sentence:

(25) a. When did he say he sang

This can mean either when he said it or when he sang. But when there is a relative clause present, no "long" reading is possible:

(25) b. When did he say the song that he sang

Here, Example 25b only refers to when he said it, not when he sang. It would follow that the AAE children will manifest the same constraint on interpreting negation, although it is a more complex phenomenon in AAE, as the same time the constraint is evident for question formation. On the other hand, as the AAE children hear SAE as well, they may have negative-any in their lexicon as well and therefore be led into confusions similar to the SAE speaker.

HABITUAL BE

We shall now consider still another obligatory AAE feature. AAE has a habitual form with both sophisticated syntax and semantics: "habitual" be. It is a form that never corresponds to the reality of the moment, as it is an attribute of character. Very young children use "be" and apparently use it correctly (Wyatt, 1991).

The use of "be" in AAE and its early appearance in children's grammars indicates an early point of serious divergence between AAE and SAE. The form "be" in AAE has main verb properties, although SAE treats "be" as both a main verb and an auxiliary. This gives rise to an inconsistency found in SAE:

(26) a. John does not play ball
     b. John does not sing a song
     c. *John does not be tall
     d. John wasn't tall

Why is Example 26c ungrammatical? If SAE were consistently to insert "do" before negatives, then 26c should be grammatical, which it is in AAE. It is no wonder then that the AAE children acquire this form readily. Because "be" behaves more regularly in AAE than in SAE, one can predict that it is more readily acquired. In fact many SAE children produce exactly the same forms recognizing the regularity of do-insertion (Jackson & Dickey, 1996):

(27) a. Do it be colored

confirming our view that it is the irregular form in SAE that is difficult to acquire. (See Hollebrandse & Roeper, 1996 for extensive discussion of "do.")

The main verb status of "be" in AAE allows it to appear in the VP and acquire "aspectual" features unknown in SAE: habituality. This feature marks "be" as grammatically a main verb (inside VP) and allows "do" elsewhere:

(27) b. He do be singing

(Technically one must adopt an additional aspect node inside VP where both habitual and the progressive -*ing* are located.) However it now has the special reading of habituality, unlike the noncopular form:

(27) c. He singing

In fact, a study of Adam's corpus (taken from Brown's transcript, 1973) reveals AAE usage of precisely this form (Jackson & Dickey, 1996).

The issues raised about negation and aspectual "be" are rooted in acquisition theory that need to be addressed in research on child AAE. In our opinion, it is this kind of research that offers the promise of answering the many complex questions raised here.

⊔

CONCLUSION

In this chapter we have taken a principles and parameters approach in describing the grammatical acquisition of AAE. We have attempted to dispel some myths about AAE and to view it in ways consistent with current acquisition theory. Clearly, our description has raised more questions than it has provided answers. However, the very nature of many of these questions lead us in new directions necessary for a clearer understanding of child AAE. Questions such as: When do AAE and SAE diverge in acquisition? Are features of AAE optional within a single grammar or a reflection of code switching between two grammars? Is the concept "variable rule" a misnomer for AAE features that are, in fact, rule-governed rules of unidentified origins? remain to be answered. We provided some examples and suggestions for possible research to answer these questions.

These questions may, in turn, bear upon fundamental issues in how dialects interact. Are AAE and SAE converging or diverging at the moment? Is their evolution toward or away from each other a result of social factors or of grammatical internal factors? In this respect, the study of child AAE and the challenges of speech pathology contribute to the clarification of fundamental issues in linguistics.

🏷

REFERENCES

Abdulkarim, L., & Roeper, T. (1996). Ellipsis as a mirror of Case and economy of representation in child grammars. VIIth International Congress of Child Language, Istanbul, Turkey.

Atkinson, M. (1992). *Children's syntax.* Oxford: Blackwell.

Bailey, C. N. (1973). *Variation and linguistic theory.* Washington, DC: Center for Applied Linguistics.

Baugh, J. (1980). A re-examination of the Black English copula. In W. Labov (Ed.), *Locating language in space and time* (pp. 83–106). New York: Academic Press.

Bereiter, C. & Engelmann, S. (1966). *Teaching disadvantaged children in the preschool.* Englewood Cliffs, NJ: Prentice-Hall.

Bland, L., Seymour, H., Beaghley, M., & Frank, D. (1996). Speech and language development in African American toddlers exposed to cocaine. 1966 Memphis Research Symposium: Communication in African-American Children and Youth. Memphis, TN.

Bloom, L., & Lahey, M. (1978). *Language development and language disorders.* New York: John Wiley.

Brown, R. (1973). *A first language: The early stages.* Cambridge, MA: Harvard University Press.

Brown, R., & Hanlon, C. (1970). Derivational complexity and the order of acquisition in child speech. In J. R. Hayes (Ed.), *Cognition and the development of language.* New York: John Wiley.

Cairns, H. S. (1996). *The acquisition of language* (2nd ed.). Austin, TX: PRO ED.

Cedergren, H., & Sankoff, D. (1974). Variable rules: Performance as a statistical reflection of competence. *Language, 50,* 333–355.

Chomsky, N. (1957). *Syntactic structures.* Mouton: The Hague.

Chomsky, N. (1972). *Language and Mind* (Enlarged ed.). New York: Harcourt Brace Jovanovitch.

Chomsky, N. (1995). *The minimalist program.* MIT Press.

Cole, L. (1980). *A developmental analysis of social dialect features in the spontaneous language of preschool Black children.* Unpublished doctoral dissertation, Northwestern University, Evanston, IL.

Cook, V. J. (1987). *Chomsky's universal grammar: An introduction.* Cambridge: Blackwell.

Craig, H. K., & Washington, J. A. (1994). The complex syntax skills of poor, urban, African-American preschoolers at school entry. *Language, Speech, and Hearing Services in Schools, 25,* 181–190.

Demetras, M. J., Post, K. N., & Snow, C. E. (1986). Feedback to first language learners: The role of repetitions and clarification questions. *Journal of Child Language, 13,* 275–292.

Green, L. (1993). *Topics in African American English: The verb system analysis.* Unpublished doctoral dissertation, University of Massachusetts, Amherst.

Green, L. (1995). Study of verb classes in African American English. *Linguistics and Education: An International Research Journal, 7,* 1.

Hollebrandse, B., &. Roeper, T. (1996). The concept of Do-Insertion and the theory of INFL in acquisition. In C. Koster & F. Wynen (Eds.), *Proceedings of GALA.* Groningen, Holland.

Hyams, N. M. (1986). *Language acquisition and the theory of parameters.* Boston: Reidel.

Jackson, J. E., & Dickey, M. (1996). Development of habitual aspect in African American children: A CHILDES search. 1996 Memphis Research Symposium: Communication in African-American Children and Youth, Memphis, TN.

Kaufman, A. A., & Kaufman, N. L. (1983). *Kaufman Assessment Battery for Children.* Circle Pines, MN: American Guidance Service.

Kovac, C. (1980). *Children's acquisition of variable features.* Unpublished doctoral dissertation, Georgetown University, Washington, DC.

Labov, W. (1969). Contraction, deletion, and inherent variability of the English copula. *Language, 45,* 715–762.

Lahey, M. (1988). *Language disorders and language development.* New York: Macmillan Co.

Lebeaux, D. (1988). *Language acquisition and the form of the grammar.* Unpublished doctoral dissertation, University of Massachusetts, Amherst.

Leonard, L. (1995). Functional categories in the grammars of children with specific language impairment. *Journal of Speech and Hearing Research, 38,* 1270–1283.

Leonard, L., Bortolini, U., Casselli, M. C., McGregor, K., & Sabbadini, L. (1992). Morphological deficits in children with specific language impairment: The status of features in the underlying grammar. *Language Acquisition, 2,* 151–179.

Lund, N., & Duchan, J. (1993). *Assessing children's language in naturalistic contexts.* (3rd ed.). Englewood Cliffs, NJ: Prentice-Hall.

MacWinney, B. (1991). *The CHILDES project: Tools for analyzing talk.* Hillsdale, NJ: Lawrence Erlbaum.

Maratsos, M. P. (1974). Preschool children's use of definite and indefinite articles. *Child Development, 45,* 446–455.

McNeill, D. (1966). Developmental psycholinguistics. In F. Smith & G. A. Miller (Eds.), *The genesis of language.* Cambridge: MIT Press.

McNeill, D. (1970). *The acquisition of language: The study of developmental psycholinguistics.* New York: Harper & Row.

Miller, J. F. (1981). *Assessing language production in children, experimental procedures.* Baltimore: University Park Press.

Morehead, D., & Ingram, D. (1973). The development of base syntax in normal and linguistically deviant children. *Journal of Speech and Hearing Research, 16,* 330–352.

Myhill, J., & Harris, W. A. (1986). The use of the verbal -s inflection in BEV. In Sankoff (Ed.), *Diversity and diachrony.* Amsterdam: John Benjamins.

Owens, R. E. (1988). *Language development* (2nd ed.). Columbus,OH: Merrill.

Penner, S. (1987). Parental responses to grammatical and ungrammatical child utterances. *Child Development, 58,* 376–384.

Pinker, S. (1984). *Language learnability and language development.* Cambridge, MA: Harvard University Press.

Pinker, S. (1989). *Learnability and cognition: The acquisition of argument structure.* Cambridge, MA: MIT Press.

Poeppel, D., & Wexler, K. (1993). The full competence hypothesis of clause structure in early German. *Language, 69,* 1–33.

Poplack, S., & Tagliamonte, S. (1989). There's no tense like the present: Verbal -s inflection in early Black English. *Language Variation and Change, 1,* 47–84.

Radford, A. (1990). *Syntactic theory and the acquisition of English syntax.* Oxford, UK: Blackwell.

Ramos, E., & Roeper, T. (1996). Pronoun case assignment by an SLI child. University of Wisconsin conference on child language, Madison, WI.

Reveron, W. W. (1978). The acquisition of four Black English morphological rules by Black preschool children. *Dissertation Abstract International, 40*(1), 27A (University Microfilms No. AAC7916019).

Rice, M., & Wexler, K. (1996). Toward tense as a clinical marker of specific language impairment in English-speaking children. *Journal of Speech and Hearing Research, 39,* 1239–1257.

Roeper, T. (1987). The acquisition of implicit arguments in the distinction between theory process and mechanism. In B. MacWhinney (Ed.) *Mechanisms of language acquisition* (pp. 309–345). Hillsdale, NJ: Lawrence Erlbaum.

Roeper, T., & Rohrbacher, B. (in press). In S. Powers, & C. Haaman (Eds.), *The acquisition of scrambling.* Dordrecht: Kluwer.

Schutze, C., & Wexler, K. (1996). Subject case licensing and English root infinitives. In A. Stringfellow, D. Cahana-Amitay, E. Hughes, & A. Zukowski (Eds.), *Proceedings of the 20th Annual Boston Conference on Language Acquisition*, Boston, MA.

Seymour, H. (1986). Clinical intervention for language disorders among nonstandard speakers of English. In O. Taylor (Ed.), *Treatment of communication disorders in culturally and linguistically diverse populations* (pp. 135–152). San Diego: College Hill Press.

Seymour, H., & Bland, L. (1991). A minority perspective in the diagnosing of child language disorders. *Clinics in Communication Disorders, 1*(1), 39–50.

Seymour, H., Bland, L., deVilliers, J., Roeper, T., & Champion, T. (1992, November). *Long distance wh-movement in children of divergent language backgrounds.* Paper presented at the annual meeting of the American Speech-Language-Hearing Association, San Antonio, TX.

Seymour, H., & Ralabate, P. (1985). The acquisition of a phonological feature of Black English. *Journal of Communication Disorders, 18,* 139–148.

Stockman, I. (1986). *The development of linguistic norms for nonmainstream populations.* In F. Bess, B. Clark, & H. Mitchell (Eds.), (ASHA Rep. No. 16). Washington, DC: ASHA.

Stockman, I., & Vaughn-Cooke, F. (1986). Implications of semantic category research for the language assessment of nonstandard speakers. *Topics in Language Disorders, 6*(4), 15–25.

Stokes, N. H. (1976). A cross-sectional study of the acquisition of negation structures in Black children. *Dissertation Abstracts International, 38*(2), 767A. (University Microfilms No. AAC7716846).

Weissenborn, J., deVilliers, J. & Roeper, T. (1996). The acquisition of superiority. Utrecht Conference on what language acquisition says to linguistic theory, Holland.

Weverink, M. (1989). Inversion in the embedded clause. In T. Maxfield & B. Plunkett (Eds.), *Papers in the acquisition of WH* (pp. 19–42). Amherst: University of Massachusetts. Department of Linguistics, GLSA Publications.

Wexler, K. (1994). Optional infinitives. In D. Lightfoot & N. Hornstein (Eds.), *Verb movement* (pp. 305–350). New York: Cambridge University Press.

Wolfram, W., & Fasold, R. (1974). *The study of social dialects in American English.* Englewood Cliffs, NJ: Prentice Hall.

Wyatt, T. A. (1991). *Linguistic constraints on copula production in Black English child speech.* Unpublished doctoral dissertation, University of Massachusetts, Amherst.

Wyatt, T. (1995). Language development in African American English child speech. *Linguistics and Education, 7,* 7–22.

Wyatt, T. A., & Seymour, H. N. (1990). The implications of code-switching in Black English speakers. *Equity & Excellence, 24*(4), 3–5.

HARRY N. SEYMOUR, PH.D.

Harry N. Seymour, Ph.D., is Professor and Chair of the Department of Communication Disorders at the University of Massachusetts at Amherst, where he also serves as Adjunct Professor of Linguistics. Professor Seymour earned his doctorate from The Ohio State University in 1971. He is a Fellow of the American Speech-Language-Hearing Association. His professional work is in the area of child language disorders. His current research objective to develop a language assessment test for children who speak African American English is supported by the National Institute of Deafness and Other Communication Disorders. He has published many articles describing the identification of language disorders among African American children.

THOMAS ROEPER, PH.D.

Thomas Roeper, Ph.D., is Professor of Linguistics at the University of Massachusetts at Amherst. He has been teaching theoretical approaches to first language acquisition for 25 years. Dr. Roeper is Editor of the *Language Acquisition Journal*. His current research involves studies in theoretical psycholinguistics.

PART III

BEYOND THE ACQUISITION OF ENGLISH: SOME REPRESENTATIVE LANGUAGES

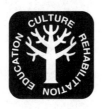

CHAPTER 6

THE ACQUISITION
OF SPANISH

LISA M. BEDORE, Ph.D.

Spanish is the third most widely spoken language after Chinese and English (Crystal, 1997). In North America Spanish is well represented; Mexico is the largest Spanish-speaking country in the world and the U.S. has the fifth largest Spanish-speaking population (Grimes, 1996). This chapter introduces general and dialect-specific features of American Spanish and provides an overview of research on the acquisition of Spanish as a first language. With this goal in mind, this chapter is organized into:

- ■ An overview of the history of Spanish in the Americas
- ■ A description of the characteristics of General Formal Spanish
- ■ Dialectal variation in American Spanish
- ■ Acquisition of Spanish as a first language

⊔

THE HISTORY OF SPANISH IN AMERICA

Within approximately 50 years of Columbus' arrival in Santo Domingo in 1492, Spain had established itself throughout the Americas. As the Spanish explored and established settlements, the use of Spanish spread west and northward across the territory that is currently Mexico and the southern U.S. (Ramírez, 1992). Major cities in North America founded during the 1500s include Santo Domingo in the Dominican Republic, La Havana in Cuba, San Juan in Puerto Rico, Panama City, Guadalajara and Mexico City in Mexico, and St. Augustine in Florida. Settlements in Texas and New Mexico were founded in the 1600s. Between 1769 and 1823, a series of missions was established in California. At the point of its greatest extension, New Spain, which became Mexico, extended from what is now Panama to the southwestern U.S. (Chang-Rodríguez, 1991).

This period of active colonization coincided with the spread of the Castilian dialect of Spanish, ordered by Queen Isabel after the Moors were driven from Spain (Heath, 1972). It was believed that establishing a single dialect would provide a means of unifying and civilizing the country. Castilian was designated the language for use in the Americas as well. In practice, however, Spanish did not spread as quickly as the rulers in Spain had hoped. Although Spanish settlers and their families used Spanish, missionaries found it more efficient to learn and preach in the Indian languages. The Spaniards taught Spanish to selected individuals from indigenous groups with the plan that these individuals would spread the language to their communities. However, many Indian groups did not appear to accept that Spanish was a necessary language for them. Thus, the selected individuals often became translators who facilitated the conduct of business between Spanish and Indian communities.

During the colonial period, Spain maintained constant contact with major cultural centers that could be easily reached, such as Mexico City or Lima, Peru. Castilian Spanish was the dialect of prestige (Chang-Rodríguez, 1991). Settlers in the Caribbean islands and coastal regions had ongoing contact with the shippers who mainly came from Andalucia, or Southern Spain. Consequently, the Andalucian dialect is considered a major source of input to the Spanish spoken in the coastal regions, especially around the Caribbean (Fontanella de Weinberg, 1992). Even today there are two major dialectal groups in American

Spanish (referred to as conservative and radical or Caribbean Spanish) that continue to reflect, to some extent, the geographical origins of the settlers. Parallel patterns of development between Peninsular (i.e., the dialects of Spain) and American Spanish also contribute to these similarities (Frago Gracia, 1996).

In the early 1800s, Spain began to lose control over America. Venezuela, Colombia, Ecuador, Peru, and Bolivia were the first countries to gain their independence from Spain (Chang-Rodríguez, 1991). In 1819, Florida became part of the U.S. Mexico gained independence in 1821. Texas gained independence from Mexico in 1836 and was annexed by the U.S. in 1845. The territories that are currently the states of California, Arizona, New Mexico, and parts of Colorado, Kansas, Nevada, Oklahoma, and Wyoming were ceded to the U.S. in the Guadalupe Hidalgo Treaty in 1848.

Gradually Spanish influence lessened. Some linguistic changes that occurred in Spain after that date are not reflected in American Spanish. One example is the /θ/ - /s/ contrast employed in some peninsular dialects. In American Spanish, the word pair *coser* "to sew" and *cocer* "to cook" are homophones; in peninsular Spanish the pair is distinct because the second "c" of *cocer* "to cook" is realized as a /θ/ (i.e., [koθér]) (Penny, 1991). As the U.S. settled those regions that had been under Spanish and Mexican control, English displaced Spanish in most regions. In remote areas, such as some fishing communities in southern Louisiana and mountain communities in northern New Mexico and southern Colorado, Spanish-speaking communities became isolated and patterns of old Spanish continue to influence current use of Spanish. For example, some Old Spanish verb forms are a part of the Spanish of New Mexico. Constant migration to states such as California, Arizona, and Texas has modernized the Spanish of these regions and the Spanish is more similar to that spoken in Mexico.

Settlement patterns differed across Latin America and relationships between settlers and indigenous groups differed. The practical result is current variation in the population demographics, language usage patterns, and cultural practices. For example, in some countries such as Mexico and Honduras, approximately 90% of the population are classified as "mestiza" (i.e., mixed Spanish and Native Indian origins). In other countries, such as Argentina, Uruguay, and Costa Rica, the majority of the population is of European heritage. In Bolivia and Ecuador the majority of the population has indigenous roots. In some Caribbean countries (e.g., Cuba, Dominican Republic) between 30 and 85% of the population has African ancestry, tracing their roots to the slaves who were brought to work on the plantations in the Caribbean.

TABLE 6–1

Countries in which Spanish is spoken and percentage of the population that is Spanish-speaking (based on Grimes, 1996).

Countries	Percentage of the Population That Speaks Spanish As a First Language
Argentina	96
Belize	43
Bolivia	41
Chile	96
Columbia	97
Costa Rica	97
Cuba	94
Dominican Republic	86
Ecuador	77
El Salvador	99
Guatemala	43
Honduras	97
Mexico	88
Nicaragua	95
Panama	78
Paraguay	2
Peru	38
Puerto Rico	67
Uruguay	92
U.S.A.	8
Venezuela	96

A list of the countries in which Spanish is currently spoken and the percentage of self-identified Spanish speakers in each country is listed in Table 6–1. Spanish is reported to be the first language of most speakers in Latin American countries. However, many indigenous languages are spoken as well. In Mexico, 8% of the population speaks one of the approximately 60 Indian languages (Grimes, 1996). Examples of more widely spoken languages include Mayan, Mixtec, and Nahuatl. Other languages spoken in Latin America include Portuguese in Brazil, Guaraní in Paraguay, and English in Belize. It cannot be assumed then that people coming from Latin America will necessarily speak Spanish.

Current immigration patterns influence the use of Spanish in the U.S. Based on the 1990 census (Current Population Reports, 1990), approximately 61% of the U.S. Hispanic population identifies itself as being of Mexican origin, 12% of Puerto Rican origin, and 5% of Cuban origin. Approximately 8% of the Hispanic population comes from Central America and the Caribbean; the countries most represented are Guatemala, Nicaragua, and El Salvador. Another 5% of the population comes from South America; Columbia is the country with the largest number of emigrants to the U.S. Approximately 38% of the U.S. Hispanic population are first generation immigrants (Current Population Survey, March 1994). Thus, a discussion of Spanish in the U.S. is incomplete if the features of Spanish throughout Latin America are not considered.

Many cultural features are shared across Latin America. Family relationships are very important. Young children are likely to spend time with their extended family on a daily or weekly basis. Another important social relationship is with a child's *compadres,* or godparents. Extended family and godparents may play an important role in child-rearing decisions. If a child has a birthday party, it is likely to include family, family friends, and godparents, as well as children of the child's age. Verbal interactions are highly valued. People admire those who can express themselves eloquently, and the ability to tell jokes or stories well is considered to be a special gift. Young children are likely to be coached to recall family members' names and to interact with adults in social conversations. Teasing interactions are one type of interaction in which children may be coached to participate. Children are likely to be introduced to stories and discourse through oral stories, including traditional or folk tales or stories about the child's family or town. In spite of these general similarities, it is important to remember that Latin America is culturally and linguistically diverse. Thus, we should expect to see variation in intersectional style between parents and children and the social and geographical dialects that children acquire. These factors need to be taken in to account in considering the language a child is acquiring and the context in which language is learned.

ᒪᖴ

LINGUISTIC CHARACTERISTICS OF GENERAL FORMAL SPANISH

In this section, the characteristics of General Formal Spanish are discussed. General Formal Spanish represents an abstraction of those features that are common in formal speech across dialects rather than the specific features of any particular dialect. As the focus of this chapter is on American Spanish, features that are restricted to peninsular Spanish are identified, but not discussed in detail. This general framework provides a base from which dialectal variations can be presented and understood and from which the structures to be acquired can be determined.

PHONOLOGY

In General Formal American Spanish there are 18 consonant and 5 vowel phonemes. The place and manner features of these consonants are described in Table 6–2. Both /y/ and /ʎ/, represented as "y" and "ll" orthographically, are realized as /y/ or /j/ in most American Spanish dialects. Thus, in these dialects, the medial sounds of words such as *cayó* [kaiyó] "he or she fell" and *calló* [kaiyó] "he or she kept quiet" are the same. A number of phonological and phonetic features characterize the phonetic inventory of Spanish and are common across dialects; these are summarized in Table 6–3.

Spanish has a five-vowel system, two front vowels /i, e/, a central vowel /a/, and two back vowels /u, o/. In addition, there are a number of permissible diphthongs: /ye, ya, yo, yu, we, wa, wo, ey, ay, oy, ew, aw/. The distribution of vowels is stable across dialects (Navarro, 1968).

Spanish is usually characterized as a syllable-timed language, meaning that stressed and unstressed syllables have approximately the same duration (e.g., Barrutia & Terrell, 1982). This contrasts with a stress-timed language such as English in which stressed and final syllables are lengthened and unstressed and word-medial syllables are shortened. However, syllable and stress timing are probably better characterized as a continuum rather than discrete categories. In Spanish, stressed syllables are of greater duration than unstressed syllables and word-medial syllables are briefer in duration than word-final syllables (Delattre, 1966; Toledo, 1988). Thus, it would be expected that the stressed final syllable in *pasó* "happened-third singular past tense" would be longer than the same syllable when it is unstressed in *páso* "step" and that the syllable *to* would be longer in *zapato* "shoe" than in *jitomate* "tomato" where it is word medial. However, the differences in duration are not as great as they are in a language such as English.

At the word level, stress must fall on one of the last three syllables. In most words, the penultimate syllable is stressed (e.g., *cása* "house"

TABLE 6–2

The consonants of General Formal Spanish.

	Labial	Labiodental	Interdental	Dental	Alveolar	Palatal	Velar	Glottal
Stops								
Voiceless	p			t			k	
Voiced	b			d			g	
Fricatives		f	θ[a]		s	y	x[c]	h[c]
Affricates						tʃ		
Nasals	m				n	ɲ		
Liquids					l	ʎ[b]		
Vibrants								
Simple					ɾ			
Multiple					r			

[a]The /θ/ is only used in dialects in Spain, not in American Spanish; in American Spanish /s/ or a variant of /s/ is employed.

[b]The palatal liquid /ʎ/ contrasts with the alveolar liquid /l/ in some dialects; however, this contrast is gradually being lost and the palatal liquid is usually not heard.

[c]Either the /x/ or the /h/ occur as a phoneme in any given dialect but not both.

Note: The phonemes included here are based on Barrutia and Terrell (1982), Bjarkman and Hammond (1989), and Canfield (1981).

TABLE 6–3

Characteristics of Spanish phonological and phonetic system.

■ The fricatives /β, ð, and (ɣ are allophones of the voiced stops /b, d, and g/. The stop variant is produced after pauses and after nasals (e.g., [kandáðo] *candado* "lock"); the stop /d/ is also produced after /l/ (e.g., [fálda] *falda* "skirt"). The fricative variants occur in all other contexts.

■ Voiceless stops are unaspirated and do not have a fricative allophone as do the voiced stops.

■ There are a number of acceptable variants of /r/ in Spanish. In General Formal Spanish, the trilled /r/ is used in word-initial position and after /r, l, or s/. It contrasts with flap /ɾ/ in word medial position (e.g., *carro* "car or wagon" versus *caro* "expensive"). As a general rule the flap /ɾ/ or a variant is produced in most running speech contexts and the trilled /r/ is more likely to be produced in formal or emphatic speech.

■ When /s/ is produced, the tongue apex may contact the lower teeth and the predorsal region of the tongue is near the upper teeth or alveolar ridge.

■ Nasals assimilate to the place of articulation before consonants within words (e.g., [bláŋko] *blanco* "white") and across word boundaries (e.g., [undéðo] *un dedo* "a finger"; and [umbeβé] *un bebé* "a baby").

■ Most syllables are open syllables (CV); closed syllables (CVC) are far less common (58% versus 27%, respectively, according to Navarro (1968).

■ Bisyllabic or multisyllabic words outnumber monosyllabic words.

■ The same consonant clusters occur in word-initial position in words like *tren* "train" or *fruta* "fruit" and in word medial position (e.g., *patrón* "boss" or *refresco* "soft drink"). Permissible consonant clusters include /pr, pl, br, bl, tr, dr, kr, kl, gr, gl, fr, fl/. Additional heterosyllabic sequences, which do not occur as word-initial clusters, may occur within words. Some examples include *escuela* "school" and *tambor* "drum"; in these cases the syllable boundary falls between the consonants. Unlike English in Spanish, clusters do not occur in word-final position and are infrequent in syllable-final position (e.g., *obstáculo* "obstacle").

■ The only single consonants that occur word finally are /l, n, r, s, d/. Although there are a few words in which /x/ occurs in final position (e.g., *reloj* "clock"), the word-final /x/ is virtually never produced in any Spanish dialect.

and *zapáto* "shoe"), stress on the final syllable is also a common pattern (e.g., *corazón* "heart" and *abrió* "opened"). Words with antepenultimate stress, such as *teléfono* "telephone" and *música* "music," are relatively less common. Lexical stress differentiates word pairs such as *pápa* "potato" and *papá* "father." Stress also interacts with the verbal inflection system. For example, with the exception of the first person plural forms, stems of present tense forms are stressed, but for forms preterite (past completed actions), the morphological markers, not the stems, are stressed.

When an affix is added to a word, penultimate stress is maintained. For example, when a diminutive is formed by attaching a suffix, indicated here in bold, stress continually shifts to the penultimate syllable (e.g., *chíco* "little," *chiquíto* "very little," *chiquitíto* "very very little"). However, if the affix is stressed, as in the case of a number of verbal inflections, then the stress pattern of the word changes (e.g., *córro* "I run present" versus *corrí* "I run past" versus *correría* "I would run"). When unstressed clitic elements are attached to a word, stress does not change because these elements cannot be stressed e.g., *láva* "wash"-imperative, *lávalo* "wash it"-imperative, *lávamelo* "wash it for me"-imperative). When clitics precede nouns or verbs, stress patterns are unaffected because of the direction of stress assignment.

ᓚ

MORPHOSYNTAX

NOUN MORPHOLOGY

Spanish nouns are marked for gender and number. The majority of nouns end in –o and are masculine or end in –a and are feminine. Thus gender is highly predictable. There are, of course, exceptions. Some examples include *la mano* "the hand" that ends in –o but is feminine and *el día* "the day" that is masculine, although it ends in –a. Nouns may also end in other vowels (e.g., *el cisne* "the swan"), or consonants (i.e., *el árbol* "the tree," *la paz* "peace"). These nouns also follow patterns in regard to gender. Nouns ending in -*d*, -*n*, and -*z* are usually feminine and nouns ending in -*l*, -*r*, or -*e* are most often masculine. Plurality is marked with /s/ except for those that end in a consonant. In those cases the ending is /es/ so as to meet the phonotactic constraints of Spanish syllable structure (e.g., *jardín* "garden," jardines "gardens").

TABLE 6–4
Spanish determiner system.

| | | Articles | | Demonstratives | | |
		Indefinite	Definite	Near	Middle	Far
Singular	Masculine	un	el	este	ese	aquel
	Feminine	una	la	esta	esa	aquella
	Neutral		lo	esto	eso	aquello
Plural	Masculine	unos	los	estos	esos	aquellos
	Feminine	unas	las	estas	esas	aquellas

The Spanish determiner system, represented in Table 6–4, includes definite and indefinite articles as well as demonstratives that code relative distance between the speaker and the referred to object. Within noun phrases, determiners and adjectives agree in number and gender with the noun they modify, as illustrated in Examples 1–3. When an adjective ends in a vowel other than *a* or *o* or in a consonant, only number agreement is observed as in Examples 4 and 5.

(1) La camisa roja
    "The red shirt"

(2) Aquel carro rojo
    "That red car"

(3) Estos zapatos rojos
    "Those red shoes"

(4) Los platos verdes
    "The green plates"

(5) Sus zapatos azules
    "Their blue shoes"

Pronouns, listed in Table 6–5, are often classified into stressed and unstressed groups. Subject, possessive, and prepositional pronouns are stressed. Subject pronouns are used in the same contexts as nouns. They are likely to be dropped when meaning is recoverable from context as in Example 6, but are employed in a more emphatic context such as Example 7.

TABLE 6–5
Stressed and unstressed pronouns.

			Stressed		Unstressed	
		Subject	Possessive	Prepositional	Object-Direct	Object-Indirect	Reflexive
Singular	1	yo	mio/a	mí	me	me	me
	2	tu/	tuyo/a	ti/	te/	te/	te/
		usted	suyo/a	sí	se	se	se
	3	él/ella	suyo/a	él/ella	se	le	se
Plural	1	nosotros/as	nuestro/a	nuestros	nos	nos	nos
	2	ustedes	suyo/a	ustedes	los	les	se
	3	ellos/ellas	suyo/a	ellos/ellas	los/las	les	se

(6) (Yo) tomo café en la mañana.
"(I) drink-first person singular present coffee in the morning."

(7) Yo como espárragos pero él no.
"I eat asparagus but he (does) no(t)."

Constructions of Examples 8 and 10 with possessive pronouns alternate with constructions with possessive adjectives in Example 9 and prepositional constructions in Example 11. Possessive pronouns agree in number and gender with the item possessed regardless of the gender of the possessor. The possessive in Example 8 refers to *el carro* "the car," but the possessive in Example 10 refers to *las bolsas* "the bags." In Example 9, the possessive adjective agrees in number with the object possessed. However, the prepositional pronoun in Example 11 refers to and agrees with the possessor, in this case for example, "my brother and I." Thus, the focus of Example 11 is on the possessors rather than on the item possessed as in constructions in Examples 8–10.

(8) Es suyo.
"(It) is his or hers."

(9) Es su carro.
"(It) is his or her car."

(10) Son nuestras.
"(They) are ours."

(11) Son las bolsas de nosotros.
"(They) are the bags of ours."

The unstressed pronouns serve as direct and indirect objects as well as reflexives (also listed in Table 6–5). These unstressed forms are classified as clitics. Clitics are forms that cannot stand on their own. In proclitic constructions, the clitic depends on the following word. With finite verbs and negative imperatives proclitic forms are required (e.g., *lo abrí* "it (I) opened"). In enclitic constructions, the clitic is attached to the preceding word. These are used with nonfinite forms such as infinitives, gerunds, and imperatives (i.e., *¿Puedes terminar antes de irte?* "Can (you) finish before to leave-infinitive-you?" *dámelo* "give-imperative it to me").

A characteristic of indirect object clitics is doubling. In the case of indirect objects, the clitic is the obligatory element as in Example 12 and doubling via an overt noun phrase in Example 13 is optional. However, the full noun phrase without the indirect object clitic as in Example 14 is judged to be questionable by some speakers and ungrammatical by others. Recently, the nature of object clitics has been a subject of debate. Franco (1992) argued that because of word order restrictions on clitics, they are more like verbal agreement inflections than pronouns.

(12) Le_i compré una $camisa_i$.
"Him_i I bought a $shirt_i$."

(13) Le_i compré una camisa a mi $hijo_i$.
"For him_i I bought a shirt for my son_i."

(14) ?Compré una camisa a mi hijo.
"I bought a shirt for my son."

Direct object clitics, Example 15, replace the full noun phrase, but cannot duplicate it as is illustrated in Example 16. When the direct object is a person rather than an object *le* is used instead of *lo* or *la* as in seen in Example 17. This is further marked by the accusative *a* "to" that precedes the direct object noun phrase. In this case the direct object can be doubled.

(15) Preparé el $pastel_i$.
"I prepared the $cake_i$."
Lo_i preparé.
"It_i I prepared."

(16) *Lo_i preparé un $pastél_i$.
"It_i I prepared a $cake_i$."

(17) Le pegó a la niña con su bicicleta.
"(She) hit-past to (accusative) the girl with her bicycle."

VERB MORPHOLOGY

There are three conjugational classes of verbs in Spanish, *–ar, –er,* and *–ir*. Tense, aspect, and mood considerations, as well as person/number agreement and conjugational class of the verb dictate choice of verbal inflection. In regard to tense selection, aspect is the predominant feature that guides a speaker's choice (Bybee, 1994). Perfective conjugations code events or situations viewed as bounded wholes; imperfective conjugations code events that can be construed as continuously ongoing or repeated. Progressive conjugations emphasize ongoing actions. Many constructions that would be conveyed through the progressive in English are conveyed through the imperfective conjugations in Spanish.

TABLE 6–6
Tense and aspect markers and their interpretations.

Tense	Perfective	
Present perfect	Ha leído todas las lecturas.	She has already read all the readings.
Imperfect perfect	Había terminado su tarea.	She had already finished her homework.
Past perfect	Hubo comido tres helados.	He had eaten three ice creams.
Conditional perfect	Hubieran levantado todas las sillas.	They would have picked up all of the chairs.
Future perfect	Habré escrito tres páginas.	I will have written three pages.
	Imperfective	
Present	Como manzanas.	I eat apples.
Imperfect	Leía el periódico.	I used to read the paper.
Preterite	Terminaron la tarea.	They finished the homework.
Conditional	Compraríamos una casa.	We would buy a house.
Future	Iré de vacaciones.	I will go on vacation.
	Progressive	
Present	Están corriendo muy rápido.	They are running very fast.
Imperfect	Estaba caminando dos millas diario.	She was walking two miles everyday.
Preterite	Estuve jugando tenis.	I was playing tennis.
Conditional	Estaría viajando.	I would be travelling.
Future	Estaremos visitando muchas ciudades.	We will be visiting many cities.

Table 6–6 contains a list of perfective, imperfective, and progressive conjugations, plus sample sentences that illustrate differences in interpretation between these conjugations. The combination of aspect and tense allows a speaker to precisely situate events in time as illustrated in Example 18.

(18) Mientras caminaba a la escuela, estaba pensando en el examén cuando me caí y me rompí el brazo.

"While I walked to school, I was thinking about the exam when I fell and broke my arm."

Indicative versus subjunctive mood is the other factor taken into account in the selection of verbal inflection. The indicative-subjunctive contrast may be made in the present, past, and future tenses. Schane (1995) characterized the contrast between indicative and subjunctive mood in terms of the illocutionary force of a verb. When the interpretation of a verb is one of assertion, declaration, or expression of a belief that is likely to be shared, then the indicative is employed (e.g., *Creo que hay abejas en el coche.* "I think that there are [indicative] bees in the car."). However, if the speaker expresses a directive or a description of emotion, that may not be shared or accepted by the listener then the subjunctive is employed (e.g., *Dudo que haya abejas en el coche.* "I doubt that there are [subjunctive] bees in the car.").

Person and number agreement is obligatory for all finite forms as is illustrated in Example 19. However, nonfinite forms (i.e., infinitive, gerunds, and participles) do not demonstrate person and number agreement as seen in Example 20. Each of the conjugational classes has its own verbal markings. The markers for the –er and –ir verbs are quite similar in most of the conjugations with the exception of first person plural forms. The Appendix (at the end of this chapter), contains a complete listing of all the conjugations for regular –ar, –er, and –ir verbs.

(19) Nosotros nadamos, ellas corren pero él duerme.
"We swim [first plural present], they run [third plural present] but he sleeps [third singular present]."

(20) Tienen que hablar por teléfono.
"(They) have [third plural present] to call [infinitive] by telephone."

The final point to be considered is stem change. Irregularity in verbal inflection in Spanish is more often marked by stem changes or irregular stems, than by irregular inflections. There are four types of stem changes: insertion of diphthongs, vowel changes, irregular stems, and consonant changes. Examples of each of these types of changes are illustrated with representative verbs in Table 6–7. These changes are predictable to some extent, as small groups of verbs follow the same

TABLE 6–7
Examples of stem changing verbs.

Change:	Diphthong (present)	Vowel Weakening (present)	Irregular Stem (preterite)	Consonant Change (present)
Sample verb:	jugar	pedir	andar	tener
Yo	juego	pido	anduve	tengo
Tú	juegas	pides	anduviste	tienes
Usted/él/ella	juega	pide	anduvo	tiene
Nosotros	jugamos	pedimos	anduvimos	tenemos
Ustedes/ellos/ellas	juegan	pidan	anduvieron	tienen

patterns. Furthermore, in the case of verbs that require the insertion of a diphthong, stem changes only occur when the stem is stressed. A verb that is typical of this pattern is *jugar* "to play" as seen in Table 6–7. Some verbs undergo more than one type of change. *Tener* "to have," for example, has three stems for present tense as well as an irregular stem that is employed for preterite conjugations.

SYNTAX

Spanish is classified as a pro-drop language, permitting null subjects. Word order variations are also acceptable. Examples 21–24 illustrate these characteristics.

(21) Los niños juegan ajedrez.
"The children play chess."

(22) Juegan ajedrez.
"(They) play chess."

(23) Juegan ajedrez los niños.
"Play chess the children."

(24) Juegan los niños ajedrez.
"Play the children chess."

Although all these sentences are equally acceptable from a grammatical standpoint, deviations from the basic S-VO word order in Spanish do not all carry exactly the same meaning. The specific syntactic construction employed, semantics, and pragmatic focus all place constraints on word order.

One syntactic construction that involves obligatory movement of elements is Wh-question formation as in Example 25 (Torrego, 1984).

(25) ¿Qué comen los pájaros?
      "What eat the birds?"
      *¿Qué los pájaros comen?
      "What the birds eat?"

Subject inversion is also obligatory in constructions when any wh-element occurs as part of a subordinate clause as in Example 26.

(26) No sé donde está el hospital.
      "(I) don't know where is the hospital."
      *No sé donde el hospital está.
      "(I) don't know where the hospital is."

There are some constraints on movement in subject inversion. In a two-verb construction such as Example 27, the subject may be placed after either of the verbs. However, if the construction contains an auxiliary (*estar* "to be" or *haber* "to have"), the subject must be placed after the verb phrase as in Example 28 (Torrego, 1984).

(27) ¿Terminó Juan de preparar la cena?
      "Finished John to prepare supper?"
      ¿Terminó de preparar Juan la cena?
      "Finished to prepare John supper?"
      ¿Terminó de preparar la cena Juan?
      "Finished to prepare supper John?"

(28) ¿Ya ha terminado Juan de preparar la cena?
      "Already has finished John to prepare supper?"
      *¿Ya ha Juan terminado de preparar la cena?
      "Already has John finished to prepare supper?"

Once subject inversion has taken place there are some limitations of ordering of other elements within the utterance. Of course the whole noun phrase must move together. There are also limitations on where the adverb may occur in sentences with subject inversion as seen in Example 29 (Torrego, 1984).

(29) Mi mamá siempre toma café.
"My mother always drinks coffee."
Mi mamá toma café siempre.
"My mother drinks coffee always."
Siempre mi mamá toma café.
"Always my mother drinks coffee."
*Toma café siempre mi mamá.
"Drinks coffee always my mother."

Within phrases, there are also ordering constraints. In noun phrases, articles always precede nouns. Adjectives typically follow the nouns they modify. Some adjectives may precede the nouns they modify but these adjectives change meaning when they are placed before the noun as in Example 30.

(30) Un chofer malo
"An evil driver"
Un mal chofer
"A bad driver"

Finally, pragmatic focus impacts word order (Azevedo, 1992). Typically, new information is placed at the end of a sentence, with old or shared information usually occupying the subject position in the sentence and can be either omitted or pronominalized as in Example 31.

(31) ¿Qué hace tu hermana ahora?
"What does your sister do now?"
(Ella) acaba de abrir un restaurante.
"(She) just opened a restaurant."

SEMANTICS

Spanish makes use of many of the same semantic distinctions that are made in other languages. For example, gender and number are incorporated into the agreement system in Spanish. Also, subjunctive mood is commonly used. An area of difference that stands out is in the verb lexicon. Spanish has been described as a verb-framed language (Talmy, 1991). Spanish verbs inherently encode directionality (e.g., *subir* "to go up," *meter* "to put in"). This contrasts with English, a satellite-framed language, in which motion verbs convey manner but not directionality. In English, directionality is expressed through the use of particles.

From a crosslinguistic perspective, Spanish offers several interesting challenges to the language learner, particularly in relation to its status as a pro-drop language. Person and number agreement in noun phrases and tense and number marking on the verb may be relatively early acquisitions, as these systems are highly regular. Furthermore, verbal inflections are syllabic and some are stressed (i.e., preterite, imperfect) thus they are easily identified. This is likely to facilitate acquisition of verbal inflection. Forms that may be challenging are articles and direct and indirect object pronouns. These forms are all clitics; being unstressed they will not be perceptually salient and may be more difficult to learn. The number of tense and aspect distinctions made in Spanish are extensive. These too could be challenging, as tense and aspect are differentiated by mental state and temporal distinctions, not physical referents.

One of the consequences of Spanish being a pro-drop language, as has already been mentioned, is that subjects can appear in several sentence positions. Because this frees up word order, the cues for constraints on word order may be less transparent to children acquiring Spanish. Thus, children may have more difficulty learning constraints on syntactic structure.

DIALECTAL VARIATION

Spanish dialects vary to some extent in each of the general areas discussed in the description of General Formal Spanish. In this section, some examples of the ways in which regional and social dialects differ from the description of General Formal Spanish are discussed to highlight the potential range of normal variation in American Spanish.

PHONOLOGICAL VARIATION

The dialects of Spanish have been described as falling into two classes, conservative and radical (Guitart, 1978). The principle difference between these dialect groups is that conservative dialects tend to maintain syllable-final consonants (e.g., syllable-final /s/ and /r/) and radical dialects tend to delete syllable-final consonants. The Spanish spoken in the central region of Mexico, Guatemala, Costa Rica, and western Argentina are all examples of conservative dialects. Examples of radical dialects include the dialects spoken in Puerto Rico, Cuba, the Dominican Republic, coastal Venezuela, Panama, and Veracruz, the eastern coastal region of Mexico (these are also often referred to as Caribbean Spanish). Within these areas, there are some differences in the ways that phonemes are produced.

Dialects of Spanish spoken within the U.S. are representative of both these groups. For example, the majority of Spanish speakers in California and Texas are of Mexican origin and their Spanish retains many of the Mexican dialectal features, with the Spanish speakers in Florida of Cuban descent and their Spanish tending toward the features of Caribbean dialects.

CONSERVATIVE DIALECTS

Conservative dialects tend to retain the majority of the phonemes described as forming part of General Formal Spanish. The syllable-final /s/ and /r/ are generally produced in both casual and formal speech. In word-initial position the /x/ alternates with /h/. Thus articulations such as [xáwla] and [háwla] are both acceptable productions of *jaula* "cage." However, there are differences in the distribution of allophones of some sounds. For example, in central Mexico and Costa Rica in addition to the flap /r/ and trilled /r/, assibilated (e.g., [řópa] *ropa* "clothes") and fricative (e.g., [káloɹ] *calor* "heat") productions are also common (Lope Blanch, 1972; Cardenas, 1975). In Northern Mexico and in Argentina /tʃ/ is frequently replaced by /ʃ/ (Fontanella de Weinberg, 1992). A word such as *lechuga* "lettuce" [letʃúga] is realized as [leʃúga].

Vowels seem to be somewhat more vulnerable among individual speakers independent of region and/or social class in Mexico. Unstressed vowels, especially /e/, are weakened or lost in words such as [əstán] *están* "they are" or [pəskáðo] *pescado* "fish." This phenomena is most common before /s/ as in CV /s/ sequences and in the context of dental stops (Lope Blanch, 1972).

RADICAL DIALECTS

Radical dialects differ from General Formal Spanish in several ways: When /b, d, g/ occur as word-initial singletons (in words such as *gato* "cat" or *dos* "two") they are realized as fricatives in rapid running speech (Hammond, 1976). The /d/ is frequently omitted in intervocalic contexts and in word-final position (Guitart, 1978). Thus *pescado* "fish" would be produced as [pekáw] and *pared* "wall" as [*paré*]. In rapid speech the velar glide may be weakened to the point that it is no longer perceptible; thus a word like *abuela* "grandmother" would be heard as [awéla] (López Morales, 1971).

Final /s/ is particularly weak in radical dialects. It is normally realized in syllable-initial position in words like *mesa* "table" or *silla* "chair." In these instances, the articulation of [s] is dorsoalveolar rather than alveolar (Guitart, 1978). However, in syllable-final position the /s/ is usually elided or aspirated; the word *este* "this" could be produced as [éte] or [éhte]. When the /s/ is produced in a word such as *asma* "asthma," there is no voicing assimilation so that it could be pronounced as [ásma] or [áhma] but not [ázma] (López Morales, 1971).

Some variations are restricted to certain groups of speakers within these dialects. For example, in Puerto Rico the /r/ is often produced as [R] or [Ŗ], a voiced or unvoiced velar vibrant that shares the features of the /r/ except for place (i.e., the /R/ is [+back] [-coronal]). Words that would be expected to be produced with the trilled /r/ in General Formal Spanish are produced with the velar vibrant in Puerto Rican Spanish (e.g., [rósa] *rosa* "rose" would be produced [Rósa]). In a survey by López Morales (1971) this velarized production of /r/ was most often identified as a characteristic of rural dialects.

Among some speakers of Cuban Spanish, liquids are subject to neutralization in syllable-final position. For example, the /r/ is assimilated before dentals as in [bédda] *verdad* "truth" or [bédde] *verde* "green." In word-final position /r/ and /l/ may both be realized as /h/. Thus [máh] could be *mar* "sea" or *mal* "bad" (López Morales, 1971). The /l/ may also be substituted for /r/ in word-final position or before alveolar consonants (e.g., *pintor* "painter" is realized as [píntol]). These patterns are not observed among more highly educated speakers of Cuban Spanish (Guitart, 1976).

In General Formal Spanish, /n/ is the only nasal which occurs in word-final position. In many of the radical dialects, the velar nasal [ŋ] replaces the /n/ in word-final position. Thus *pan* "bread" will be produced as [páŋ]. If the final [ŋ] is deleted then the final consonant may be realized as nasalization of the preceding vowel (e.g., [pã]). This process may also occur across word boundaries in expressions like [beŋaká] *ven acá* "come here" (Hammond, 1979).

One of the consequences of loss of syllable-final consonants, particularly –s, is that meaning contrasts are lost. The singular-plural distinction and the second person familiar marker may be lost when the speaker does not produce /s/. Third person plural forms may also be lost if the speaker does not produce word-final /n/. Several compensatory strategies have been documented that presumably reduce potential confusions of meaning. In rapid connected speech there is compensatory vowel lengthening so that a minimal pair *pescado* "fish" and *pecado* "sin" is differentiated by vowel length [pe:káw] and [pekáw] (Hammond, 1978). This pattern is observed in medial position but not in word-final position (Hammond, 1980). Poplack (1986) found that if a confusion of meaning would result, that –s and other final consonants were less likely to be omitted.

MORPHOSYNTACTIC VARIATION

PRONOUNS

The use of pronouns also varies in a number of Central and South American countries (described by Quesada Pacheco, 1996). In all Spanish-speaking countries, *usted* "you" (formal) is the form that is employed as a marker of courtesy or respect in formal contexts. However, the form tú "you" (familiar) that denotes familiarity or affection is not used in the same way in all Spanish-speaking countries. In some dialects, an alternative *vos* is employed and replaces *tú* and *tí* as in Example 32.

> (32) Te hablé a *tí* ayer para ver si *tú* me acompañabas al cine.
>   Te hablé a *vos* ayer para ver si *vos* me acompañabas al cine.
>   "I called you yesterday to see if you would go to the movies with me."

In some dialects *vos* replaces *tú* as a marker of familiarity or solidarity (e.g., Peru [Caravedo, 1996]; Argentina and Uruguay [Donni de Mirande, 1996]; Chile [Wagner, 1996]). In Costa Rica, however, the respectful form *usted* is employed with family members (e.g., between husbands and wives or children and parents) and *vos* is used for friends or in other informal situations. In Guatemala and El Salvador both *tú* and *vos* are employed; *tú* marks solidarity and vos marks familiarity (Quesada Pacheco, 1996).

Some speakers of Southern Cone Spanish (i.e., southern region of South America) demonstrate different patterns of direct and indirect object clitic usage. The pronouns *lo* and *la* are used for indirect and direct objects and direct object pronouns may be doubled. These pronouns demonstrate gender agreement, not animacy as is dominant with the use of *le* and *les* in General Formal Spanish. A sample of a form that is reported as grammatical is *La$_i$ comí la torta$_i$* "It (feminine$_i$) (I) ate the cake (feminine$_i$)" (Franco, 1992). Some speakers of Peruvian Spanish prefer the production of full noun phrases and judge the use of clitics to be ungrammatical (Caravedo, 1996).

VERB MORPHOLOGY

Verb morphology does not vary greatly across dialects. In American Spanish, the preterite is preferentially used for past tense marking, with present perfective forms preferred in Peninsular Spanish. Some dialects report increased use of conditional over subjunctive forms. There is some variability in the inflections used with the pronoun *vos*. In some dialects a stressed vowel is employed, although in others a stressed diphthong is employed (e.g., *comés* versus *coméis*). Among some speakers, the stressed diphthong is employed with the *tú* pronominal form (e.g., Wagner, 1996). Although it does not effect the meaning or selection of verb tenses, there are some differences in the phonetic realization of some morphological markers (e.g., *corriste* becomes *corristes* or *comprábamos* is realized as *comprábanos*) (e.g., Cardenas, 1975; Sedano & Bentivoglio, 1996). Changes of this type are typically classified as overgeneralizations and are observed in dialects in the U.S., Mexico, and other parts of Latin America.

SEMANTIC VARIATION

Lexical variation is extensive across Spanish dialects. Various dialects adopted different words for local products, such as foods. For example, there are two names for "peanut": *cacahuate* and *maní*. In other cases, the same words have different meanings across dialects. One example is *pantalla* that is "earring" for speakers of Puerto Rican Spanish but "television screen" or "movie screen" in Mexican and other dialects of Spanish.

The aspects of dialectal variation that have the most potentially generalized impact on language acquisition are phonological variants. For example, the verbal agreement system that children acquiring Caribbean Spanish hear is somewhat different than that heard by children acquiring conservative dialects. In particular, children may not learn the same things about number agreement as Caribbean Spanish is less regular. For example, instead of hearing *los perros* "the dogs," the child might hear plural marked as *lo perro* "the dogs" (in contrast to the singular form *el perro* "the dog"). Differences in clitic usage may also emerge because speakers of all dialects may not use clitics to the same extent or in the same ways.

⅃

ACQUISITION OF SPANISH AS A FIRST LANGUAGE

PHONOLOGICAL DEVELOPMENT

In the prelinguistic phase, children acquiring Spanish are like children acquiring other languages. Spanish-learning infants' babbling inventories are similar to those of infants from other language backgrounds. For example, there are no significant differences in the voice onset time of initial stop consonants such as those observed in adult speakers (Eilers, Oller, & Benito García, 1984; Macken & Barton, 1980). Neither monolingual English-speaking adult listeners nor bilingual Spanish-English listeners could accurately identify the language background of infants acquiring Spanish or English as a first language based on samples of babbled utterances (Thevenin, Eilers, Oller, & Lavoie, 1985).

As children begin to produce recognizable, phonetically consistent forms to express the words of their language, individual strategies are used to produce more complex syllable structures that are characteristic of Spanish (Lleó, 1996). One strategy is spreading or assimilation of consonantal features (such as place of articulation). Children employing this strategy start by producing the same point of articulation, usually labial, but sometimes coronal or dorsal, in each of the syllables of the word (e.g., [papápo] for /sapáto/ *zapato* "shoe" or [noníno] for /dormíðo/ *dormido* "asleep" [Lleó, 1996]). Gradually children begin to vary the point of articulation within words, incorporating coronal and dorsal articulations. Consonant vowel interaction is another strategy that children frequently employ. For example, palatalization of those sounds that adjoin /i/ provide evidence of this pattern (e.g., [gadʒíta] for /kasíta/ *casita* "house" or [ʔakɔcinə] for /kosína/ *cocina* "kitchen" [Lleó, 1996]). Another difference in strategy is in the number of syllables produced by the children. For all three children studied by Lleó (1996) in this study, the majority of their productions were disyllabic. However, one child tended to produce shorter words with segments produced accurately. The others used somewhat longer words but were less accurate in terms of adult-like production of segments.

Studies of phonological development in Spanish have focused on the acquisition of consonants. In Table 6–8 the results of studies of phonemic acquisition in children who are speakers of conservative (i.e., Mexican and U.S. Mexican) and radical (Puerto Rico and Dominican Republic) dialects are summarized.

Differences in the criterion level for accepting phonemes as acquired and differences in the phonemes studied complicate comparisons of the results of these studies. However, the pattern of acquisition of Spanish consonants appears to be similar across these samples of speakers from different dialectal groups. The same consonants seem to be acquired early and late by all children. Many of the studies have not included children under the age of 3. However, based on Fantini's (1985) case study of his son's bilingual development and Anderson and Smith's (1987) study of 2-year-old Puerto Rican children, it appears that a number of speech sounds emerge before age 3.

Jiménez (1987a) analyzed the error patterns present in her participants' productions and found that the most commonly misarticulated sounds were /r, ɾ, s, g, ñ, and x/. The /r/ and /s/ were also late acquisitions in other groups (see Acevedo, 1993; Linares, 1981; Melgar de González, 1976 in Table 6–8). In interpreting these results, it is important to consider the syllable position in which the sounds were tested. In the case of /s/, for example, there are differences in syllable-initial and syllable-final position. The /s/ is more likely to be produced in syllable-initial position than in syllable-final position. The prolonged acquisition of this sound could reflect the difference in word position.

Analyses of phonological process use suggest that by 4 years of age, Spanish-speaking children have acquired the phonological rules of their native language, although there may still be individual phonemes that are produced inaccurately or inconsistently. Hodson and Paden (1991), for example, reported on the use of phonological processes in the speech of 4-year-old Mexican-American children with intelligible speech. The four most frequently occurring processes in this population were deviations in production of flap /ɾ/ and trill /r/ (referred to as tap/trill deviation by Hodson & Paden) (13%), consonant sequence reduction (8%), lateral /l/ deviations (6%), and glide deviations (6%). Goldstein and Iglesias (1996) examined the use of phonological processes in typically developing children of Puerto Rican origin. Among typically developing 3-year-olds the most frequently occurring phonological processes were liquid simplification (6.1%) and cluster reduction (15.2%) in contexts where the liquid or consonant cluster would be expected (e.g., flor "flower"). For 4-year-olds, the only two processes that occurred more than 5% of the time were cluster reduction and final

TABLE 6–8

The age of acquisition of Spanish consonants.

Study:	Acevedo (1993)	Fantini (1984)	Jimenez (1987b)	Linares (1981)	Melgar (1976)	Anderson & Smith (1987)	de la Fuente (1985)
Origin of Participants:	Texas	Texas	California	Chihuahua, Mexico	Mexico City	Puerto Rico	Dominican Republic
Criterion:	90%	Produced	50%	90%	90%	75%	50%
p	3;6	1;6	<3;0	3	3–3½	2	2.0
b	3;6	1;6	<3;0	6	4–4½		2.0
t	3;6	1;6	<3;0	3	3–3½	2	2.0
d	4;0		3;3	4			
k	4;0	2;0	<3;0	3	3–3½	2	2.0
g	5;11+	1;6	3;3	3	4–4½		2.5
β		2;0		6			
f	3;6	2;6	<3;0	4	3–3½		2.0
ð		1;6		4			
ɣ							2.0
s	4;0	1;6	3;3	6	6–6½		3.0
x	4;0	2;6	3;3				3.0
tʃ	4;6	2;0	<3;0	4	3–3½	2	2.0
m	3;6	1;6	<3;0	3	3–3½	2	2.0
n	3;6	1;6	<3;0	3	3–3½	2	2.0
ñ	3;6	2;6	3;7	3	3–3½		2.0
l	3;6	2;0	3;3	3	3–3½		2.5
ɾ	4;6	4;5	3;7	4	4–4½		3.0
r	5;11+	5;0	4;7	6	6–6½		3.5
w	3;6	1;6	<3;0	5		2	
j	3;6	1;6	<3;0		3–3½	2	2.5
h-x				3			

consonant deletion; all other processes occurred in fewer than 3% of the children's productions.

Dialect did, however, appear to influence the errors manifested by these groups of children. For example, in the Jiménez (1987a) study, children who did not produce /r/ substituted /ɾ, d, or l/, but the 2-year-olds in Anderson and Smith's (1987) study substituted /l/ or /h/ for /R/. These substitutions reflect the features of the target phonemes. For example, Mexican children's substitution of the flap /ɾ/ or /d/ share the placement features of /r/ but differ in the feature [tense]. The /h/ produced in place of /R/ by the Puerto Rican children shares the posterior placement for the velar vibrant /R/.

Substitution patterns for /s/ are also reported to differ across dialects. Children of Mexican origin substituted a /t/, /θ/, /tʃ/ or omitted it (Eblen, 1982; Jiménez, 1987b). It is interesting to consider the source of these substitutions as some seem quite unlikely given the ambient language. For example, the substitution of /θ/ for /s/ seems quite unusual if it is viewed as the substitution of a nonnative sound for a native language sound (i.e., /θ/ does not occur in Mexican Spanish). It is much more likely that this production results from a distortion in the production of /s/ rather than as a substitution. The /tʃ/ substitution also seems unusual, given that in some languages affricates are relatively late acquisitions (see Eblen, 1982, for further discussion). In Spanish, however, /tʃ/ is acquired as early as or earlier than /s/ (see Table 6–8). Puerto Rican children tended to substitute a /ʃ/ or /h/ for /s/ (Anderson & Smith, 1987). These productions seem to reflect the place of articulation that is prevalent in the target dialect.

Children must also acquire nonsegmental aspects of phonology, such as stress. To explore how children acquire stress in Spanish, Hochberg (1988b) compared the accuracy of 3- to 5-year-old children's spontaneous and imitated words with varying stress patterns. In spontaneous speech, children produced words with regular stress more accurately than words with irregular stress. In the imitation task, children were 78% accurate for regular words, 57% accurate for irregular words, and 44% accurate for words with prohibited stress patterns. Errors consisted of overregularization of irregular stress patterns. These findings provide evidence that even at 3 years of age, children appear to have learned the stress patterns of Spanish.

In a longitudinal study, Hochberg (1988a) explored the process of production of stress in children from 1;7 to 2;2 years of age. At the beginning of data collection, children showed no overall difference between their production of words with final or penultimate stress. One child was more accurate with words with final stress and two of the children were more accurate on final stress in spontaneous production, but imitated words with penultimate stress more accurately. By the final data point, three out of the four children studied produced penultimate-stressed words more accurately, which indicated a growing awareness of regular stress patterns in Spanish. That it was no easier for children to produce words with one stress pattern than another suggested that children start off "neutral" toward stress. Gradually children acquired and refined rules.

COMMUNICATIVE INTENTS AND PRAGMATIC FUNCTIONS

Jackson (1989) documented the communicative intents of four Mexican Spanish-speaking children during the one-word stage. In her case studies of these toddlers, the communicative intent categories described by Dore (1975) adequately captured the variety of communicative intents used by these children (e.g., request for action, request for information, protest). However, there were individual differences in the ways that the participants expressed these intents. For example, two of the children preferred to point out and describe objects to request objects. Another child achieved this by pointing out objects she wanted with phrases such as *mira* "look" and *a ver* "let's see." Jackson's findings are similar to those reported by Pérez and Castro (1988) for slightly younger children acquiring Spanish and/or Gallego in a Spanish/ Gallego bilingual context.

LEXICAL ACQUISITION

In terms of overall number of words acquired, there appear to be few differences in vocabulary acquisition patterns of children acquiring Spanish and learners of English or Italian (Jackson-Maldonado, Thal, Marchman, Bates, & Gutierrez-Clellen, 1993). As in these other language groups, children demonstrated steady climbs in the number of words acquired in the period from 8 to 20 months of age. The number of words acquired by the Spanish-learning children never differed greatly from the median levels for children acquiring English as a first language. The distribution of vocabulary items by syntactic class was also similar for these groups. The largest portion of their vocabularies was made up of nouns followed by verbs and then closed class items. Early on, children's learning curve for nouns was steeper—later verbs and closed-class morphemes were added more quickly. At all points, children's noun vocabulary was larger than other word classes.

However, Spanish-learning children may demonstrate some unique patterns of vocabulary acquisition strategies and use. As a language, Spanish offers the learner different grammatical cues than English and this may influence how children interpret new words they hear. One example is provided by Waxman's (1994) crosslinguistic study of children's interpretation of novel adjectives. In an experimental task children were shown an object with a novel characteristic, taught a novel adjective (e.g., *una pelota tiza* "a 'tiza' ball" referring to a spike-covered ball) and then asked to find another one. Spanish-learning children tended to point out another object (i.e., another ball) suggesting that they interpreted the novel word as a noun. Waxman indicated that this might be because adjectives in Spanish occur in constructions that are on the surface identical to noun phrase constructions (e.g., *Dame la pelota roja.* "Give me the red ball." *Dame la roja.* "Give me the red [one]."). Children learning English and French, on the other hand, hear a construction with a dummy element replacing the noun (i.e., *Give me the red one.*). Thus, for Spanish-learning children there is no overt cue to help them differentiate a noun and adjective in such a context.

Verb semantics may also play a role in what information the child expresses. Sebastián and Slobin (1994) studied Spanish-learning children's use of verbs in discourse. Some 3-year-olds use simple verbs (e.g., *se cayó* "(she) fell"-third singular past reflexive or *lo tiró* "(she) it threw"-third singular past) while others increased complexity of the verb phrase by using adverbs such as *arriba* "up" or *dentro* "inside." Frequently these adverbs were used redundantly (i.e., *se metió adentro* "(she) got in"-reflexive inside). After age 5, children marked changes in direction by describing the scene (e.g., *De repente el monstruo se cayó del árbol. Por suerte había un colchón ahí.* "Suddenly the monster fell from the tree. Luckily there was a mattress right there."). Over time, children relied increasingly on this strategy.

A semantic distinction between copular forms emerges early. *Ser* and *estar* are among the first verbs employed by young children; 2-year-olds use both. *Ser* is appropriately used with nominal expressions as in Example 33 and *estar* is used in locative expressions (Example 34). *Estar* as an auxiliary emerges slightly later in progressive constructions as in Example 35.

(33) Es eso Isabel? "Is that Isabel?" (23 months; in MacWhinney, 1995; Montes, 1987, 1992).

(34) Aquí está mi Mickey "Here is my Mickey" (28 months; Radford & Ploennig-Pacheco, 1995).

(35) Está volando. "It is flying" (29 months; Radford & Ploennig-Pacheco, 1995).

Several researchers (González, 1978; Jacobsen, 1986; Sera, 1992) have documented correct early productions of copula forms. Sera (1992) also employed an elicitation task with children aged 3 to 9 years with adult controls to determine if all child uses of *ser* and *estar* were adult-like. All groups performed similarly, confirming that children generally use copula forms in an adult-like manner. One exception that was observed for all the child groups, including the 9-year-olds, was the use of *estar* to discuss the location of events rather than *ser*.

MORPHOSYNTAX

NOUN MORPHOLOGY

A look at the utterances in Example 36 of very young Spanish speakers, who are beginning to combine words, reveals that from very early on children acquiring Spanish make use of grammatical morphology.

(36) Otro sucio "Another dirty (one)" (19 months; in MacWhinney, 1995; Montes, 1987, 1992)

Ese sienta en la camita "That one sits on the little bed" (19 months; in MacWhinney, 1995; Montes, 1987, 1992)

El pato allá "The duck over there" (19 months; in MacWhinney, 1995; Montes, 1987, 1992)

From the time that children are producing words, vowels *e, a,* and *u* appear to emerge as proto-articles (e.g., [epá] for *el pan* "the bread," [ukéka] for *una muñeca* "a doll") (López-Ornat, 1997; Pérez & Castro, 1988). López-Ornat (1997) traced the development of proto-articles into full articles in one girl acquiring Spanish in Madrid between 1;7 to 2;3 years to evaluate the premorphological status of these forms. Over time, the percentage of nouns with omissions of articles (i.e., vowels or proto-articles) before nouns decreased from approximately 40% at 1;7

years to 8% by age 2;1. The percentage of nouns with correctly produced articles increased from 2% at 1;7 to 71.5% by 2;1. These vocalic forms did not occur with any of the verb forms used by López-Ornat's subject except for infinitive constructions (e.g., *a ver* "to see") and before participles in perfective constructions (i.e., *ha roto* "has broken"). This was taken as evidence that these vowels only occurred in grammatically relevant positions and served a pregrammatical function.

These studies focused only on the presence of the article, not on gender agreement. From the time that Spanish-learning children begin to produce words, nouns usually end with the appropriate vowel. As articles emerge, gender errors are occasionally observed. These tend to be limited to those nouns that end in consonants or *–e* (e.g., *una pez* "a-feminine fish-masculine," *un llave* "a-masculine key-feminine," Hernández-Pina, 1984). Gender errors also result from overgeneralization of the masculine article (e.g., *otro sopa* "another-masculine soup-feminine" [Radford & Ploennig-Pacheco, 1995]). Masculine appears to be the default gender marker, as children do not produce feminine articles with nouns that end in *o* (Radford & Ploennig-Pacheco, 1995). When children combine words, adjectives are usually produced with correct gender agreement as in (i.e., *otra gelatina* "another-feminine jello-feminine"). Sometimes, however, overgeneralizations such as *mota rota* "broken motorcycle" or *tierra azula* "blue dirt" are produced, leading to questions about the source of correct gender agreement (Hernández Pina, 1984). In these productions, the child has changed the gender of the noun and adjective in *mota rota* and added a vowel to the end of *azul* that is not needed.

Pérez-Pereira (1990, 1991) explored the nature of gender agreement in a novel word production task with children aged 4 to 11 years. Children were taught names for novel objects and were asked to describe other objects employing color terms. For example, they were shown a novel object or creature that was referred to as, for example, a *linólo* and asked to describe a red one. This was used to elicit adjective agreement; in this case, the correct descriptor would be *rojo* not *roja*. A variety of morphophonological and gender cues were manipulated. Gender agreement errors such as *la linolo rojo* (when the novel, irregular form *una linolo* was taught and *la linolo roja* was expected) occurred very infrequently and only in 4- and 5-year-old children. Natural gender influenced the use of agreement, but gender cues were not necessary to generate correct responses. The most reliable cue was morphophonological marking on the noun (e.g., *tica* versus *talaz*), although children were able to make use of the article and produce correct gender agreement. It appears that children begin by focusing on phonological cues

and that later they learn that morphosyntactic cues can override phonological cues in the case of irregular words. Initially, children tend to
assign masculine gender.

The first distinction to emerge in the production of subject pronouns is the first-second person distinction. Muñoz and Vila (1986) and
Shum, Conde, and Diaz (1992) documented correct usage of *yo* "I" and
tú "you"-familiar in the speech of children aged 2 and younger. These
forms were used in deictic expressions more often than as subjects (e.g.,
ahora yo "now me" or *a tú* "to you"). Subject forms substituted for prepositional forms before these emerged, as in the second example (i.e.,
a tú should be *a tí*). Subject pronouns were also frequently placed in the
postverbal position (i.e., *corro rápido yo* "[I] run fast I"), an appropriate
position in certain pragmatic contexts (Muñoz & Vila, 1986). The same
patterns of person distinction were observed for other pronouns. For
example, *mí* "me" and *tí* "you" were also the first prepositional pronouns used. Third person forms, *él* "he" and *ella* "she" emerged closer
to age 3 years.

Unstressed pronouns were also present in the samples of children
around 2 years of age as seen in Example 37. These forms were sometimes omitted in obligatory or expected contexts such as in Example 38
in which the accusative pronoun *lo* "it" is missing. There are also some
examples of overuse in which dative pronouns were doubled, with this
not allowed in the adult language in Example 39.

(37) Cárgame. "Carry me." (29 months; Radford & Ploennig-
Pacheco, 1995)
Yo te pongo a tí. "I (to) you put on to you." (29 months; Radford
& Ploennig-Pacheco, 1995)

(38) Te quito. "Off you (it-omitted) I take." (26 months; Shum et al.,
1992)

(39) Un niño pequeñito que me ha tirado a mí la torre mía. "A little
child that (to) me has knocked-over to me the tower of mine."
(27 months; Shum et al., 1992)

Very young children may omit number agreement early on. For
example, possessive forms are used as fixed forms (e.g., *mi brazos* "my-
singular arms-plural") (Radford & Ploennig-Pacheco, 1995). Some instances of plural marking and number agreement are observed before
2½ years of age (Aparici, Díaz, & Cortés, 1996; Kvaal, Shipstead-Cox,
Nevitt, Hodson, & Launer, 1988). The majority of nouns end with vowels and take /s/; this form appears to be established by age 3 years

(Pérez-Percira, 1989). The /es/ is not mastered until age 4 and children continued to have trouble with it on a novel word inflection task through age 6 (Pérez-Pereira, 1989). School-aged children sometimes produce errors in number agreement in complex sentences that contain a considerable amount of material between, for example, a clitic and the agreeing element as in Example 40.

(40) Le$_i$ tengo más miedo a los tiburones$_j$. "To it-singular$_i$ (I) have more fear to the sharks-plural$_j$." (First grader; Rodríguez, 1992).

VERB MORPHOLOGY

Group and case studies (Cortés & Vila, 1991; González, 1978, 1983; Jacobsen, 1986; Kvaal et al., 1988; Morales, 1989; Vivas, 1979) have all reported on acquisition of verb morphology in children acquiring Spanish as a first language from approximately 2 years of age. It is difficult to compare the results of these studies because both age and MLU (calculated using different rules) have been used to describe the levels of the children. Nevertheless, these studies provide a converging picture of the order of emergence of verbal markers among children acquiring Spanish. Initially children make heavy use of third singular present tense, sometimes substituting third singular forms for others as in the Example of 41.

(41) No sale. "(It does) not come out-third singular." (26 months; Radford & Ploennig-Pacheco, 1995)

Venga mi amigos a escuela. "Come-third singular present my-singular friends to school." (31 months; Radford & Ploennig-Pacheco, 1995)

¿Qué me pone yo? "What myself put-third singular I? (27 months; Radford & Ploennig-Pacheco, 1995)

Before 2½ years of age, children are reported to begin to produce the preterite and gerund forms in present progressive constructions. Between the ages of 2½ and 3 years, the imperfect and periphrastic future forms are usually reported. Progress between the ages of 3 and 4 years is marked by an increase in the usage of tenses that have already been acquired (i.e., preterite), and increases in correct person and number marking with those forms. Dialectal differences are apparent at this point. Children exposed to American dialects acquire perfective constructions at age 4 or somewhat later (Johnson, 1996;

Morales, 1989; Slobin & Bocaz, 1988); these are among the earliest forms for children acquiring peninsular Spanish (Cortés & Vila, 1991; Slobin & Bocaz, 1989). The subjunctive is observed in children between the ages of 3½ and 4½ years (González, 1983; Naharro, 1996).

Although a number of tenses emerge early, it is not clear when tense marking and person and number agreement become productive for children acquiring Spanish. In children of 2 and 3 years of age, progressive constructions occur more often with activity verbs and preterites are produced with state and change of state verbs (Jacobsen, 1986; Slobin & Bocaz, 1988). Present and preterite forms frequently are reported to occur first in the third person singular (e.g., González, 1983; Vivas, 1979). González (1983) suggested that this also appears to be true for later acquired forms as well. Past progressive, imperfect, and present perfect all emerge in the third person singular initially. Pérez-Pereira (1989) explored the question of productivity of verbal inflection with children aged 3–6 years using a novel verb inflection task. The ability to inflect a novel verb provides evidence of a productive rule, because a child will never have heard the form previously, thus it cannot have been memorized. The majority of real verbs were inflected correctly by 3-year-olds in this study, but novel verbs were not correctly inflected until age 4 years or later.

Errors in verbal inflection are uncommon among children acquiring Spanish (e.g., Sebastián & Slobin, 1994). Where children produce errors in verbal inflection, these tend to be extensions of –ar endings to –er and –ir verbs (e.g., *saló* for *salió* or *escondó* for *escondió*). By age 5½, this type of error almost never occurs in the speech of monolingual Spanish-speaking children (Friedenberg, 1991). Children also tend to overgeneralize the roots of irregular verbs (i.e., *yo sabo* for *yo sé* or *cabo* for *quepo*). As children acquire more complex tenses, these errors continue to emerge (e.g., *ponían el dibujo para que lo hacieramos [hiciéramos] nosotros*; Rodríguez, 1992). Errors in stem changing verbs (such as the substitution of *ruedamos* for *rodamos* or *rodo* for *ruedo*) are the most common verb error. When children overregularize the stems, they either produce stem changes unnecessarily (e.g., *juegamos* for *jugamos*) or fail to produce them in obligatory contexts (i.e., *juga* for *juega*). A group of Mexican first graders produced stem change errors approximately 36% of the time (Rodríguez, 1992). Children rarely inserted a diphthong in those verbs which did not require stem changes (Friedenberg, 1991); this suggests that children did not have difficulty identifying stem changing verbs but did have trouble identifying the rules for stem changes.

SYNTAX

One syntactic phenomenon of interest in Spanish is grammatical subjects, because Spanish is a pro-drop language. In early word combinations between approximately 1½ and 2 years of age, children frequently
place the subject after the verb (López-Ornat, 1990) and make use of
morphologically and contextually redundant subjects (Radford &
Ploennig-Pacheco, 1995). These findings seem to suggest that children
have only limited knowledge of subject use. However, Austin, Blume,
Parkinson, Núñez del Prado, and Lust (1997) suggested that Spanish-
learning children are aware of the pro-drop nature of subjects. In the
free speech samples of 1- and 2-year-olds, regardless of the presence or
absence of an overt subject, verbal inflection was correctly used over
90% of the time. The only cases in which verbal inflection was omitted
was when an auxiliary was omitted (e.g., *te dicho* "told you" for *te he
dicho* "[I] have told you" [Austin et al., 1997]). However, these children's
awareness of discourse constraints on null subjects was not adult-like.
Up to 68% of the null subjects produced by these children were pragmatically inappropriate.

Another area of recent interest in the area of syntax is the emergence of functional categories. Evidence for the functional category *Inflection* (INFL) is obtained through the evaluation of children's
production of morphological elements. Torrens (1995), for example, explored the emergence of INFL in four children acquiring Spanish and
Catalán. Between the ages of 1;9 and 2;2, these children produced singular verb forms primarily. However, the forms that were produced
were virtually error free and the productions suggested that the children differentiated finite and infinite contexts. Torrens took this as evidence of early emergence of the functional category INFL.

If, following Franco's (1992) arguments that object clitics are verbal
agreement morphemes, then clitic doubling also provides evidence of
the acquisition of the functional category INFL. Correct production of
constructions with clitic doubling require the child to differentiate finite
and nonfinite verb contexts. In the examples cited by Torrens and Wexler (1996) children between 2 and 3 years of age produced clitic-doubled
expressions in contexts in which they were obligatory such as te_i *he
regañada a* ti_i "you$_i$ I have scolded to you$_i$." These constructions were
also produced in contexts that were appropriate but optional such as se_i
lo digo a mi mamá, "to her$_i$ it (I) tell to my mother$_i$." They also produced
dative experiencers, *a* $mí_i$ *si* me_i *gusta* "to me$_i$ yes me$_i$ (it) pleases," and
left dislocations with clitics, *ese* $cochecito_i$ lo_i *ha comprado* "that little car$_i$
it$_i$ (he/she/you) has-third singular bought." Only one omission was

found in the samples of this child and there were no instances of use in contexts that an adult would not use a clitic. Finally, the correct placement of negative elements also corresponds to the acquisition of INFL (Bel, 1996); children begin to correctly place negative elements at the same time that they correctly use inflections.

The development of complex syntax has been documented in conjunction with studies of the development of discourse. Gutierrez-Clellen and colleagues studied discourse production in a story retelling task with children aged 4 to 8 years. There were several indices of increased syntactic complexity in the language of these children including increased use of clause sequences and greater complexity of narrative statements (Gutierrez-Clellen & Iglesias, 1992). Syntactic structures with subordination, including relative clauses, adverbials, and prepositional phrases also increased over time (Gutierrez-Clellen & Hofstetter, 1994). Finally, children made increased use of referential devices such as appropriately detailed phrases and less ambiguous phrases (Gutierrez-Clellen & Heinrichs-Ramos, 1993).

LANGUAGE SOCIALIZATION

Some cultural preferences have been reported in terms of language socialization. Studies of language socialization have focused on those features that characterize language learning interactions in Hispanic families primarily in the U.S. and Mexico. Blount and Padgug (1977) explored what features marked the infant-directed speech of Spanish-speaking parents as compared to English-speaking parents. Features such as exaggerated intonation and high pitch were frequent in both groups of parents. However interactional features, including repetition and interpretation of a child's utterance were more common in the speech of the Spanish-speaking parents with English-speaking parents using more paralinguistic features, such as breathiness and raised volume.

Field and Widemayer (1981) evaluated mother-infant interactions to determine if differences that are reported in other countries are maintained in families who have immigrated to the U.S. Low socioeconomic (SES) families of Cuban, Puerto Rican, and South American origins participated in this study. It was believed that these groups of parents might have similar child-rearing habits, because they were homogenous in terms of employment, educational levels, and religious beliefs. Parent-child behaviors, such as talking and gazing, were observed during mealtimes. Cuban mothers spent 82% of the time talking to their infants and used relatively long utterances. South American and Puerto Rican mothers spoke less of the time and used somewhat shorter utterances with their infants. The pattern for gaze was reversed. Cuban infants spent the least amount of time looking at their mothers with Puerto Rican infants spending the most time gazing at their mothers. The Cuban mothers engaged in more teaching games, whereas the Puerto Rican mothers engaged in more social games. Planos, Zayas, and Busch-Rossnagel (1995) addressed a similar question to explore the relationship between maternal teaching behaviors and acculturation to Anglo culture. Participants were U.S.-born Puerto Rican and Dominican-born women. Even when acculturation was controlled, groups differed significantly in their preferred interaction styles with their infants. Puerto Rican women used more inquiry and praise, whereas the Dominican women modeled new behaviors and were more directive with their infants.

Parents may continue to play active roles, such as is reported for infants in the examples mentioned above, in play and language activities. In a task that compared Spanish- and English-speaking mothers' teaching styles on a construction activity, Laosa (1980) found that Spanish-speaking mothers used more directives and modeled, with English-speaking mothers asking questions and praising more often. In play activities with toys, such as cars and kitchen sets, parents asked many questions (Tenenbaum & Leaper, 1997). Mothers tended to ask a number of causal questions that demanded conceptual answers and fathers asked more yes-no questions. This contrasts with what has been observed in European-descent families (i.e., fathers ask more conceptually demanding questions). Parental beliefs and educational level may also impact what types of parent-child interactions are observed. Zukow (1987) found that rural parents with minimal education tended to believe that language was a skill that developed gradually and could not be taught. Parents from the same area, but with an "elevated" educational level believed that language was a skill to be stimulated. In a U.S. Mexican community, Pease-Alvarez and Vasquez (1994) asked parents how young children learned to talk. This group of parents emphasized the role they played in shaping children's babbling to language through their responses to their children. These beliefs seemed to have an effect on the amount of language stimulation that the parents provided for their infants and toddlers.

Parents may also employ different teaching strategies with their infants and young children in different contexts. Gutierrez-Clellen (1995) observed that parents provided direct instruction to facilitate symbolic play events, such as bathing or feeding a baby, for children who were between the one- and two-word stages of development. Parent-initiated events were more frequent at the one-word level. With older children who produced more multiword utterances, parents initiated somewhat less.

Zukow (1989) documented siblings' roles in teaching slightly older children in rural families in Central Mexico. In this context, the mother provided verbal instructions to the older siblings. Siblings modeled and talked about what a younger child was expected to do. In this way they provided simplified linguistic input to the children. For example, an older child showed a younger one how to make a tortilla or explained how and where to sweep (e.g., *¡Mira! ¡Mira, barre por allá! ¡Por allá!* "Look! Look! Sweep over there! Over there!"). Pérez-Granados and Callanan (1997) questioned Mexican-descent parents about the roles that siblings play in young children's learning. Parents reported that older siblings directly taught or modeled for their younger siblings skills in the areas of play, language comprehension, and social skills, among others. For example, the older children taught the younger ones how to play games, sing songs from school, and showed them what to say and how to say it. Thus, all members of the family may become involved in language teaching.

The events and topics around which adult-child conversation center also vary (Heath, 1986). In Mexican American families, children may be encouraged to label objects in the immediate environment and recall family names. Questions between children and adults are more likely to focus on new information than on shared events. However, the whole family may participate in discussions planning future events such as a picnic or a trip to visit relatives. One type of interaction in which children may be encouraged to participate is teasing (Eisenberg, 1986). Adults may initially help a child identify teasing or provide a response that a child may imitate (e.g., *Dile que estás muy bonita.* "Tell him/her you are very pretty."). Through scaffolding of this type, children learn to initiate teasing interactions.

Eisenberg (1985) followed two girls between their second and third birthdays and documented how children learned to talk about past experiences. The parents facilitated the girls' talking about experiences to recount new information to other adults in their environment rather than to talk about shared events (see also Heath, 1986). For example, the child was asked to tell her father about a trip to school (i.e., *Dile a tu papí que fuistes a la escuela de Laura.* "Tell your daddy that you went to Laura's school.") or to tell someone what was happening at the time a photo was taken. Communicating about past experiences provided an opportunity to integrate the child into his or her social environment.

Early on, the parents elicited many of the stories using yes-no questions. Later the use of yes-no questions dropped as the girls were able to provide more information spontaneously. When wh-questions were asked, these tended to be how, what, or why questions.

⊔

SUMMARY AND CONCLUSIONS

The results of these studies provide an emerging picture of Spanish language acquisition. However, many interesting questions remain to be explored. For example, in regard to the acquisition of verbal inflection the results seen thus far are sometimes in disagreement. Researchers who have studied the order of acquisition of verbal inflections observe that verbal morphemes emerge early. However, sometimes children aged 3 to 5 years overgeneralize or do not produce all conjugations equally accurately, especially when they are required to inflect real or novel verbs in an elicited production task (i.e., Pérez-Pereira, 1989). This contrasts with claims of consistently correct usage as evidence of functional categories in syntactic acquisition by very young children (e.g., Austin et al., 1997; Torrens, 1995). Studies that employ a variety of tasks to probe children's morphosyntactic knowledge will provide insights into the nature of Spanish-learning children's use of verbal inflection.

More research into syntactic acquisition as it relates to morphology, as well as how it relates to discourse, will shed light on the path to Spanish-learning children's becoming competent communicators. For example, Austin et al. (1997) observed that in the context of discourse many preschool-aged children's null subjects were illicit. Gutierrez-Clellen and Heinrichs-Ramos (1993) discussed 4- and 8-year-old children's growing competence with the use of referential devices and the increasing clarity of their use of referents. These findings suggest that some aspects of syntax, particularly in the context of discourse demands, may be learned over an extended period of time.

Language socialization is another area that needs to be investigated in greater detail. The studies up to now have focused on the patterns of immigrants or individual parent's strategies. These findings cannot be generalized to the diverse elements of Hispanic culture at large. Looking at how parents and children interact has implications for questions about the role of input in language acquisition. It also has practical implications for application in the area of education where we may wish to develop culturally and linguistically appropriate teaching strategies in regular or special education.

Methodological concerns are another factor to be considered in interpreting studies of Spanish language acquisition. Many of the studies to date are based on single subjects or very small groups. There are also differences in the language backgrounds of children studied in America and Spain. For example, throughout the Spanish-speaking world, bilingualism is common. In America, Spanish-speaking children are learning Indian languages or English. In Spain, children are acquiring other Romance languages (e.g., Catalán or Gallego) or Basque. To understand children acquiring American Spanish, it is particularly important to follow large groups of children who are acquiring Spanish in similar linguistic and cultural circumstances. This would shed light on common aspects of Spanish language acquisition and on the effects of language contact. Documentation of competence in each of a child's languages might facilitate the interpretation of the data for bilinguals if the languages impact one another. It would also be helpful to employ standard measures in Spanish (e.g., the use of MLU in words) to be able to more readily compare results across studies.

Continued study of Spanish is important from several perspectives. The U.S. Hispanic population continues to grow and a large proportion of this population speaks Spanish. Thus, information about Spanish has practical implications for education and related fields. Furthermore, the study of language systems that differ in terms of morphological richness, syntactic flexibility, or semantic characteristics help us identify and understand universal and language-specific aspects of language acquisition. Crosslinguistic studies of Spanish can make significant contributions in this regard.

⊔

REFERENCES

Acevedo, M. (1993). Development of Spanish consonants in preschool children. *Journal of Childhood Communication Disorders, 15*, 9–15.

Anderson, R., & Smith, B. (1987). Phonological development of two-year-old monolingual Puerto Rican Spanish-speaking children. *Journal of Child Language, 14*, 57–78.

Aparici, M., Díaz, G., & Cortés, M. (1996). El orden de adquisición de morfemas en Catalán y Castellano [The order of acquisition of morphemes in Catalan and Spanish]. In M. Pérez-Pereira (Ed.), *Estudios sobre la adquisición del Castellano, Catalán, Eusquera y Gallego* (pp. 165–174). Santiago, Spain: Universidad de Santiago de Compostela.

Austin, J., Blume, M., Parkinson, D., Núñez del Prado, Z., & Lust, B. (1997). The status of pro-drop in the initial state: Results for new analyses of Spanish. In A. Pérez-Leroux & W. Glass (Eds.), *Contemporary perspectives on the acquisition of Spanish: Volume 1. Developing grammars* (pp. 37–54). Somerville, MA: Cascadilla.

Azevedo, M. (1992). *Introducción a la lingüística Española* [Introduction to Spanish linguistics]. Englewood Cliffs, NJ: Prentice Hall.

Barrutia, R., & Terrell, T. (1982). *Fonética y fonología Españolas* [Spanish phonetics and phonology]. New York: John Wiley.

Bel, A. (1996). La adquisición de la negación en Catalán y Castellano [The acquisition of negation in Catalan and Spanish]. In M. Pérez-Pereira (Ed.), *Estudios sobre la adquisición del Castellano, Catalán, Eusquera y Gallego* (pp. 231–240). Santiago, Spain: Universidad de Santiago de Compostela.

Bjarkman, P., & Hammond, R. (1989). Introduction: Modern phonological approaches to American Spanish pronunciation. In P. Bjarkman & R. Hammond (Eds.), *American Spanish pronunciation* (pp. 1–8). Washington DC: Georgetown University Press.

Blount, B., & Padgug, E. (1977). Prosodic, paralinguistic, and interactional features in parent-child speech: English and Spanish. *Journal of Child Language, 4,* 67–86.

Bybee, J. (1994). Spanish tense and aspect from a typological perspective. In P. Hashemipour, R. Maldonado, & M. van Naerssen (Eds.), *Studies in language learning and Spanish linguistics in honor of Tracy D. Terrell* (pp. 442–457). New York: McGraw-Hill.

Canfield, D. L. (1981). *Spanish pronunciation in the Americas.* Chicago: University of Chicago Press.

Caravedo, R. (1996). Perú. In M. Alvar (Ed.), *Manual de dialectología Hispánica: El Español de América* (pp. 152–168). Barcelona, Spain: Ariel.

Cardenas, D. (1975). Mexican Spanish. In E. Hernández-Chávez, A. Cohen, & A. Beltram (Eds.), *El lenguaje de los Chicanos* (pp. 1–6). Arlington, VA: Center for Applied Linguistics.

Chang-Rodríguez, E. (1991). *Latinoamérica, su civilización y su cultura* [Latin America, her civilization and culture]. New York, NY: Harper Collins Publishers.

Cortés, M., & Vila, I. (1991). Uso y función de las temporales en el habla infantil [Use and function of tenses in infantile speech]. *Infancia y Aprendizaje, 53,* 14–43.

Cressey, W. (1989). A generative sketch of Castilian Spanish pronunciation: A point of reference for the study of American Spanish. In P. Bjarkman &

R. Hammond (Eds.), *American Spanish pronunciation* (pp. 48–70). Washington DC: Georgetown University Press.

Crystal, D. (1997). *The Cambridge encyclopedia of language* (2nd ed.). Cambridge, UK: Cambridge University Press.

Current Population Reports. (1990). *1990 census of population and housing* [Summary Tape File 3C]. Washington DC: U.S. Census Bureau. Available URL: http://www.census.gov/cdrom/lookup

Current Population Survey. (1994, March). *Hispanic origin* [On-line data file]. Washington DC: U.S. Census Bureau. Available URL: http://www.census.gov/population

de la Fuente, M. (1985). *The order of acquisition of Spanish consonant phonemes by monolingual Spanish-speaking children between the ages of 2;0 and 6;5.* Unpublished doctoral dissertation, Georgetown University, Washington DC.

Delattre, P. (1966). A comparison of syllable length conditioning among languages. *International Review of Applied Linguistics, 4,* 183–198.

Donni de Mirande, N. (1996). Argentina-Uruguay. In M. Alvar (Ed.), *Manual de dialectología Hispánica: El Español de América* (pp. 209–221). Barcelona, Spain: Ariel.

Dore, J. (1975). Holophrases, speech acts, and language universals. *Journal of Child Language, 2,* 21–40.

Eblen, R. (1982). A study of the acquisition of fricatives by three-year-old children learning Mexican Spanish. *Language and Speech, 25,* 201–220.

Eilers, R., Oller, K., & Benito-García, C. (1984). The acquisition of voicing contrasts in Spanish and English learning infants and children: A longitudinal study. *Journal of Child Language, 11,* 313–336.

Eisenberg, A. (1985). Learning to describe past experiences in conversation. *Discourse Processes, 8,* 177–204.

Eisenberg, A. (1986).Teasing: Verbal play in two Mexicano homes. In B. Schieffelin & E. Ochs (Eds.), *Language socialization across cultures* (pp. 182–198). Cambridge, UK: Cambridge University Press.

Fantini, A. (1985). *Language acquisition of a bilingual child: A sociolinguistic perspective.* San Diego, CA: College-Hill Press.

Field, T., & Widemayer, S. (1981). Mother-infant interactions among lower SES Black, Cuban, Puerto Rican, and South American immigrants. In T. Field, A. Sostek, P. Vietze, & P. Leiderman (Eds.), *Culture and early interactions* (pp. 41–62). Hillsdale, NJ: LEA.

Fontanella de Weinberg, M. B. (1992). *El Español de América* [Spanish in America]. Madrid, Spain: Mapfre.

Frago Gracia, J. (1996). Formación del Español de América [Formation of American Spanish]. In M. Alvar (Ed.), *Manual de dialectología Hispánica: El Español de América* (pp. 11–23). Barcelona, Spain: Ariel.

Franco, J. (1992). *On object agreement in Spanish.* Unpublished doctoral dissertation, University of Southern California, Los Angeles.

Friedenberg, J. (1991). The acquisition of Spanish as a first and second language: Learner errors and strategies. In L. Malavé & G. Duquette (Eds.), *Language, culture, and cognition* (pp. 55–80). Clevedon, UK: Multilingual Matters.

Goldstein, B., & Iglesias, A. (1996). Phonological patterns of normally developing Spanish-speaking 3- and 4-year olds. *Language, Speech, and Hearing Services in the Schools, 27,* 82–90.

González, G. (1978). *The acquisition of Spanish grammar by native Spanish-speaking children.* Rosslyn, VA: National Clearinghouse for Bilingual Education.

González, G. (1983). Expressing time through verb tenses and temporal expressions in Spanish: Age 2;0–4;6. *NABE Journal, 7,* 69–82.

Grimes, B. (Ed.). (1996). *Ethnologue: Languages of the World* (13th ed.). Dallas, TX: Summer Institute of Linguistics. Available URL: http://www.sil.org/ethnologue

Guitart, J. (1976). *Markedness and a Cuban dialect of Spanish.* Washington DC: Georgetown University Press.

Guitart, J. (1978). A propósito del Español de Cuba y Puerto Rico: Hacia un modelo no sociolingüístico de lo sociodialectal [Regarding the Spanish of Cuba and Puerto Rico: Toward a non-sociolinguistic model of the social dialectic]. In H. López Morales (Ed.), *Corrientes actuales en la dialectología del Caribe Hispánico* (pp. 77–92). Río Piedras: Editorial Universitaria, Universidad de Puerto Rico.

Gutierrez-Clellen, V. (1995). Narrative development and disorders in Spanish-speaking children: Implications for the bilingual Interventionist. In H. Kayser (Ed.), *Bilingual speech-language pathology* (pp. 97–127). San Diego: Singular Publishing Group.

Gutierrez-Clellen, V., & Heinrichs-Ramos, L. (1993). Referential cohesion in the narratives of Spanish-speaking children: A developmental study. *Journal of Speech and Hearing Research, 36,* 559–567.

Gutierrez-Clellen, V., & Hofstetter, R. (1994). Syntactic complexity in Spanish narratives: A developmental study. *Journal of Speech and Hearing Research, 37,* 645–654.

Gutierrez-Clellen, V., & Iglesias, A. (1992). Causal coherence in the oral narratives of Spanish-speaking children. *Journal of Speech and Hearing Research, 35,* 363–372.

Hammond, R. (1976). Phonemic restructuring of voiced obstruents in Miami-Cuban Spanish. In F. Aid, M. Resnick, & B. Saciuk (Eds.), *1975 Colloquium on Hispanic linguistics* (pp. 42–51). Washington DC: Georgetown University Press.

Hammond, R. (1978). An experimental verification of the phonemic status of open and closed vowels in Caribbean Spanish. In H. López Morales (Ed.), *Corrientes actuales en la dialectología del Caribe Hispánico* (pp. 93–143). Río Piedras: University of Puerto Rico Press.

Hammond, R. (1979). The velar nasal in rapid Cuban Spanish. In J. Lantolf, F. Frank, & J. Guitart (Eds.), *Colloquium on Spanish and Luso-Brazilian linguistics* (pp. 19–36). Washington DC: Georgetown University Press.

Hammond, R. (1980). Las realizaciones fonéticas del fonema /s/ en el Español Cubano de Miami [Phonetic realizations of the phoneme /s/ in Miami Cuban Spanish]. In G. Scavnicky (Ed.), *Dialectología Hispanoaméricana: Estudios actuales* (pp. 8–15) Washington DC: Georgetown University Press.

Heath, S. (1972). *Telling tongues.* New York: Teachers College Press.

Heath, S. (1986). Sociocultural contexts of language development. In *Beyond language: Social and cultural factors in schooling language minority children* (pp. 143–186). Los Angeles: Evaluation, Dissemination, and Assessment Center.

Hernández Pina, F. (1984). *Teorías psicosociolingüísticas y su aplicación a la adquisición del Español como lengua materna* [Psycho-sociolinguistic theory and its application to the acquisition of Spanish as a first language]. Madrid, Spain: Siglo XXI de España Editores.

Hochberg, J. (1988a). First steps in the acquisition of Spanish stress. *Journal of Child Language, 15,* 273–292.

Hochberg, J. (1988b). Learning Spanish stress: Developmental and theoretical perspectives. *Language, 64,* 683–706.

Hodson, B., & Paden, E. (1991). *Targeting intelligible speech* (2nd ed.). Austin, TX: PRO-ED.

Jackson, D. (1989). *Una palabra: Multiplicidad de intenciones y funciones* [One word: A multiplicity of intentions and functions]. Unpublished doctoral dissertation, El Colegio de Mexico, Mexico City, Mexico.

Jackson-Maldonado, D., Thal, D., Marchman, V., Bates, E., & Gutierrez-Clellen, V. (1993). Early lexical development in Spanish-speaking infants and toddlers. *Journal of Child Language, 20,* 523–549.

Jacobsen, T. (1986). ¿Aspecto antes de tiempo? Una mirada a la adquisición temprana del Español [Aspect before tense? A look at the early acquisition of Spanish]. In J. Meisel (Ed.), *Adquisición de lenguaje* (pp. 97–114). Frankfurt, Germany: Vervuert.

Jiménez, B. (1987a). Articulation error patterns in Spanish-speaking children. *Journal of Childhood Communication Disorders, 10,* 95–106.

Jiménez, B. (1987b). Articulation of Spanish consonants in children aged 3–5 years, 7 months. *Language, Speech, and Hearing Services in the Schools, 18,* 357–363.

Johnson, C. (1996). Desarrollo morfosintáctico del verbo Español: Marcaje del tiempo y aspecto en Mexico y Madrid [Morphosyntactic development of the verb in Spanish: Marking of tense and aspect in Mexico and Madrid]. In M. Pérez-Pereira (Ed.), *Estudios sobre la adquisición del Castellano, Catalán, Eusquera y Gallego* (pp. 147–156). Santiago, Spain: Universidad de Santiago de Compostela.

Kvaal, J., Shipstead-Cox, N., Nevitt, S., Hodson, B., & Launer, P. (1988). The acquisition of 10 Spanish morphemes by Spanish-speaking children. *Language, Speech, and Hearing Services in the Schools, 19,* 384–394.

Laosa, L. (1980). Maternal teaching strategies in Chicano and Anglo-American Families: The influence of culture and education on maternal behaviors. *Child Development, 51,* 759-765.

Linares, T. (1981). Articulation skills in Spanish-speaking children. In R. Padilla (Ed.), *Ethnoperspectives in bilingual education research: Bilingual education technology* (pp. 363–367). Ypsilanti: Eastern Michigan University Press.

Lleó, C. (1996). To spread or not to spread: Different styles in the acquisition of Spanish phonology. In B. Bernhardt, J. Gilbert, & D. Ingram (Eds.), *Proceedings of the UBC International Conference on Phonological Acquisition* (pp. 215–228). Somerville, MA: Cascadilla Press.

Lope Blanch, J. (1972). *Estudios sobre el Español de México* [Studies on the Spanish of Mexico]. México: Universidad Nacional Autónoma de México.

López Morales, H. (1971). *Estudio sobre el Español de Cuba* [Study on the Spanish of Cuba]. New York: Las Américas.

López-Ornat, S. (1990). La formación de la oración simple: Las omisiones sintáctica (S-V-O) en la adquisición del Español [The formation of the simple sentence: syntactic omissions (S-V-O) in the acquisition of Spanish]. *Estudios de Psicología, 41,* 41–72.

López-Ornat, S. (1997). What lies in between a pre-grammatical and a grammatical representation? Evidence on nominal and verb form-function mappings in Spanish from 1;7 to 2;1. In A. Pérez-Leroux & W. Glass (Eds.), *Contemporary perspectives on the acquisition of Spanish Volume 1: Developing grammars* (pp. 3–20). Somerville, MA: Cascadilla.

Macken, M., & Barton, D. (1980). The acquisition of the voicing contrast in Spanish: A phonetic and phonological study of word-initial stop consonants. *Journal of Child Language, 7,* 433–458.

MacWhinney, B. (1995). The CHILDES Project: Tools for analyzing talk (2nd ed.). Hillsdale, NJ: Lawrence Earlbaum.

Melgar de González, M. (1976). *Como detectar al niño con problemas del habla* [How to detect the child with speech problems]. Mexico City, Mexico: Trillas.

Montes, R. (1987). Sequencias de clarificación en conversaciones de niños. *Morphe,* 3–4.

Montes, R. (1992). *Achieving understanding: Repair mechanisms in mother child conversations.* Unpublished doctoral dissertation, Georgetown University, Washington, DC.

Morales, A. (1989). Manifestaciones de pasado en niños Puertorriqueños de 2–6 años [Manifestations of the past tense in Puerto Rican children from 2–6 years of age]. *Revista de Lingüística Teórica y Aplicada, 27,* 115–131.

Muñoz, C., & Vila, I. (1986). Adquisición y uso de los pronombres de primera y segunda persona en Castellano [Acquisition and use of pronouns of the first and second person in Spanish]. In F. Fernández (Ed.), *Pasado, presente y futuro de la lingüística aplicada en España* (pp. 331–338). Valencia, España: Asociación Española de Lingüística Aplicada.

Naharro, M. (1996). La adquisición del subjuntivo Español en lengua materna [The acquisition of the Spanish subjunctive in first language]. In M. Pérez-Pereira (Ed.), *Estudios sobre la adquisición del Castellano, Catalán, Eusquera y*

Gallego (pp. 217–230). Santiago, Spain: Universidad de Santiago de Compostela.

Navarro, T. (1968). *Studies in Spanish phonology* (R. Abraham, Trans.). Coral Gables, FL: University of Miami Press.

Pease-Alvarez, C., & Vasquez, O. (1994). Language socialization in ethnic minority communities. In F. Genesee (Ed.), *Educating second language children* (pp. 82–102). Cambridge, UK: Cambridge University Press.

Penny, R. (1991). *A history of the Spanish language.* Cambridge, UK: Cambridge University Press.

Pérez, M., & Castro, J. (1988). Fenómenos transicionales en el acceso al lenguaje [Transitional phenomenea in the access to language]. *Infancia y Aprendizaje, 43,* 13–36.

Pérez-Granados, D., & Callanan, M. (1997). Parents and siblings as early resources for young children's learning in Mexican-descent families. *Hispanic Journal of Behavioral Sciences, 19,* 3–33.

Pérez-Pereira, M. (1989). The acquisition of morphemes: Some evidence from Spanish. *Journal of Psycholinguistic Research, 18,* 289–312.

Pérez-Pereira, M. (1990). Cómo determinan los niños concordancia de género? [How do children determine gender agreement?]. *Infancia y Aprendizaje, 50,* 73–91.

Pérez-Pereira, M. (1991). The acquisition of gender: what Spanish-speaking children tell us. *Journal of Child Language, 18,* 571–590.

Planos, R., Zayas, L., & Busch-Rossnagel, N. (1995). Acculturation and teaching behaviors of Dominican and Puerto Rican mothers. *Hispanic Journal of Behavioral Sciences, 17,* 225–236.

Poplack, S. (1986). Acondicionamiento gramatical de la variación fonológica en un dialecto Puertorriqueño [Grammatical conditioning of phonological variation in a Puerto Rican dialect]. In R. Nuñez-Cedeño, I. Páez-Urdaneta, & J. Guitart (Eds.), *Estudios sobre la fonología del Español del Caribe* (pp. 95–107). Caracas, Venezuela: La Casa de Bello.

Quesada Pacheco, M. (1996). El Español de América Central [The Spanish of Central America] In M. Alvar (Ed.), *Manual de dialectología Hispánica: El Español de América* (pp. 101–115). Barcelona, Spain: Ariel.

Radford, A., & Ploennig-Pacheco, I. (1995). The morphosyntax of subjects and verbs in child Spanish: A case study. *Essex Research Reports in Linguistics, 5,* 23–67.

Ramírez, A. (1992). *El Español de los Estados Unidos: El lenguaje de los Hispanos* [The Spanish of the United States: The language of the Hispanics]. Madrid, Spain: Mapfre.

Rodríguez, O. (1992). Rasgos sui generis en el habla de niños Mexicanos de seis años [Individual characteristics of the language of six-year-old Mexican children]. In R. Barriga Villanueva & J. García Fajardo (Eds.), *Reflexiones lingüísticas y literarias, Volumen I* (pp. 115–137). México, DF: El Colegio de México, Centro de Estudios Lingüísticos y Literarias.

Schane, S. (1995). Illocutionary verbs, subject responsibility, and presupposition: The indicative vs. the subjunctive in Spanish. In P. Hashemipour, R. Maldonado, & M. van Naerssen (Eds.), *Studies in language learning and Spanish linguistics in honor of Tracy D. Terrell.* (pp. 360–374). New York: McGraw-Hill.

Sebastián, E., & Slobin, D. (1994). Development of linguistic forms: Spanish. In R. Berman & D. Slobin (Eds.), *Relating events in narrative: A crosslinguistic developmental study* (pp. 239–284). Hillsdale, NJ: LEA.

Sedano, M., & Bentivoglio, P. (1996). Venzuela. In M. Alvar (Ed.), *Manual de dialectología Hispánica: El Español de América* (pp. 116–133). Barcelona, Spain: Ariel.

Sera, M. (1992). To be or to be: Use and acquisition of the Spanish copulas. *Journal of Memory and Language, 31,* 408–427.

Shum, G., Conde, A., & Díaz, C. (1992). Pautas de adquisición y uso del pronombre personal en lengua Española. Un estudio longitudinal [Models of acquisition and use of the personal pronoun in the Spanish language]. *Estudios de Psicología, 48,* 67–86.

Slobin, D., & Bocaz, A. (1988). Learning to talk about movement through time and space: The development of narrative abilities in Spanish and English. *Lenguas Modernas, 15,* 5–24.

Talmy, L. (1991). Path to realization: A typology of event conflation. *Proceedings of the Seventeenth Annual Meeting of the Berkeley Linguistics Society* (pp. 480–519). Berkeley, CA: Berkeley Linguistics Society.

Tenenbaum, H., & Leaper, C. (1997). Mothers' and fathers' questions to their children in Mexican-descent families: Moderators of cognitive demand during play. *Hispanic Journal of Behavioral Sciences, 19,* 318–332.

Thevenin, D., Eilers, R., Oller, K., & Lavoie, L. (1985). Where's the drift in babbling drift? A crosslinguistic study. *Applied Psycholinguistics, 6,* 3–15.

Toledo, G. (1988). *El ritmo en el Español: Estudio fonético con base computacional* [Rhythm in Spanish: A phonetic study with a computational basis]. Madrid, Spain: Editorial Gredos.

Torrego, E. (1984). On inversion in Spanish and some of its effects. *Linguistic Inquiry, 15,* 103–127.

Torrens, V. (1995). The acquisition of the functional category inflection in Spanish and Catalan. *MIT Working Papers in Linguistics, 26,* 451–472.

Torrens, V., & Wexler, K. (1996). Clitic doubling in early Spanish. In A. Stringfellow, D. Cahana-Amitay, E. Hughes, & A. Zukowski (Eds.), *Boston University Child Language Development Conference 20 Proceedings* (pp. 780–791). Somerville, MA: Cascadilla Press.

Vivas, D. (1979). Order of acquisition of Spanish grammatical morphemes: Comparison to English and some crosslinguistic methodological problems. *Kansas Working Papers in Linguistics, 4,* 77–105.

Wagner, C. (1996). Chile. In M. Alvar (Ed.), *Manual de dialectología Hispánica: El Español de América* (pp. 152–168). Barcelona, Spain: Ariel.

Waxman, S. (1994). The development of an appreciation of specific linkages between linguistic and conceptual organization. *Lingua, 92,* 229–257.

Zukow, P. (1987). Teorías populares sobre lo que niños comprenden y prácticas interactivas en una población rural de Méjico Central [Folk theories of comprehension and caregiver practices in a rural-born population in Central Mexico]. *Infancia y Aprendizaje, 39–40,* 151–158.

Zukow, P. (1989). Siblings as effective socializing agents: Evidence from central Mexico. In P. Zukow (Ed.), *Sibling interaction across cultures: Theoretical and methodological considerations* (pp. 79–105). New York: Springer-Verlag.

⌐ᴚ

APPENDIX

COMPLETE LISTING OF INFLECTIONAL MARKERS FOR –AR, -ER, AND –IR VERBS

AR Indicative

	Present	Preterite	Imperfect	Future	Conditional
Yo	hablo	hablé	hablaba	hablaré	hablaría
Tú	hablas	hablaste	hablabas	hablarás	hablarías
Usted/él/ella	habla	habló	hablaba	hablará	hablaría
Nosotros	hablamos	hablamos	hablabamos	hablaremos	hablaríamos
Ustedes/ellos/ellas	hablan	hablaron	hablaban	hablarán	hablarían

ER Indicative

	Present	Preterite	Imperfect	Future	Conditional
Yo	como	comí	comía	comeré	comería
Tú	comes	comiste	comías	comerás	comerías
Usted/él/ella	come	comió	comía	comerá	comería
Nosotros	comemos	comemos	comíamos	comeremos	comeríamos
Ustedes/ellos/ellas	comen	comieron	comían	comerán	comerían

IR Indicative

	Present	Preterite	Imperfect	Future	Conditional
Yo	duermo	dormí	dormía	dormiré	dormiría
Tú	duermes	dormiste	dormías	dormirás	dormirías
Usted/él/ella	duerme	durmió	dormía	dormirá	dormiría
Nosotros	dormimos	dormimos	dormíamos	dormiremos	dormiríamos
Ustedes/ellos/ellas	duermen	durmieron	dormían	dormirán	dormirían

AR Perfective

	Present	Imperfect	Preterite	Conditional	Future
Yo	he hablado	había hablado	hube hablado	habría hablado	habré hablado
Tú	has hablado	habías hablado	hubiste hablado	habrías hablado	habrás hablado
Usted/él/ella	ha hablado	había hablado	hubo hablado	habría hablado	habrá hablado
Nosotros	hemos hablado	habíamos hablado	hubimos hablado	habríamos hablado	habremos hablado
Ustedes/ellos/ellas	han hablado	habían hablado	hubieron hablado	habrían hablado	habrán hablado

ER Perfective

	Present	Imperfect	Preterite	Conditional	Future
Yo	he comido	había comido	hube comido	habría comido	habré comido
Tú	has comido	habías comido	hubiste comido	habrías comido	habrás comido
Usted/él/ella	ha comido	había comido	hubo comido	habría comido	habrá comido
Nosotros	hemos comido	habíamos comido	hubimos comido	habríamos comido	habremos comido
Ustedes/ellos/ellas	han comido	habían comido	hubieron comido	habrían comido	habrán comido

IR Perfective

	Present	Imperfect	Preterite	Conditional	Future
Yo	he dormido	había dormido	hube dormido	habría dormido	habré dormido
Tú	has dormido	habías dormido	hubiste dormido	habrías dormido	habrás dormido
Usted/él/ella	ha dormido	había dormido	hubo dormido	habría dormido	habrá dormido
Nosotros	hemos dormido	habíamos dormido	hubimos dormido	habríamos dormido	habremos dormido
Ustedes/ellos/ellas	han dormido	habían dormido	hubieron dormido	habrían dormido	habrán dormido

AR Subjunctive

	Present	Past	Future
Yo	hable	hablara	hablare
Tú	hables	hablaras	hablare
Usted/él/ella	hable	hablara	hablare
Nosotros	hablemos	habláramos	habláremos
Ustedes/ellos/ellas	hablen	hablaran	hablaren

ER Subjunctive

	Present	Past	Future
Yo	coma	comiera	comiere
Tú	comas	comieras	comieres
Usted/él/ella	coma	comiera	comiere
Nosotros	comamos	comíeramos	comiéremos
Ustedes/ellos/ellas	coman	comieran	comieren

IR Subjunctive

	Present	Past	Future
Yo	duerma	durmiera	durmiere
Tú	duermas	durmieras	durmieres
Usted/él/ella	duerma	durmiera	durmiere
Nosotros	durmamos	durmíeramos	durmiéremos
Ustedes/ellos/ellas	duerman	durmieran	durmieren

LISA M. BEDORE, Ph.D.

Lisa M. Bedore, Ph.D., is a Research Associate in the Department of Communicative Disorders at San Diego State University. She completed her graduate work at San Diego State University and Purdue University. Her research focuses on aspects of morphological and phonological development in Spanish-speaking and English-speaking children with typically developing language skills and with specific language impairment. She has extensive experience working with Spanish-speaking preschoolers in Mexico, Indiana, and California.

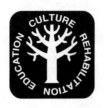

CHAPTER 7

FRENCH LANGUAGE ACQUISITION IN NORTH AMERICA

JOSÉE FORTIN, Ph.D.
MARTHA B. CRAGO, Ph.D.

I n exploring the acquisition of French in North America, this chapter opens with an overview of the characteristics of North American French and a description of its use from a political and demographic perspective. In particular, the chapter is concerned with French spoken in Canada, specifically in Quebec. This language, hereafter referred to as Quebec French, is the focus of the chapter, as Quebec is the only Canadian province where the majority of the population speaks French. There are certain Canadian cities outside of the province of Quebec where a substantial portion of the population may speak French. However, even in situations where the majority of the population of a particular city speaks French, it is important to remember that this same population of French speakers composes only a small minority of those living in a province in which such a city is located.

North American and European French are not extensively compared or contrasted in this chapter, as these two "dialects" are structurally similar. Still, a few distinguishing features are found and these are discussed in the second section of the chapter. Before our exploration into the structure of Quebec French, Canadian demographics and politics are examined.

ᄂ

POLITICAL AND DEMOGRAPHIC PERSPECTIVES ON FRENCH SPOKEN IN CANADA

The following information on the demographic distribution of French-speaking Canadians is taken from the 1991 Canadian census (Statistiques Canada, 1991). However, before examining these demographics, some definitions from Statistics Canada are in order. "First language" refers to the first language that a person has learned in childhood and has maintained into adulthood. If this language, mastered prior to attending school, is no longer understood, then a second language must be identified. If a person was exposed to two languages simultaneously, the person is asked to specify which language was spoken most often in the home. If both languages are used equally, it is considered that both languages have been mastered. "Language spoken in the home" is the language spoken most often in the home at the time of the census. If two languages are used equally, the person can specify that both are used. "Metropolitan census region" is the urban center, as well as adjacent urban and rural areas with close economic and social ties to the urban center. A metropolitan census region is defined when the urban center has at least 100,000 residents, based on the previous census.

The vast majority of Canadian French speakers, or francophones, as they are referred to in Canada, are from Quebec (see Table 7–1). Outside of Quebec there are only relatively small pockets of francophones.

STATUS OF THE FRENCH LANGUAGE OUTSIDE OF QUEBEC

The small numbers of francophones outside of Quebec can be viewed as evidence of language assimilation (see the map in Figure 7–1). The phenomenon of language assimilation in Canada is no different from that seen elsewhere (Maheu, 1970). Sauvy (1966) has described the process of language assimilation as unfolding in the following manner.

TABLE 7–1

Number and proportion of francophones by metropolitan census region, and by province and territory based on 1991 census data (Sample: 20%).

Metropolitan Census Region or Province	Speakers of French as First Language		Speakers of French in the Home		People With Knowledge of Both French and English	
	Number	%	Number	%	Number	%
Vancouver	21,375	1.35	5,455	0.34	114,165	7.21
Victoria	4,340	1.53	1,180	0.42	21,800	7.69
British Columbia	**48,835**	**1.50**	**12,120**	**0.37**	**207,175**	**6.38**
Calgary	11,385	1.52	3,100	0.41	52,370	7.00
Edmonton	20,360	2.45	6,255	0.75	64,000	7.69
Alberta	**53,715**	**2.13**	**17,805**	**0.71**	**167,155**	**6.64**
Regina	2,830	1.49	740	0.39	10,605	5.60
Saskatoon	3,725	0.65	1,110	0.53	13,165	6.33
Saskatchewan	**20,885**	**2.14**	**6,350**	**0.65**	**50,800**	**5.21**
Winnipeg	31,115	4.83	14,210	2.20	67,925	10.52
Manitoba	**49,130**	**4.55**	**23,545**	**2.18**	**98,800**	**9.15**
Hamilton	4,180	1.56	2,930	0.49	39,020	6.57
Kitchener	2,530	1.50	1,485	0.42	23,720	6.72
London	2,135	1.19	1,045	0.28	24,105	6.40
Oshawa	2,465	2.15	2,215	0.93	15,660	6.58
Ottawa-Hull	307,130	33.67	273,810	30.02	388,100	42.55
St-Catherines-Niagara	14,770	4.10	6,160	1.71	28,865	8.02
Sudbury	45,245	28.98	30,605	19.60	60,050	38.46
Thunder Bay	3,075	2.50	1,160	0.94	8,330	6.78
Toronto	22,865	1.34	18,230	0.47	309,255	8.00
Windsor	13,685	5.28	4,030	1.55	27,685	10.68
Ontario	**485,395**	**4.87**	**300,085**	**3.01**	**1,136,245**	**11.39**
Chicoutimi-Jonquiere	156,910	98.31	157,500	98.68	24,020	15.05
Montreal	2,080,980	67.32	2,108,525	68.21	1,492,280	48.28
Quebec	613,930	96.26	620,835	97.35	176,415	27.66
Sherbrooke	123,955	90.67	125,465	91.77	49,720	36.37
Trois-Rivieres	131,810	97.72	132,785	98.44	29,095	21.57
Quebec	**5,556,105**	**81.58**	**5,604,020**	**82.29**	**2,412,985**	**35.43**
St-John's	535	0.32	225	0.13	7,990	4.70
Newfoundland	**2,770**	**0.49**	**1,230**	**0.22**	**18,495**	**3.29**
Prince-Edward Island	**5,590**	**4.36**	**2,935**	**2.29**	**12,950**	**10.11**
Halifax	9,490	2.99	3,150	0.99	30,540	9.61
Nova Scotia	**36,635**	**4.11**	**21,585**	**2.42**	**76,465**	**8.58**
St-Jean	5,555	4.49	2,080	1.68	13,090	10.59
New Brunswick	**241,565**	**33.71**	**220,590**	**30.79**	**211,525**	**29.52**
Yukon	**865**	**3.13**	**360**	**1.30**	**2,570**	**9.29**
Northwest Territories	**1,375**	**2.39**	**610**	**1.06**	**3,495**	**6.09**
CANADA	6,502,865	24.09	6,211,235	23.01	4,398,655	16.29

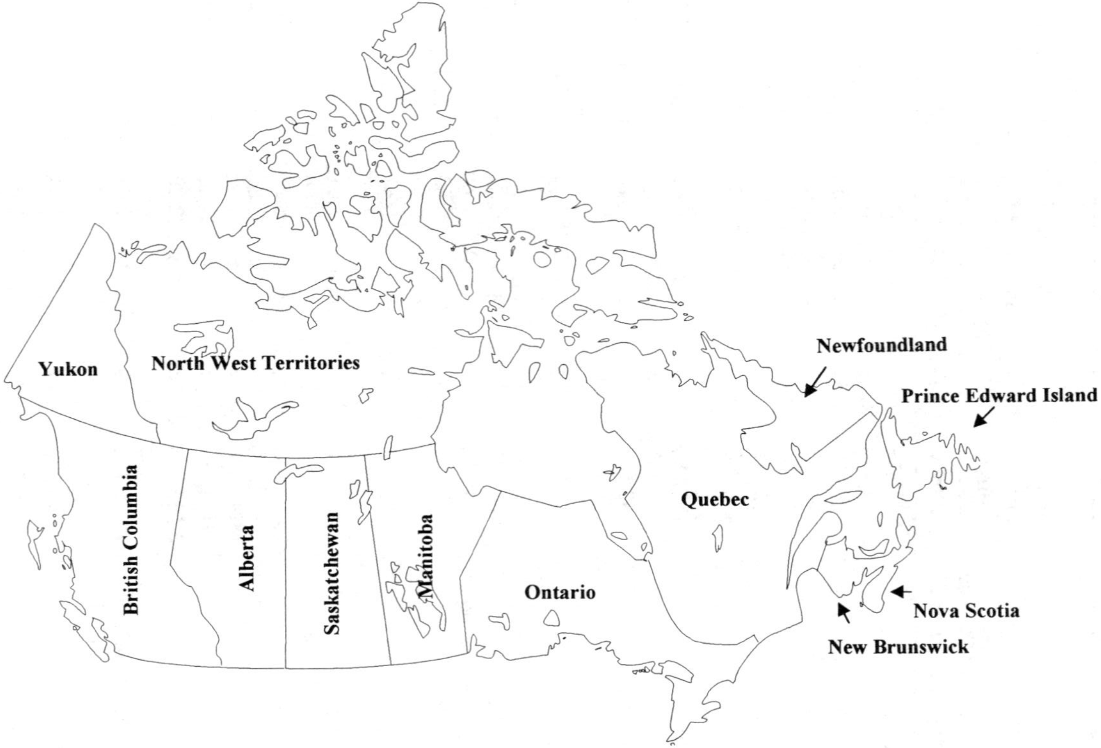

FIGURE 7-1
Canada.

A language becomes dominant by getting a foothold in business, the civil service, the armed services, publishing, and the media, forcing speakers of the nondominant language (whether or not they are a majority of the population) to adopt the dominant language to survive economically. Thereafter, within mixed language situations, the dominant language takes precedence. Furthermore, speaking the dominant language on a daily basis at work may become a habit and eventually spill over outside the workplace. A dominant language can also take over in a mixed marriage or even in households including speakers of the nondominant language. Schools and their playgrounds are other venues that facilitate the loss of a first nondominant language among children. In Canada, historically, the assimilation of francophones by the anglophone culture has occurred in all provinces, except in Quebec (Maheu, 1970).

Even in a city such as Sudbury, Ontario, where approximately one third of the residents are francophone by birth (*Statistics Canada*, 1991), nearly all of the population, whether francophone or anglophone, speaks English the majority of the time, falling in line with the domination of the English language throughout the province (Gilbert & Langlois, 1994). French is the language of about 19% of the population of Sudbury, at least in the home. However, on the street, English predominates even among the francophones. There is a paucity of commercial and civic signs in French (Leblanc, 1996a, 1996b). In fact, Leblanc points out that French in Sudbury owes much of its survival to its local bilingual university. Nevertheless, despite the influence of this university and despite the sheer number of French speakers, anglicization is strong and threatens the survival of the French language in this city.

The situation is different in the province of New Brunswick, partly because of its proximity to the province of Quebec. In New Brunswick, most mother tongue French speakers use their first language at home. Bilingualism in certain areas of that province is common, even in advertising. French appears to be less threatened than in areas like Northern Ontario, which are geographically more remote from Quebec.

Another pertinent phenomenon has been referred to as neutralization (Gilbert & Langlois, 1994). Without a clearly defined territory, francophones in the provinces outside of Quebec, often few in number, become a somewhat disenfranchised minority. As shown in Figure 7–2, this appears to be the fate of most French Canadians living outside of Quebec, Ontario, and New Brunswick. With proportions below 6%, their lack of political power can act to severely limit their linguistic possibilities.

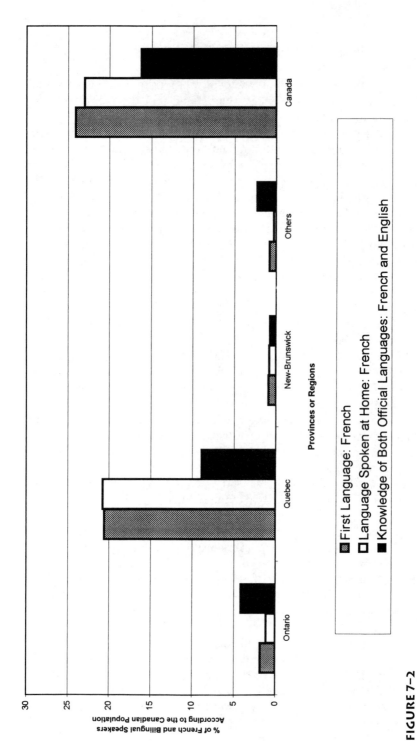

FIGURE 7–2

Percentage of French speakers according to mastery of the language. (Data from "Donnees du recensement, 1991," Ottawa: Statistiques Canada.)

Legend:
- First Language: French
- Language Spoken at Home: French
- Knowledge of Both Official Languages: French and English

X-axis (Provinces or Regions): Ontario, Quebec, New-Brunswick, Others, Canada

Y-axis: % of French and Bilingual Speakers According to the Canadian Population (0, 5, 10, 15, 20, 25, 30)

The percentages in Figure 7–2 may, in some cases, represent an overlap of population groups. For instance, a person may have French as a first language and may also know English. Alternatively, a person may have English as a first language and also be bilingual. In any case, approximately 20% of the population of Canada are francophones living in Quebec. In total, the 1991 census (Table 7–1) revealed that 24.09% of Canadians have French as their first language and 23% speak French in the home. This suggests that the difference between French-speaking Canadians living in Quebec and those living elsewhere in Canada is only 3 or 4%. Excluding information from the few francophone cities of Ontario and New Brunswick, these figures reveal that the distribution of francophones in the remaining provinces and territories falls below 1%. Furthermore, French/English bilingualism is centered in the provinces of Quebec, Ontario, and New Brunswick. Individuals with knowledge of both French and English account for 8.94% of the population of Quebec, 4.1% in Ontario, and 0.78% in New Brunswick, leaving another 2.37% of French/English bilinguals in the rest of the country. These data are surprising considering that the predominant image of Canada is of a bilingual country with two official languages, French and English. Although there is a legal obligation to provide services in either of the official languages, bilingualism in Canada is not so widespread. For example, even in a metropolitan census region such as Sudbury, Ontario where 20–30% of the population is French speaking, requesting services in French is not a common practice. One can imagine, then, the impossibility of realistically expecting such services to be delivered in French in other areas of the country where there are even fewer French speakers (Leblanc, 1996a, 1996b). In fact, in most parts of Canada outside of Quebec and certain regions of Ontario and New Brunswick, very few people speak or even understand any French at all. One of the authors has noted that in large tourist attractions in western Canada, signs are more likely to be in Chinese than in French, especially in British Columbia which counts around 5% Chinese, who represent almost 20% of the immigrants in that province (*Statistics Canada*, 1991).

The processes of assimilation and neutralization of the French language in areas of Canada outside of Quebec help to explain why Quebec represents such a special situation in North America. We now examine the situation of French in Quebec.

THE SITUATION OF FRENCH IN QUEBEC

In Quebec, French is spoken by 80% of the population or even as much as 90% of the population, if Montreal is excluded (see Table 7–1). To understand the complex political phenomenon of the French language in Quebec, a brief historical overview of the last 20 years is helpful.

In the 1960s, the people of Quebec (the *Quebecois*) had to face two difficult facts (Termote & Gauvreau, 1988). First, there was a striking decrease in the birth rate in the province, and, second, most immigrants to Quebec tended to register their children in English schools. Furthermore, the 1971 census confirmed the decline of French as a first language, with more than a third of francophones outside Quebec having been assimilated (Charbonneau & Maheu, 1973). To deal with these realities, the Quebec government set up commissions and passed several language laws (Bill 22; 1974; Bill 101; 1977). In essence, the Quebec government decided it was necessary to establish a policy to protect and promote the growth of French in the province.

The French Language Charter, passed in 1977, marked the beginning of the enhanced status of French in Quebec. Shortly before this charter was legislated in 1976, a new political party, the Parti Quebecois, had come to power led by René Lévesque. This party, as a part of the sovereignist movement, advocated that Quebec be seen as a distinct society due to its preponderance of French speakers. The French Language Charter, promoted by the Parti Quebecois, was designed to protect Quebec from a number of threats to the French language. Among these threats were the diminishing number of French speakers, the domination of English in businesses, the perception of low esteem for the French language in the Canadian confederation and the unsatisfactory transmission of the language in schools (Masse et al., 1996). The charter's preamble stated that it would recognize the will of the Quebecois to ensure the quality and growth of the French language, and that it resolved to make French the language of the state and the law, as well as the everyday language of the workplace, education, communications, business, and trade. The overall aim of such a linguistic policy was to make French the official language of Quebec, and the language common to all Quebecois (Chartre de la langue française, cited in Masse et al., 1996).

The French Language Charter has had several implications. Businesses with more than 50 employees have had to "francisize" their work environment. The charter gave employees the right to be supervised in French and protected them from being fired or suffering wage reductions for not speaking or not having mastered a language other than French. Professionals cannot receive a license to practice in Quebec unless they can prove their competency in French. Commercial signs have to be written only in French. In addition, immigrants were obliged to enroll their children in French schools.

However, by means of the Blaikie rulings (1978–1979), the Quebec Superior Court and the Supreme Court of Canada ruled that certain provisions of the charter were unconstitutional by virtue of Article 133 of the Canadian Constitutional Act of 1867. Article 133 imposed official bilingualism on federal and Quebec courts and parliaments, but not on those of other provinces (Mandel, 1992). As a result, in 1979 the Quebec government reinstated institutional bilingualism in legislation and in the courts. This seemed somewhat incoherent, as it gave the French and English languages equal status in Quebec public life. It assumed that Quebec residents who do not understand French necessarily understand English. Furthermore, it granted English the status of a language common to all Quebecois.

In much the same way, another law, Bill 178 (1988) modified the rulings about the French language on commercial signs. Certain businesses were allowed to post signs indoors in a language other than French, as long as French held a predominant position on the sign. Unless otherwise noted, outdoor signs still had to be in French only.

In the face of mounting internal and international political pressures from the United Nations that declared Bill 178 in contradiction to the International Bill of Human Rights, this law was replaced in December 1992. At the present time, outdoor commercial signs can be bilingual, as long as French predominates in size and placement on the sign. In addition, certain other legislative changes have affected the language of education. Immigrant children may now attend English-speaking schools, if at least one of their parents attended primary school in English. In all other cases, French has remained as the obligatory language of education. In terms of health and social services, Bill 142, passed in December 1986, recognized the right of an English-speaking person to receive health and social services in English. Such ongoing legal changes underscore the constantly changing nature of the situation of French in Quebec.

In fact, the French Language Charter has undergone more than 200 revisions. The Quebec National Assembly made some changes voluntarily, with Canadian Constitutional laws of 1867 and 1982, the Quebec Human Rights Charter (1975) and the Canadian Charter of Rights and Freedoms (1982) imposing others. Although the principles of the French Language Charter are still valid today, the situation and the attitudes are no longer those of 1977. Moreover, Quebec's language situation is subject to ongoing influences by both national and international economic forces. For instance, the North American Free Trade Agreement (NAFTA) has increased sales of unilingual English products in Quebec.

The demographic threat to French in Quebec also continues to be a social reality. According to demographic and linguistic studies by Termote (1994, 1995), a decline in the number of francophones in Quebec will take place in the foreseeable future. In fact, Termote estimates that the proportion of French-speaking individuals will fall just below 80% before the year 2016. Furthermore, the phenomenon of urban spread and the concentration of francophones outside of Montreal is important (see Table 7–1). Throughout Quebec, the percentage of Quebecois with French as a first language hovers around 90%, except in the Montreal area. Such a situation may conceivably create a cultural and sociolinguistic rift between the Montreal urban community and the rest of the province. The fate of French, therefore, in some ways depends on Montreal, home to about half of the population of the province (Lessard, 1996).

In sum, Quebec remains the stronghold of French in Canada, but the status of the language is in flux. Enforcing language laws, integrating immigrants into the francophone community, a rich French culture in Montreal, and esteem for the French language, in general, are key elements required to keep this particular minority language of North America alive and well in the 21st century.

⊐

CHARACTERISTICS OF FRENCH SPOKEN IN NORTH AMERICA

Although the linguistic characteristics of French spoken in North America are numerous, we highlight only certain aspects in the next part of the chapter.

WORD ORDER

In French, word order depends on a pivot word, namely the verb (V). The verb can stand alone when giving an order to someone, but it is most often accompanied by a subject (S) and/or an object (O) or an attribute (A). Usual word order is subject-verb-object. This produces the following types of sentences:

   (1) Bois   "Drink"
      V

   (2) Bois (du) lait   "Drink milk"
      V   O

   (3) Mon chat boit   "My cat drinks"
          S   V

   (4) Mon chat boit (du) lait   "My cat drinks milk."
          S   V   O

   (5) Mon chat est content   "My cat is happy."
          S   V   A

These characteristics are examined later.

In French, articles, numerals, possessives, indefinite or definite articles, or demonstrative pronouns (represented by D for determiner in French), as well as adjectives (Aj), must precede a noun in both the subject position and object position (Grévisse, 1986).

   (6) Mon petit chat boit du lait   "My little cat drinks milk."
      D   Aj S   V   O

Certain adjectives may either precede or follow a noun. Their position alters the meaning of the adjective (Hénault & Piccard, 1991).

   (7) Un grand homme   "A great man"
       Un homme grand   "A big man"

WORD ORDER IN RELATIVE CLAUSES

Whereas determiners and prepositions precede a noun, words or structures modifying a noun like colour adjectives (AjC) and relative clauses (Rel) usually follow a noun (Grévisse, 1986).

   *(8) Le chat blanc, **qui dort,** est le mien.*
       S   AjC /Rel V/ V   O
      "The white cat, that is sleeping, is mine."

Relative clauses may be introduced by different pronouns, each with a different role: *qui/* "who" is a subject (S); *que* or *qu'/* "that" is a direct object (DO); and *dont/* "of which" is an indirect object (IO). The form, *dont,* is now falling into disuse in spoken Quebec French (Fortin, 1996). In France, however, this pronoun is still very much in use, both in written and spoken language.

WORD ORDER WITH OBJECT OR REFLEXIVE PRONOUNS

French word order is affected when the direct or indirect objects are replaced by pronouns. In this case, the object precedes the verb. Therefore, a S-V-O sentence becomes a S-O-V sentence (Grévisse, 1986). If both objects are replaced by personal pronouns, the structure is longer and more complex, yet follows the same form: S-DO-IO-V.

(9) *L'enfant la lui donne.*   "The child gives it to her."
    S   DO IO V

The position of the reflexive (Ref) follows similar rules.

(10a) *Elle se brosse les dents.*   "She brushes her teeth."
      S   Ref V   DO

(10b) *Elle se les brosse.*   "She brushes them."
      S   Ref DO V

For verbs in the imperative, the same principles apply that the objects must follow the verb rather than precede it.

(11a) *Donne une fleur à ta maman.*   "Give a flower to your mom."
       V   DO   IO

(11b) *Donne-la lui.*   "Give it to her."
       V   DO IO

First or second person pronouns used as objects are more complicated because their order is reversed, depending on mood. If utterances are declarative, an indirect object pronoun (IO) must precede a direct object pronoun (DO), but in the imperative mood this same indirect object pronoun is placed at the end of the sentence (Grévisse, 1986).

(12a) *L'enfant me donne la main.*   "The child gives me his hand."
       IO V   DO

(12b) *L'enfant me la donne.*   "The child gives it to me."
       IO DO V

(13a) *Donne-moi la main.*   "Give me your hand."
     V IO DO

(13b) *Donne-la moi.*   "Give it to me."
     V DO IO

WORD ORDER IN THE FORMATION OF QUESTIONS

Word order is also variable in the formation of questions (Grundstrom & Léon, 1973). There are four different ways to form a yes-no question. In the first of these forms, the word order is identical to producing a declarative sentence. A rising intonation at the end of the sentence indicates a question (Grévisse, 1986). Although acceptable, this form is rare in Quebec French. No instance of this form was found in 54 speech samples analysed by Fortin (1996). It seems that this question form is more common in France.

(14a) *Tu vas à l'école?*   "You go to school?"
     S V   O

In two other forms of questions, a change in word order takes place in the subject and verb positions (Labelle & Valois, 1996). This reversal can be either the interrogative verbal phrase *Est-ce que* followed by the declarative sentence or the inversion of the subject and verb positions without any other change. These two interrogative forms are common both in written and spoken French (Grévisse, 1986).

(14b) *Est-ce que tu vas à l'école?*   "Do you go to school?"
     Interr. S V   O

(14c) *Vas-tu à l'école?*   "Do you go to school?"
     V S   O

A final question form is one that is typical of Quebec French. In it, a question marker /*tu*/ "you" follows the verb. This pronoun marker does not have a grammatical function (Morin, 1985). Analysis of spontaneous language samples (Fortin, 1996) revealed that this form of question represents 89.3% of question forms in individuals below age 15. Although this percentage is lower for individuals between 15 and 27 years of age, it remains the most common form of question used in conversation. In more formal contexts, this form is replaced by the simple subject-verb reversal or by the interrogative verbal phrase *Est-ce que* as in Example 14b.

(14d) *Elle vas-tu à l'école?*   "Does she go to school?"
        S   V   O

WORD ORDER IN WH-QUESTIONS

There are two question forms that use wh-question words. The first of these forms occurs in questions beginning with an interrogative (wh-word), such as *quoi* or *que*/ "what," *où*/ "where," *quand*/ "when," *comment*/ "how," *combien*/ "how much," *pourquoi*/ "why," *quel*/ "which." These may undergo subject-verb inversion (Grévisse, 1986; Labelle, 1990; Labelle & Valois, 1996) or, alternatively, in spoken language the inversion often does not take place and the interrogative form is denoted by intonation.

(15a) *Où   vas-tu?*   "Where are you going?"
       Wh V S

(15b) *Où tu vas?*   "Where you are going?"
       Wh S V

The interrogative pronoun *qui*/ "who," however, does not follow this rule because it becomes the subject.

(15c) *Qui va là?*   "Who is going there?"
       Wh V

Another question form typical of Quebec French is the use of the verbal phrase *C'est* / "It is" followed by a relative pronouns *qui* / "who" preceding a relative phrase *qui* + *V* + *O* / "who" + V + O. The redundancy of the relative pronoun is particular to Quebec French. In Fortin's samples (1996), 68.5% of the subjects produced this structure at least one time. No occurrence of that form was noted with any other pronoun.

(15d) *C'est qui qui vient souper?* "It is who who is coming for dinner?"
　　　V-phrase O Wh-S V

A second form of a wh-question uses the verbal phrase *Est-ce que* at the beginning of the sentence, followed by the interrogative, the subject, and verb.

(15e) *Qui est-ce qui vient?* "Who is coming?"
　　　Wh-phrase S V

MORPHOLOGY

In French, morphological markers occur on nouns, pronouns, determiners, adjectives, and verbs. All these elements may be inflected for gender and number. For verbs and pronouns, a third inflection exists for person (Grévisse, 1986).

AGREEMENT IN GENDER AND NUMBER FOR NOUN

In French, nouns have a gender. For instance, *poupée* / "doll" is a feminine noun while *ballon* / "ball" is masculine. Nouns can also be singular or plural. Articles, adjectives, and verbs must agree in gender and number with the noun. Nouns are preceded by a determiner (Grévisse, 1986). Gender in French is completely arbitrary, except in the case of animate beings who are classified according to sex, such as *chien-chienne* / "dog" or *patron-patronne* / "boss." Some words may be used as either masculine or feminine words, yet others will take on a different meaning when they take on a different gender (Hénault & Piccard, 1991).

(16a) *Un responsable de projet* "A project manager"
　　　Une responsable de projet "A project manager"

(16b) *Un livre* "A book"
　　　Une livre "A pound"

The arbitrariness of gender and its inherent variability in some words are often sources of confusion to both first- and second-language speakers of French.

Plural is marked when referring to more than one object, person, or idea. Pluralization can be problematic, because there are many rules for plural formation in French. Such rules are too numerous to explain in detail here. Suffice it to say that the most common form of the plural is made by adding "s" to the singular form.

AGREEMENT IN GENDER AND NUMBER FOR PRONOUN

French pronouns can be personal, possessive, demonstrative, indefinite, relative, or interrogative (see Table 7–2). Unlike other pronouns, personal pronouns not only agree in number and gender, but also in person with the word they replace. Their form varies depending on the individual(s) they represent, or the thing(s) to which they refer. They also change depending on their grammatical function within the sentence (Moignet, 1965).

AGREEMENT IN GENDER AND NUMBER FOR ADJECTIVE AND DETERMINER

The words modifying nouns and pronouns deserve special attention. Both adjectives and determiners must agree with the noun or pronoun. *Le, la, les*/ "the" are the definite articles in French (Hénault & Piccard, 1991). They agree in gender and number with the words they modify (see Table 7–3).

(17) *Le chat*   "the cat"
     Les chats   "the cats"

Contracted articles are formed by combining definite articles with prepositions *à* or *de: au (à le)* / "at the," *du (de le)* / "of the" or "from the," *aux (à les)* / "at the," *des (de les)* / "of the" or "from the" (Grévisse, 1986).

(18a) *La cabane des (de les) enfants*   "the children's hut"

(18b) *Je vais au (à le) magasin.*   "I am going to the store."

TABLE 7–2
French pronouns as a function of grammatical roles.

		Subject	Direct Object	Indirect Object	Adverbial Clause (of space)	Apposition and After Prepositions
Singular	1st person	Je	Me	Me		Moi
	2nd person	Tu	Te	Te		Toi
	3rd person	Il,elle, on	Le, la, en	Lui, en, y	En, y	Lui, elle
Plural	1st person	Nous	Nous	Nous		Nous
	2nd person	Vous	Vous	Vous		Vous
	3rd person	Ils, elles	Les	Leur, en, y	En, y	Eux, elles

TABLE 7–3
French articles.

	Singular		Plural	
	Masculine	**Feminine**	**Masculine**	**Feminine**
Definite	Le	La	Les	Les
Contracted	Au (à le)	À la	Aux (à les)	Aux (à les)
Contracted	Du (de le)	De la	Des (de les)	Des (de les)
Indefinite	Un	Une	Des	Des
Partitive	Du	De la	Des (de les)	Des (de les)

Un, une, des/ "a" are the indefinite articles of French (Grévisse, 1986). They agree in person and number with the words they modify.

(19) *Un chat*   "A cat"
     Des chats   "Cats."

Du, de la, des / "some" are the partitive articles in French (Damourette & Pichon, 1971).

(20) *Du pain, de la viande et des légumes*   "Some bread, meat, and vegetables"

Possessive adjectives in French agree in gender and number with the modified noun and in person with the possessor (Grévisse, 1986) (see Table 7–4).

TABLE 7–4
French possessive adjectives.

		Possessed			
		Singular		Plural	
		Masculine	**Feminine**	**Masculine**	**Feminine**
Possessor	**Singular**	Mon	Ma	Mes	
		Ton	Ta	Tes	
		Son	Sa	Ses	
	Plural	Notre		Nos	
		Votre		Vos	
		Leur		Leurs	

TABLE 7–5
French demonstrative adjectives.

	Masculine	**Feminine**
Singular	Ce, cet	Cette
Plural	Ces	Ces

(21a)	*Son père*	"His father"
(21b)	*Sa mère*	"His mother"

Demonstrative adjectives that identify the being or object they precede have gender and number agreement. *Ce, cet, cette, ces* / "this, these" are demonstrative adjectives (Grévisse, 1986). Often, in Quebec French, the demonstrative adjectives are reinforced by hyphenating *-ci* or *-là* to the noun (see Table 7–5).

(22a)	*Cette femme*	"This woman"
(22b)	*Ce garçon*	"This boy"
(22c)	*Cet animal*	"This animal"
(22d)	*Ce manteau-ci*	"This coat"

VERB AGREEMENT

The verb agrees in person and number with the subject, which may be either present or implied as in the imperative form. The verb has several morphological markers: person, tense and aspect, number, mood, and occasionally gender. Person is noted by the pronoun, with which the verb must agree (Grévisse, 1986). The agreement for person on the verb may be audible or, at times, inaudible. The following example is the conjugation of the verb *travailler* / "to work." In the conjugation of this verb, the first, second, and third persons singular and the third person plural are all pronounced the same way. Person can only be identified audibly by the pronoun. The agreement on the verb for number is equally difficult to hear. For instance, the second person plural, although pronounced differently from its singular form, is homophonous with the infinitive form *travaillez* /travaje/ or *travailler* /travaje/. Only the first person plural provides some audible clue as to the person and number. Occasionally, the plural of the third person pronoun is audible, because a liaison is made with those verbs that begin with a vowel. This verb belongs to what is referred to as the first group of verbs, those whose infinitive forms end in *-er*.

(23) First group verb: *travailler* / "to work"

Person	Singular	Plural
1	*je travaille*	*nous travaillons*
2	*tu travailles*	*vous travaillez*
3 masculine	*il travaille*	*ils travaillent*
3 feminine	*elle travaille*	*elles travaillent*

The above conjugation cannot be generalized to all verbs, as French verbs fall into three different conjugation classes, each of which is characterised by a particular infinitive form and its specific endings. The first group, typified by Example 23, composes about 90% of French verbs and consists of verbs ending in *-er* in the infinitive. The second group consists of about 300 verbs ending in *-ir* in the infinitive. The third group of irregular verbs includes the remaining 175 verbs (Bescherelle, 1980). By grouping the verbs into three groups, it is possible to make generalizations about their endings.

(24) Second group verb: *finir* / "to finish"

Person	Singular	Plural
1	*je finis*	*nous finissons*
2	*tu finis*	*vous finissez*

3 masculine	*il finit*	*ils finissent*
3 feminine	*elle finit*	*elles finissent*

(25) Third group verb: *prendre* / "to take"

Person	Singular	Plural
1	*je prends*	*nous prenons*
2	*tu prends*	*vous prenez*
3 masculine	*il prend*	*ils prennent*
3 feminine	*elle prend*	*elles prennent*

In both of Examples 24 and 25 conjugations, the singular forms are pronounced the same way, which does not allow for any auditory distinction between different persons. The plural endings, however, provide information on both person and number, with the infinitive form distinguishable from the second person plural.

TENSE AND ASPECT

Morphemes of tense and aspect in French are almost identical. In fact, the tense marker places the event in terms of the moment in which it is related. Aspect markers suggest that the event being talked about is strictly connected to the moment in which the speaker is talking (Vet, 1980). In French, aspect may be manifested by semiauxiliaries, such as *aller* / "to go" plus the verb, *avoir à* / "to have to" plus the verb (Roy, 1976) or by suffixes and prefixes (Grévisse, 1986).

(26a) *Regarde, je t'ai apporté un cadeau!*   "Look, I brought you a gift!"

(26b) *Je m'en vais acheter du lait.*   "I am going to buy milk."

In these two examples, the action is neither past nor future, but rather it is inextricably linked to the present moment. Example 26a refers to completed aspect, with 26b referring to a future aspect.

Of the seven moods in French, the indicative, subjunctive, imperative, and conditional moods are conjugated, with the other three: the infinitive, participial, and gerund, not conjugated (Imbs, 1960).

INDICATIVES AND CONDITIONALS

There are eight tenses in the indicative mood. Four are referred to as simple tenses and the other four are compound tenses (Larochette, 1980). The tenses are listed in Table 7–6. Generally, the present is used

TABLE 7–6
French verb tenses.

Simple Tenses	Examples	Composed Tenses	Examples
Present	J'aime	**Past Perfect**	J'ai aimé
Past Historic	J'aimai	**Past Anterior**	J'eus aimé
Imperfect	J'aimais	**Pluperfect**	J'avais aimé
Future	J'aimerai	**Future Perfect**	J'aurai aimé

to show that an action is being undertaken in the here and now. Imperfect and perfect past tenses are generally used to refer to recent, continuous, or recurring event. Vet (1980) and Labelle (1994) provide an excellent summary of the past tense of French verbs. Very simply, the imperfect tense has two temporal connotations. It can be used to express a finished action or an action progressing within a narration or description. The past perfect tense, on the other hand, is used to express the result or consequence of an action, suggesting that the action has been completed and is formed with the auxiliary *avoir* / "to have" or *être* / "to be" and a past participle. The following example is a common type of narration in which the imperfect is used first to depict an incomplete action, and then the perfect tense is used to show completed actions.

(27) *Les enfants couraient, ont trébuché, puis sont allés retrouver leur mère en pleurant.*

"The children ran, fell down, and went to their mother, crying."

The future tense can be used in two ways, either by inflecting the verb stem with a future ending or by adding the semiauxiliary verb *aller* / "to go" followed by an infinitive. These two forms are interchangeable in almost any context (Grévisse, 1986).

(28a) *Je vais souper au restaurant ce soir.* "I am going to have supper at restaurant tonight."

(28b) *Je souperai au restaurant ce soir.* "I will have supper at restaurant tonight."

French makes use of many other compound tenses to convey that a long time has elapsed since an action has taken place (pluperfect) as in Example 29a, to convey that an action has been accomplished prior to another past event (past anterior) as in Example 29b, or that an action will take place prior to another (anterior future) as in Example 29c. These tenses are formed with an imperfect, perfect, and future auxiliary followed by the past participle (Grévisse, 1986).

(29a) *J'étais au rendez-vous, comme convenu.*   "I went to the appointment, as agreed."

(29b) *Je fus rendu avant toi.*   "I was there before you."

(29c) *J'aurai terminé mon verre de lait avant toi.*   "I will have finished my glass of milk before you."

The conditional conveys wishes and suppositions. Used in its past tense form, it includes an auxiliary verb conjugated in the present conditional along with a past participle (Hénault & Piccard, 1991).

(30a) *J'aurais aimé vous accompagner, mais j'étais malade.*   "I would have liked to go with you, but I was sick."

(30b) *Il vaudrait mieux vous abstenir.*   "It would be better not to say anything."

IMPERATIVES AND SUBJUNCTIVES

The last two verb forms to be discussed are the imperative and subjunctive. The imperative is used for commands, requests, and wishes, with the subjunctive used to express thoughts, desires, doubts, wills, wishes, fears, and a feeling for an unaccomplished, possible but uncertain action. Both may be used in the present or past. An imperative may therefore be constructed with either a present or a past form. A past imperative is formed by combining the auxiliary in its present imperative form with a past participle (Grévisse, 1986). The past of the subjunctive is formed in much the same way (Bescherelle, 1980).

(31a) *Donne-moi la poupée.*   "Give me the doll."

(31b) *Sois rendue à temps.*   "Be there on time."

(31c) *Il faut que je fasse mes devoirs.*   "I have to do my homework."

(31d) *Que je sois arrivé à l'heure lui a plu.*   "Being on time pleases him."

WORD FORMATION

Although there are two ways to form new words in French—by derivation and compounding—the former is more common (Grévisse, 1986). Most derivations in French consist of adding a suffix to the word stem. In French, there are several ways to form nouns: from a verb as in Example 32a, from another noun with the same root as in Example 32b, or by nominalizing the verb as in Example 32c. The following are examples of noun formation in French:

(32a)	*Porter*	"To carry"
	Porteur	"Someone who carries things"
(32b)	*Pâtissier*	"Baker"
	Pâtisserie	"Bakery"
(32c)	*Goûter*	"To taste"
	Goûter	"Snack"

Because suffixes play an important role in forming French words, groupings have been created to organize suffixes according to their meaning. For example, suffixes *-eur* or *-ier* usually convey a tradesperson or professional, with *-et* being a diminutive (Grévisse, 1986).

Adverbs are derived from a feminine qualifying adjective, to which the suffix *-ment* is added.

(33)	*Lent*	"Slow"
	Lent + e + ment	"Slow + ly"

Although compounding to form new words is rare, this method is seen more and more frequently in marketing and advertising. Compound words are formed with two nouns, an adjective and a noun, or a verb and a noun. The rule common to all three forms is the use of a hyphen to link the words. These words can be problematic in terms of agreement in gender and number. In most cases, however, context provides the necessary information to determine the agreement (Grévisse, 1986).

(34)	*Garde-robe*	"Closet"

In Example 34, the main word of the compound is *robe* and, as such, it provides the feminine gender to the compound word.

⌐ᄀ

DEVELOPMENTAL STAGES OF FRENCH ACQUISITION

Research into children learning Quebec French is limited to works by Lightbown (1977), Paradis and Genesee (1996), Labelle (1990, 1994), Labelle and Valois (1996), Pierce (1992), Fortin (1996), Pouliot (1996), Méthé (1996), Stanké (1996), Gauthier (1996), and Gagné and Pagé (1981) among others. This makes drawing conclusions about developmental stages of Quebec French a difficult and uncertain task. Moreover, the primary purpose of much of the research was not to study unilingual French acquisition, but rather to compare the language acquisition of unilingual children with the language acquisition of other target populations, such as bilingual children or children with specific language impairment. Bearing this in mind, this section provides an overview of the developmental stages of Quebec French and briefly presents certain ways in which developing language differs from the adult model.

FIRST WORD AND COMBINATIONS

Generally, children speaking Quebec French utter their first words at around 12 months of age. Two-word combinations start around 18 months of age . When these two-word combinations appear, verb inflections begin to be produced to mark the consequent or a particular action. Nonfinite verb forms are abandoned earlier in French than in English (Paradis & Genesee, 1996).

(35) <u>Child form</u>: *Papa parti.*   "Dad (is) gone."

Although word order is respected in the above example, this is not always the case in the early stages of development. In fact, observations gathered until now reveal variability in terms of the structure of two- or three-word utterances. The rare child will use the Subject-Verb-Object canonical form, but often Verb-Object-Subject or Verb-Subject-Object structures are produced.

(36) <u>Adult form</u>: *Le bébé a tout mangé.*   "The baby ate everything."
     <u>Child form</u>: *Tout mangé bébé.*   "Everything eaten baby."

PRONOUNS AND DETERMINERS

Pronouns, determiners, and prepositions appear at around age 2. The first pronoun to appear is usually *moi* / "me," replacing *je* / "I." In terms of determiners, possessives usually appear first, while *à* / "at," marker of possession or location, is the first preposition to appear in early syntactic structures.

(37a) <u>Child Form</u>: *Moi (je) veux*   "Me (I) want"

(37b) <u>Child Form</u>: *Mon bébé*   "My baby"

(37c) <u>Child Form</u>: *Bébé à Marie*   "Marie's baby"

Determiners, such as definite and indefinite articles (see Table 7–3) appear at around this time, but, according to Clark (1985), children are often 6 years old before they master article usage. In the early years, therefore, children will overgeneralize definite articles, without taking into account information shared among the speakers. Other findings (Stanké,1996), however, suggested that 5- and 7-year-old-children are able to use articles appropriately 96% and 98% of the time, respectively. Methé (1996) reported similar findings in use of possessives. According to Methé, 5- and 7-year-olds use possessive pronouns 99–100% of the time.

QUESTION FORMATION

Yes-no questions and <u>where</u> questions are usually the first to emerge. Questions are usually formed by using rising intonation and/or omitting the verb or auxiliary. Other interrogative markers emerge shortly after these first ones.

(38a) <u>Child Form</u>: *(Est-ce que) Papa (est) parti?*   "(Is) Dad gone?"

(38b) <u>Child Form</u>: *Où (est) papa?*   "Where (is) Dad?"

(38c) <u>Child Form</u>: *Quoi (Qu'est-ce que c'est) ça?*   "What (is) that?"

NEGATIVES

Early utterances also include various forms of negatives: *pas* / "not," *plus* / "no more," *non* / "no." These negative forms either precede or follow the noun phrase.

(39a) <u>Child Form</u>: *Le chien ne joue pas.*   "The dog is not playing."

      <u>Child Form</u>: *Pas joue le chien.*   "Not play the dog."

(39b) <u>Child Form</u>: *(Il n'y en) A p(l)us.*   "(There is) No more."

(39c) <u>Child Form</u>: *Non (je ne veux pas la)* "No (I don't want) apple."
                  pomme.

The forms seen in Examples 39a and 39b are the most common. According to Verrips and Weissenborn (1992), the most common form is *pas* "not." In fact, the existence of the third form has been disputed by Déprez and Pierce (1993). Paradis and Genesee (1996) suggested that using the negative *non* "no" in a sentence is only seen in bilingual 2-year-olds. The issue, however, has yet to be resolved.

SYNTACTIC COMPLEXITY

The second year marks the beginning of increasing syntactic complexity. The first clauses emerge, namely frequently used compound sentences (*et* / "and"; *puis* / "then"). Relative clauses beginning with *qui* / "who" are also common, but *qui* is often simplified to *i*. It is difficult to determine if this is an initial consonant deletion or pronoun *il* / "he" substitution. The latter interpretation seems more likely because 2- and 3-year-olds are able to produce /k/ at this stage.

(40) <u>Child Form</u>: *C'est moi (qu)i joue.*   "I am the one who plays."

    Throughout the second year, concepts and sentence structure become more complex. Certain locatives and prepositions are used with increasing precision, such as *sur* / "on," *dans* / "in," *de* / "of" or "from," *par* / "by." Negation becomes increasingly like the adult form, namely placed within the utterance. The omission of *ne*, common in spoken French, is also seen in children's productions of negatives.

(41) <u>Child Form</u>: *Je (ne) veux pas la pomme.*   "I do not want the apple."

Adverbial clauses, introduced by *quand* / "when" and *si* / "if," also begin to emerge at this age. Infinitive clauses follow, replacing the more difficult subjunctive form.

(42) <u>Child Form</u>: *Je veux venir.*   "I want to come."

     <u>Adult Form</u>: *Je veux que tu viennes.*   "I want you to come."

The mastery of temporal lexemes is expected close to the third year. At approximately 36 months, children begin using adverbs such as *demain* "tomorrow" and *hier* "yesterday," yet they may do so interchangeably. Their usage sometimes only marks events that are not in the present time. However starting at 42 months, the temporal lexicon typically begins to expand. Temporal adverbs like *tout de suite* "right now," *tantôt* "later" are used, but often inappropriately. Adult-like use of these adverbs only emerges at around 5 years of age. Gauthier's (1996) findings revealed that 5- and 7-year-olds use temporal adverbs appropriately 88% and 91% of the time, respectively.

Distinguishing between determiners emerges late. At age 3, the use of definite articles still predominates. At around 42 months, however, determiners such as *des* / "some" and *aux* / "to the" emerge, and the conceptual differences between definite and indefinite articles finally starts to be teased apart.

Total mastery of morphemes of tense, aspect, and mood is not expected until after age 12. Even at this age, however, children still confuse tense and mood, particularly when using the subjunctive and conditional forms. Research has focused on specific temporal forms such as the past tense (Labelle, 1994; Gauthier, 1996; Méthé, 1996). Gauthier focused on the past perfect and imperfect tenses. According to Gauthier, 5-year-olds use the perfect and imperfect appropriately 95% of the time, while 7-year-olds do so 97% of the time. Labelle has shown that the pluperfect tense is used by 5-year-olds in a different context than the one adults use it in. Children in her study used the pluperfect tense instead of the expected perfect tense. In fact, it takes several years for children to discern the exact semantic uses for various past tense forms.

STEPS ON THE WAY TO ACQUISITION: OVERGENERALIZATION AND CONFUSIONS

Children acquiring Quebec French, like children acquiring other languages, pass through a number of stages on their way to mastery. Along the way they produce several nonadult-like forms, such as; overgeneralization, morphological confusions in gender, number, person, and tense, as well as inexplicit word order and incomplete or tangled complex sentence structure.

Overgeneralizations often occur with the verb, and manifest themselves in the application of the rule for the first group of verbs (ending in -*er*) to all verbs, including irregular verbs. Found in 2- to 4-year-olds, this phenomenon affects both the infinitive and past participle forms (Hiriartborde, 1973).

(43a) Infinitive
    Adult Form: *Mettre*   "To put"
    Child Form: *Metter** "To put"

(43b) Infinitive
    Adult Form: *Dire*   "To say"
    Child Form: *Diser**   "To say"

(43c) Past Participle
    Adult Form: *Mis*   "Put"
    Child Form: *Metté**   "Put"

(43d) Past Participle
    Adult Form: *Bu*   "Drank"
    Child Form: *Buvé**   "Drank"

Frequency of occurrence has been proposed to explain these overgeneralizations resulting from the overapplication of the first verb group paradigm. An inventory of words used by young children reveals, however, that there are more verbs belonging to the third group (irregular verbs) than to the first group. Analysis of 54 clinical language samples of children aged 2;3 to 4;8 (Fortin, 1996) revealed that irregular verbs are used 61% of the time, with -*er* verbs and -*ir* verbs used 32% and 7% of the time, respectively. These data support a much earlier study by Guillaume (1927). Such results suggested, therefore, that overgeneralizations are not necessarily the result of frequency of use by children, although the usage may be related to frequency of input.

Overgeneralizations are not as frequent in the development of number or gender morphemes. Nevertheless, French does have its own peculiar developmental characteristics with regard to these morphemes, namely the inconsistent use of the appropriate gender marker. Such inconsistency may be explained by the paucity of semantic rules determining noun gender in French. Problems with gender take the form of the inconsistent selection of determiners by children under the age of 3 years. Children may use a masculine determiner for a word used in one context and choose a feminine one for another context. By age 5, children speaking Quebec French have mastered the concept of gender (Fortin, 1996; Lightbown, 1977). Stanké (1996) found that 5- and 7-year-olds had incorrect gender in only 2.2% and 0.7% of their articles, respectively. The gender of third person pronouns, however, is less readily mastered, and often the masculine pronoun is used in contexts clearly calling for the use of the feminine form. According to Fortin (1996), *il* / "he" was still used for *elle* / "she" by 4-year-olds, with Clark (1985) finding that this confusion occurred only until age 3. Clark did, however, concede that in some children the confusion could extend over a longer period.

The emergence of other pronouns is not well documented in French. Grégoire (1947) suggested that first person singular personal pronouns (*je* or *moi* / "I" or "me") are the first to emerge. The research of Fortin (1996) and Pouliot (1996) showed a somewhat different pattern of development of the first person pronoun. The strong pronoun, *moi* / "me" emerges several months earlier than the clitic, *je* / "I." Two-year-olds will say *Moi veux* / "Me want." In fact, *je* does not emerge before 30 months and is then used in combination with *moi,* such as *Moi je veux* / "Me I want." At approximately age 3, other pronouns are produced, with *il* / "he" taking precedence over other third person pronouns and plural forms. In both adult and child speakers of Quebec French the first person plural *nous* / "we" is frequently replaced by the indefinite pronoun *on* / "one."

The plural forms of pronouns and nouns are relatively easily acquired by francophone children. The only information necessary to mark the plural in spoken French occurs in the use of the appropriate determiners, as the plural of the noun in most cases is homophonous with the singular form. Number related confusions do occur in verbs. Children below the age of 4 tend to use noun and pronoun plurals, but fail to make the proper agreement with the verb, as in the following examples.

(44) <u>Adult Form</u>: *Les enfants reviennent de l'école.* "The children are coming back from school."

    <u>Child Form</u>: *Les enfants, il(s) revient de l'école.* "Children, he is coming back from school."

Although there are word order confusions in young children's spoken French, they are infrequent. Their occurrence in 2- or 3-word utterances is, in some cases, related to the use of the nonfinite form and to subject reversals and/or replacements.

Complex sentences develop slowly, going through stages of incomplete mastery. There is little research specific to the acquisition of complex forms, but Fortin's (1996) analysis of speech samples of 2- to 5-year olds revealed some characteristics of this type of development. For instance, the relative pronoun, *qui* / "who" is often overused in relative clauses. In fact, the *que* / "what" pronoun is virtually nonexistent until 42 months. Pouliot (1996) pegged the use of relative clauses using *qui* / "who" somewhat later (42 months) with the *que* / "what" clauses emerging only around 48 months.

Fortin's (1996) analysis of samples of 54 children's language revealed only a few noncanonical, ungrammatical forms. The most common ones consisted of the right or left displacement of an apposed word. The next example shows a displacement to the right.

(45) <u>Adult Form</u>: *Le canard n'est pas content.* "The duck is not happy."

     <u>Child Form</u>: *Il n'est pas content, le* "He is not happy, the
               canard. duck."

Displacements such as this are common among francophone children. According to Faïta (1974), displacements may be seen up until age 9. It must be noted, however, that many adult speakers also use the same displacement, particularly when addressing a child. This form is hardly ever observed in written French.

Errors pertaining to pronoun placement tend to endure (Pierce, 1992). In addition to displacement and emphasis difficulties, object pronouns are also a source of difficulty. In both reflexive and direct object situations, structures tend to adopt the subject-verb-object canonical form, regardless of the presence of an object pronoun.

(46a) <u>Adult Form</u>: *Le canard va se mouiller.* "The duck is going to get wet."

      <u>Child Form</u>: *Le canard va mouiller* "The duck is going to
                lui. get wet it."

(46b) <u>Adult Form</u>: *Je la lui donne ou je la* "I give it to him."
                  donne à lui.

      <u>Child Form</u>: *Je donne elle à lui.* "I give she to him."

Although the *Je la lui donne* structure exists in French, no instance of it was found in Fortin's (1996) samples. In 1977, Bautier-Castaing made similar observations in children aged 4 to 8, namely the lack of a double clitic in the object positions. Language samples taken from 5- and 7-year-old Quebec French children support these findings (Gauthier, 1996; Méthé, 1996; Stanké, 1996).

Coordinate clauses are also late in the development of Quebec French perhaps due to difficulties with tense agreement and understanding conjunctions conceptually. For instance, although *mais* / "but" appears early in children's language, it is not used appropriately until age 9.

Another distinction that seems to pose particular problems for children learning Quebec French is between definite and indefinite articles. In Stanké's (1996) study, 43% of errors made in articles by 5-year-old children pertained to distinguishing between the appropriate use of the definite or indefinite article, although this percentage dropped to 24% in 7-year-olds.

Difficulties in developing the possessive form is related to the fact that possessives agree in number and gender with the possession and not with the possessor.

(47a) *Les chatons de la fille ou ses chatons.*   "The girl's kittens or her kittens."

(47b) *La chatte du garçon et de la fille ou leur chatte.*   "The boy's and girl's cat or their cat."

⊔

CONCLUSION

This chapter has situated the acquisition of Quebec French in its unique social and political context in North America. This context is ever-evolving, but, at present, French is strongly represented by both child and adult speakers in Quebec. Despite the strength of the language and the numerous children who speak French fluently, acquisitional studies of Quebec French are all too scarce. This makes the understanding of the development of children's language incomplete and somewhat vague. We can only hope that the study of the acquisition of the French language spoken in North American will continue and flourish in future years.

⊔

REFERENCES

Bautier-Castaing, E. (1977). Acquisition comparée de la syntaxe du français par des enfants francophones et non-francophones. *Études de linguistique appliquée, 27,* 19–41.

Bescherelle, M. (1980). *Le nouveau Bescherelle: L'art de conjuguer: Dictionnaire de 12,000 verbes.* LaSalle, Canada: Hurtubise HMH.

Charbonneau, H., & Maheu, R. (1973). *Les aspects démographiques de la question linguistique au Québec.* Québec: Éditeur officiel.

Charte de la langue française. (1996). In M. Masse, N. René, H. Dorion, M. Tremblay, P. Lucier, R. Normand, M. Bouchard, A. Vieira, R. Thivierge, J. Legault, M. Plourde, G. Dumas, P. Bouchard, & P. Georgeault, *La situation de la langue française au Québec* (pp. 15–18). Bilan. Rapport remis à la Ministre responsable de l'application de la Charte de la langue française (Avant-projet).

Clark, E. V. (1985). The acquisition of romance languages with special reference to French. In D. Slobin (Ed.), *The crosslinguistic study of language acquisition* (pp. 687–782). Hillsdale, NJ: Lawrence Erlbaum.

Damourette, J., & Pichon, E. (1971). *Des mots à la pensée. Essai de grammaire de la langue française.* Paris: D'Artrey.

Déprez, V., & Pierce, A. E. (1993). Negation and functional projections in early grammar. *Linguistic Inquiry, 24,* 25–67.

Faïta, D. (1974). *Étude syntaxique du français parlé par des enfants de neuf ans.* Unpublished doctoral dissertation, Université de Provence, France.

Fortin, J. (1996). *Habiletés morpho-syntaxiques de sujets normaux franco-québécois.* Unpublished manuscript, L'Hôpital Ste. Justine, Montréal, Qué.

Gagné, G., & Pagé, N. (1981). *Études sur la langue parlée des enfants québécois, 1969–1980.* Montréal, Québec: Presses de l'Université de Montréal.

Gauthier, V. (1996). *Utilisation des morphèmes grammaticaux de temps et des adverbes de temps par des enfants avec dysphasie développementale.* Unpublished master's thesis, Université de Montréal, Montréal, Québec.

Gilbert, A., & Langlois, A. (1994). *Regard sur les nouvelles réalités franco-ontariennes.* Vanier: Association Canadienne-Française de l'Ontario.

Grégoire, A. (1947). *L'apprentissage du langage.* Liège: Droz.

Grévisse, M. (1986). *Le bon usage* (12ᵉ éd.). Paris-Gembloux: Duculot.

Grundstrom, A., & Léon, P. R. (1973). *Interrogation et intonation en français standard et en français canadien.* Paris-Bruxelles: Didier.

Guillaume, P. (1927). Les débuts de la phrases dans le langage de l'enfant. *Journal de psychologie, 24,* 1–25.

Hénault, J., & Piccard, R. (1991). *Grammaire française: de l'observation à l'objectivation.* Laval, Canada: Éditions FM.

Hiriartborde, A. (1973). Sur la généralisation de quelques marques grammaticales dans le langage d'enfants de 3 ans ½. *Études de linguistique appliquée, 9,* 101–124.

Imbs, P. (1960). *Les temps du verbe français* (2ᵉ éd.). Paris: Klincksieck.

Labelle, M. (1990). Predication: WH-movement and the development of relative clauses. *Language Acquisition, 1,* 95–119.

Labelle, M. (1994). Acquisition de la valeur des temps du passé par les enfants francophones. *Revue québécoise de linguistique, 23,* 99–121.

Labelle, M., & Valois, D. (1996). The status of post-verbal subjects in French child language. *Probus, 8,* 53–80.

Larochette, J. (1980). *L'emploi des formes de l'indicatif en français.* Munchen: Fink.

Leblanc, G. (1996a, 21 Septembre). Le bastion de Sudbury. Français à la maison et anglais dans la rue (p. B1). *La Presse.*

Leblanc, G. (1996b, 22 Septembre). Les 500,000 francophones de l'Ontario. Une minorité qui se débat pour ne pas devenir comme les autres (p. A7). *La Presse.*

Lessard, D. (1996, 23 Mars). L'avenir du français se joue à Montréal (pp. A1–A2). *La Presse.*

Lightbown, P. (1977). *Consistency and variation in the acquisition of French.* Unpublished doctoral dissertation, Columbia University, New York.

Maheu, R. (1970). *Les francophones du Canada 1941–1991.* Montréal: Éditions Parti Pris.

Mandel, M. (1992). *The charter of rights and the legalization of politics in Canada.* Toronto: Thompson Educational Publishing.

Masse, M., René, N., Dorion, H., Tremblay, M., Lucier, P., Normand, R., Bouchard, M., Vieira, A., Thivierge, R., Legault, J., Plourde, M., Dumas, G., Bouchard, P., & Georgeault, P. (1996). *La situation de la langue française au Québec.* Bilan. Rapport remis à la Ministre responsable de l'application de la Charte de la langue française (Avant-projet).

Méthé, S. (1996). *Grammatical morphology in French language-impaired children.* Unpublished master's thesis, McGill University, Montréal.

Moignet, G. (1965). *Le pronom personnel français. Essai de psycho-systématique historique.* Paris: Klincksieck.

Morin, Y. C. (1985). On the two French subjectless verbs *voici* and *voila. Language, 61,* 777–820.

Paradis, J., & Genesse, F. (1996). Syntactic acquisition in bilingual children. *Studies in Second Language Acquisition, 18,* 1–25.

Pierce, A. E. (1992). *Language acquisition and syntactic theory: A comparative analysis of French and English child grammars.* Dordrecht: Kluwer Academic Publishers.

Pouliot, J. (1996). *Développement de la morphologie et de la syntaxe.* Unpublished manuscript, Université de Montréal, Montréal.

Roy, G. R. (1976). *Contribution à l'analyse du syntagme verbal. Étude morphosyntaxique et stylistique des coverbes.* Québec: Presses de l'Université Laval.

Sauvy, A. (1966). *Théorie générale de la population*. Paris: Presses Universitaires de France.

Stanké, B. (1996). *Étude de l'emploi des articles chez des enfants dysphasiques franco-québécois âgés de 7 ans*. Unpublished master's thesis, Université de Montréal, Montréal.

Statistiques Canada (1991). *Données du recensement*. Ottawa: Statistiques Canada.

Tanase, E. (1943). *Essai sur la valeur et les emplois du subjonctif en français*. Montpellier: Rouvière.

Termote, M. (1994). *L'avenir démolinguistique du Québec et de ses régions* (Collection Dossiers, 38). Québec: Conseil de la langue française.

Termote, M. (1995). *Perspectives démolinguistiques du Québec et de la région de Montréal, 1991–2041*. Québec: Institut national de recherche scientifique.

Termote, M., & Gauvreau, D. (1988). *La situation démolinguistique du Québec* (Collection Dossiers, 30). Québec: Conseil de la langue française.

Touratier, C. (1980). *La relative: Essai de théorie syntaxique*. Paris: Klincksieck.

Verrips, M., & Weissenborn, J. (1992). Routes to verb placement in early German and French: The independence of finiteness and agreement. In J. M. Meisel (Ed.), *The acquisition of verb placement* (pp. 283–331). Dordrecht: Kluwer Academic Publishers.

Vet, C. (1980). *Temps, aspects et adverbes de temps en français contemporain*. Genève: Droz.

JOSÉE FORTIN, Ph.D.

Josée Fortin, Ph.D., is an Associate Researcher at Sainte-Justine Hospital and University of Montreal, Department of Speech and Language Pathology, and Professor of Speech Pathology at Laurentian University. Dr. Fortin's research and clinical work includes typically developing children as well as children with speech and language impairments and reading disabilities.

MARTHA B. CRAGO, Ph.D.

Martha B. Crago, Ph.D., is an Associate Professor in Communication Sciences and Disorders and the Associate Vice-Principal (Graduate Studies) at McGill University. Her research and publications span a variety of issues in child language development, including language socialization, language acquisition, and language impairment. Dr. Crago's research includes work with monolingual, bilingual, typically developing children and children with language impairment who speak English and/or French or Inuktitut. Her work appears in a number of journal articles and book chapters.

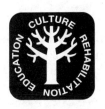

CHAPTER 8

ACQUIRING INUKTITUT

MARTHA B. CRAGO, Ph.D.
SHANLEY E. M. ALLEN, Ph.D

Inuktitut is the language spoken by Inuit people in the Canadian Arctic. There are approximately 28,000 Inuit people living across the Canadian North. Nearly 40% of this population is under the age of 15. The Inuit of Canada live in the Northwest Territories, Northern Quebec, and Newfoundland. The acquisitional properties of Inuktitut reported in this chapter are derived from research that took place in Northern Quebec.

The ancestors of the Inuit people living in Northern Quebec inhabited this arctic tundra land as early as 9000 BC. These earliest people were part of the Dorset and pre-Dorset culture originating in Alaska. By 1000 AD these very early cultures were replaced by members of the Thule culture, people who traveled nomadically to eastern Canada from Alaska. The Thule culture remains the basis for the cultural traditions of the present Inuit inhabitants of Northern Quebec (Dorais, 1992a). This culture is based on the hunting of land and sea mammals and fish as well as the gathering of vegetation, duck down, and eggs, among other things. Traditionally, Inuit lived in family groupings, traveling nomadically according to the seasons and the availability of wild-life and living in igloos, tents, and some sod and stone dwellings.

Today, life is quite different for the Inuit of Northern Quebec. For the last 30–40 years, they have lived a sedentary existence in 14 settlements located along the periphery of a vast peninsula that borders Hudson Bay on the west, the Straits of Hudson to the north, and Ungava Bay to the east. The settlements range in size from 110 people in the smallest to over 1,000 in the largest. The economy is no longer exclusively based on traditional hunting and gathering activities, but rather is divided between such traditional activities, cash jobs, and welfare support. Families now live in houses and apartments with telephones, televisions, running water, and numerous modern appliances purchased through local stores. Schools have been built in every community, some as late as the mid 1960s. At present, the schools and health care services are under local Inuit control. The Inuit of Northern Quebec also have autonomous governmental structures and a territory-wide land holding association.

With just this brief introduction to the present day situation of Inuit people in Northern Quebec, the rest of this chapter concentrates on their language and how it is acquired in the modern context. First, Inuktitut is described with reference to related languages and related populations of speakers spread across the circumpolar north from Siberia to Greenland. This is followed by a description of the cultural context for learning and speaking Inuktitut in Northern Quebec. The grammatical properties of the language are then compared to the English language with particular attention to the acquisition of some of these grammatical properties by young Inuit children. Finally, the chapter concludes with a brief look into the future of language use and acquisition in Northern Quebec.

ᕍ

WHO SPEAKS INUKTITUT AND RELATED LANGUAGES?

Inuktitut is a language in the Eskimo-Aleut family of languages. These languages are spoken around the polar regions in a vast circle extending from Siberia and Alaska through the Canadian Arctic to Greenland. There are some 137,000 people who can be considered members of the Eskimo and Aleut populations (Dorais, 1992b). Approximately 69% (94,877) of them speak their indigenous languages (see Table 8–1).

TABLE 8–1
Speakers of the Eskimo-Aleut languages.

Family	Branch	Subbranch	Population	% Speakers
Eskimo-Aleut	Aleut	Aleut	2,800	25%
	Eskimo	Inuit	105,500	72%
		Yupik	29,000	62%

Sources: Data from "Les langues autochtones d'hier à aujourd'hui," by L. J. Dorias, 1992. In J. Maurais, Ed. *Les langues autochones du Québec* (pp. 63–113). Québec: Publications du Québec; and "La situation linguistiques dans l'arctique. *Inuit Studies, 16,* 237–235.

Speakers of the Inuit group of languages include people from Alaska, the Canadian Arctic, and Greenland. There are subdivisions of the Inuit language group. People in Alaska speak a language known as *Inupiaq,* whereas people in the Western Canadian Arctic speak *Inuktun. Inuktitut* is the language of Eastern Canadian Inuit and *Kalaallisut* is the language of Greenlanders or *Kalaallit,* as they call themselves. These subdivisions of the Inuit language are somewhat but not completely mutually intelligible to speakers from the different regions.

The number of speakers of Inuit languages varies widely in each of the countries where they live (Dorais, 1990). In Siberia, for instance, the number of people who are still able to speak their indigenous language is negligible and limited to older people. Speakers of Inupiaq in Alaska range from 26% to 48% of the population, depending on the various regions of their territory. The Canadian situation is even more disparate; only 25% of the population in the Western Canadian Arctic speak Inuktun, whereas 99% of the population of Northern Quebec speak Inuktitut. Greenland presents the most salutatory indigenous language situation with a countrywide figure of 98% of the population speaking Kalaallisut.

Retention and erosion of these indigenous languages appears to be related to a set of interconnected factors. In part, there is a relationship between language erosion and the advent of second-language speakers and particularly of schools with second-language instruction. In Canada, for example, schools were established first in the Western Arctic. In turn, this is the territory with the smallest percentage of speakers of an Inuit language in Canada. Language retention, on the other hand, appears to be related to indigenous language instruction at school and literacy in the indigenous language (Dorais, 1990). The following three examples from Alaska, Northern Quebec, and Greenland show how such factors have created various patterns of language usage.

In Alaska, a writing system for Inupiaq (using the Roman alphabet) was developed in 1946 and revised in the 1960s by a native speaker of Inupiaq in collaboration with missionary linguists from the Summer Institute of Linguistics. Since the 1940s most parents have not spoken Inupiaq with their children. These parents were members of a generation of people who were taught in English in school and were punished for speaking their native language. To spare their children the same fate, and under the impression that English would help their children get ahead in the world, many parents have spoken only English in their homes. Tenacious efforts to teach Inupiaq as a second language have taken place since 1972. However, only 5,000 out of 13,000 people still use this language and only a few isolated communities have any fluent speakers under 20 years of age (Dorais, 1990).

The situations in Northern Quebec and Greenland contrast sharply with the Alaskan one. In Northern Quebec, Inuktitut orthography was developed by missionaries around 1865. A certain Reverend Peck (known also as *Uqammak*) sent religious literature in syllabics all over the region. By 1925, most Inuit in the region were literate, having learned to read at home from their parents. Schools were established very late in Northern Quebec because of provincial-federal jurisdictional misunderstandings. As a result, many communities had no schools and no second-language instruction until the mid 1960s. A scant 10 years later, a land claims settlement, the James Bay Northern Quebec Agreement, gave Inuit of this region control over their own schools. With local control came the creation of Inuktitut language instruction, the training of Inuit teachers, and the prodigious production of pedagogical materials in the native language. By 1981, 5,160 of the 5,330 people in Nunavik were still speakers of Inuktitut (Dorais, 1990, 1992a, 1992b).

The language retention situation in Greenland is even more remarkable (Dorais, 1990). Greenlandic, or Kalaallisut, has been written since the early 1700s when Danish missionaries began translating the Bible and teaching in the native language. Schools in Kalaallisut were set up over 260 years ago and today there is a university where students may study through the doctoral level at least partially in their indigenous language. This very early literacy and educational history, together with geographic isolation and long-standing political autonomy, have created the only country of Inuit speakers where the indigenous language is the official language. Despite the discrepancy between the Greenlandic situation and the impoverished language use patterns of Siberia, Alaska, and the Western Canadian Arctic, the Inuit language group is still considered to be one of the very few indigenous language groups in the world with a long-term chance of survival (Foster, 1982).

⌐ᒪ

THE CULTURAL CONTEXT FOR SPEAKING AND LEARNING INUKTITUT

Inuktitut as it is spoken in Northern Quebec is learned by children in a cultural context that is both traditional and evolving. Ethnographic studies of language socialization practices in Inuit homes and schools of Northern Quebec have documented the culturally based interactions that provide a framework for language acquisition both in family settings (Crago, 1988; Crago, 1992; Crago, Allen, & Hough-Eyamie, 1997; Crago, Annahatak, & Ningiuruvik, 1993) and in classrooms (Crago & Eriks-Brophy, 1993a, 1993b; Crago, Eriks-Brophy, Pesco, & McAlpine, 1997; Eriks-Brophy, 1992; Eriks-Brophy & Crago, 1993, 1994). The family language socialization study focused on four children (aged 1;0 to 1;9 at the outset) and their families who live in two small remote communities on Ungava Bay in Northern Quebec. These families were videotaped for 1 year every 4 months. This study also included interview data from 20 older and younger mothers. As these children became school-aged, school practices of language socialization with their Inuit teachers from kindergarten to Grade 2 were documented with classroom videotapes and teacher interviews. This study was followed by continued research with the same children, their classmates, and their non-Inuit second-language teachers in Grade 3, when the language of instruction shifted from Inuktitut to English or French. In the next part of this chapter, findings from both the home and the school studies are described.

FAMILY STRUCTURE

To begin, the Inuit of Northern Quebec still live, for the most part, in close connection with their families. These families are structured in somewhat different ways than those that have typically been associated with the North American white middle class (WMC). Often young mothers or young couples will live with their first children in their parents' home before moving out on their own. Caregiving in these homes is spread over a number of people. A child's young aunts, uncles, and grandparents are highly involved in interactions with the child. Even today, children are raised, for the most part, in multiaged, multiparty talking environments. At a young age, children are oriented toward a great deal of interaction with their age-similar peers. One- and 2-year-olds observed during the home language socialization study played daily with cousins or near-age brothers, sisters, and friends. Peer talk among the 1- to 3-year-olds involved pretend play with and without toy props and talk that accompanied physical play. A number of older women, past their own child-bearing age, raise children that they have adopted. Caregiving in their homes is often shared with older sibling caregivers. Custom adoption is, in fact, a very frequent practice in Northern Quebec for women of all ages. In the communities where our research took place, as many as 40% of the children were adopted into and out of their families. This meant that the four children in our study were being raised by women from two different age groups: those in their late 40s and those in their early 20s. Such an age differential in the mothers allowed a fortuitous historical perspective on caregiving practices and the possibility to document diachronic change.

OLDER WOMEN'S LANGUAGE SOCIALIZATION PRACTICES

Inuit language socialization practices in the homes with more traditional mothers were strikingly different from what has been documented for North American WMC homes (Crago, 1992; Crago, Allen, et al., 1997; Heath, 1983; Schieffelin & Eisenberg, 1984). Mothers over 45 years of age used language socialization practices that included a specific baby word lexicon, a special register of affectionate talk, the deliberate exclusion of young children from adult conversations, and highly frequent use of the imperative form in directives to the child. In comparison with what has been reported for North American WMC mothers, these older Inuit mothers never asked questions of the children to which they already knew the answer, they made no requests for displays of expressive language from the child, and they rarely expanded their children's utterances. In addition, young children's early vocalizations were not interpreted as meaningful. Considerable behavior, including companionship and discipline, as well as such activities of daily living as bedding, bathing, dressing, and eating were co-constructed in silence. As a result, the young children of these older women rarely had the role of conversational partners with their mothers. In fact, these mothers engaged in about one third as much conversation with their children as younger Inuit mothers and about one sixth as much as a comparison group of American WMC mothers (Hough-Eyamie, 1993; Hough-Eyamie, Pan, Crago, & Snow, in preparation). Instead, most of the children's verbal interactions took place with their peers and siblings. Sibling caregivers involved themselves in frequent repetition routines with the children in which they explicitly modelled the production of such things as Inuit greeting routines. Inuit children were also frequently in multi-age gatherings in which they were exposed to considerable overheard language. Despite such differences in language socialization, Inuit children attain developmental language milestones in much the same manner as has been reported for North American WMC children. As described later in this chapter, the acquisition of particular structural features, of course, differs from acquisition patterns in other languages and appears to be related to the typology of the Inuktitut language and the structural properties of the overheard input that Inuit children are exposed to (Allen, 1996a; Allen & Crago, 1996; Crago, Allen, et al., 1997).

DIACHRONIC CHANGE: YOUNG MOTHERS' LANGUAGE SOCIALIZATION PRACTICES

Inuit socialization practices in Northern Quebec show the effects of diachronic change. Young Inuit mothers' ways of talking to their children do not completely resemble the older, more traditional mothers' ways (Crago et al., 1993). Over time, North American WMC practices are being adopted and used by young Inuit women. Some of the young mothers stated explicitly that they talked to their children in certain ways to copy the patterns of WMC people, whom they characterized as more "educated," and to prepare their children for school and the kind of discourse that the non-Inuit second-language teachers would use in the classroom. For instance, young mothers described themselves as using less of the special baby word vocabulary, less of the register of affectionate talk, and none of the rhythmical verses that older mothers created for their young babies. In addition, they differed strikingly from the older mothers in their use of questions that elicit labeling from the child as well as in the use of repetition routines to practice second-language politeness words and counting sequences. Furthermore, certain young mothers requested verbal displays from their children in the form of recounting experiences to others. The overall pattern of change was one of younger mothers engaging with their children as conversational partners in ways that were quite different from older mothers.

This involved, in addition to the features described, an increase in conversational interactions in a given time period.

Older Inuit women sometimes complained about the changes that were happening in the ways of talking with children. They blamed some of the changes on the advent of WMC teachers into their communities—teachers they felt brought not only their language but also their culture's patterns of communicative interaction into the lives of Inuit children. Similarly, changes in child-rearing practices and language socialization have evolved in other places throughout the circumpolar region. When one of the authors reported on her findings about language socialization in older mothers' homes in Northern Quebec, a number of Inuit women in the audience echoed the diachronic nature of change in their comments. A Greenlander said, "What you have described is the way things were in my mother's house." An Inuk woman from the Western Canadian Arctic said, "Sadly, I only know what you speak of from my grandmother's house."

LANGUAGE SOCIALIZATION IN SCHOOLS

Commentary about the role of schools in inducing change in home patterns of socialization motivated a set of studies of the classroom context for language learning in communities in Northern Quebec. The same four children who were studied in their homes were followed into their classrooms, where for the first 3 years of their education they had Inuit teachers instructing them in Inuktitut. Ethnographically framed microanalysis of their language lessons demonstrated a form of instructional discourse that is quite different from what has previously been reported for North American WMC teachers (Crago & Eriks-Brophy 1993a, 1993b; Eriks-Brophy, 1992; Eriks-Brophy & Crago, 1993, 1994; Mehan, 1979). In Inuit teachers' classrooms, the children were instructed to attend to their peers, group nomination and response formats were used, students were not expected to raise their hands to be called on, modeling written work after another student's work was acceptable, teachers rarely evaluated students' responses in front of others, and individual displays of expressive language in front of the group were rarely requested from the children. Furthermore, students' initiations were frequently incorporated into the lesson by the Inuit teachers.

As the four children continued their education past Grade 2, they encountered non-Inuit teachers for the first time. Their language of instruction shifted to English or French and, at the same time, the discourse of language instruction in the classroom changed (Crago, Eriks-Brophy, et al., 1997; Eriks-Brophy, 1997). With the non-Inuit teachers, Inuit children were expected to raise their hands, wait to be called on as individuals, required to speak in front of the group, and then were publicly evaluated on their performance. The lessons were largely teacher controlled, with the children being directed to attend to the teacher and not to each other. Their initiations were rarely incorporated into the lessons. Such differences from the Inuit teachers' ways of teaching demonstrate the culturally based and culturally variable nature of classroom discourse. They also demonstrate the potential for miscommunication across the cultural lines. Such miscommunications made these Inuit children's transition to their second-language classrooms very challenging. The power differentials between the students and their teachers meant that miscommunications could result in punitive and personally unpleasant situations for the children (Crago, Eriks-Brophy, et al., 1997).

The cultural context for Inuit children who are learning language, both their mother tongue and a second language, is a complex mixture of old and new, home and school. The educational and parental patterns of adaptation bridge two worlds in a time of rapid and often disruptive change. The potential for loss of a highly valuable language as well as the cultural patterns for its use in social interaction is considerable.

Ꮤ

LINGUISTIC STRUCTURE OF INUKTITUT

Though both home and school offer rapidly changing patterns of socialization into language use, almost 100% of the Inuit children in Northern Quebec are still learning Inuktitut as their first language. Inuktitut as a language remains relatively strong overall, and is still the major if not only language used in input to Inuit children in most of this region. This section presents information about the patterns young Inuit children follow in learning the morphology and syntax of their language. First, however, some major aspects of the linguistic structure of Inuktitut are described. For purposes of clarity, they are presented in contrast with the comparable structural properties of English.

Inuktitut, like other languages in the Eskimo–Aleut family, is of rather complicated structure. It is a polysynthetic language, its case system is ergative, and it employs a large number of nominal and verbal inflections. Typical word order is subject-object-verb, though ellipsis of both the subject and object is common. In contrast, English is basically an analytic language. Its case system is accusative and it employs relatively few nominal or verbal inflections. Typical word order in English is subject-verb-object and ellipsis of subjects and objects is forbidden in most cases. The following paragraphs discuss each of these structural properties. Further details may be found in Dorais (1988).

POLYSYNTHESIS

Polysynthesis is a common property of many Native American languages and Inuktitut is one of the best known examples of a polysynthetic language. A polysynthetic language is able to express in one word of several morphemes what would require a sentence of several individual words in a more analytic language like English. Much of the syntax of the language occurs within an individual word expressed by the relationships between morphemes, rather than within a sentence expressed by relationships between words. Thus, polysynthetic languages tend to have more morphemes per word than other types of languages. In addition, many of those morphemes express syntactic functions such as adjectival or adverbial modification, negation, changing word classes, and changing valency. Examples such as that in 1 are common in terms of number, type, and function of morphemes.[1]

---

[1] The following abbreviations are used:

For nominal case: ABS = absolutive; ALL = allative (*to, with,* agentive *by*); ERG = ergative; MOD = modalis (oblique case for direct object).

For verbal modality: CSV = causative; IMP = imperative; IND = indicative; INT = interrogative; PAR = participial (functionally equivalent to indicative in Northern Quebec Inuktitut).

For word-internal morphology: ANTP = antipassive; CAUS = causative; EMPH = emphatic; FUT = future; NEG = negative; NOM = nominalizer; PASS = passive; PAST = past; PERF = perfective; POL = politeness (preceding imperative); PRES = present.

For verbal inflection: 1 = 1st person; 2 = 2nd person; 3 = 3rd person; s = singular; d = dual; S = subject; O = object.

For nominal inflection: SG = singular; PL = plural.

(1) *Illujuaraalummuulaursimannginamalittauq.*
illu-juaq-aluk-mut-uq-lauq-sima-nngit-gama-li-ttauq
house-big-EMPH-ALL.SG-go-PAST-PERF-NEG-CSV.1sS-
but-also
"But also, because I never went to the really big house."
(Dorais, 1988)

This word begins as a nominal with the noun root *illu-* "house." The
nominal part of the word includes word-internal morphemes that
express adjectival modification (*-juaq-* "big") and emphasis (*-aluk-*
"EMPH"), and ends with a case marker indicating case and number of
the nominal (*-mut-* "ALL.SG"). The word changes class to become verbal with the affixation of the verbalizer *-uq-* "go to." The verbal part of
the word is then affixed with a number of word-internal morphemes
including time or tense (*-lauq-* "PAST"), aspect (*-sima-* "PERF"), and
negation (*-nngit-* "NEG"). The grammatical part of the word ends with
a portmanteau cross-referencing inflection giving information about
the verbal modality and person and number of the subject (*-gama*
"CSV.1sS"). Finally, there are two enclitics that give additional information joining this word to other words and concepts in the discourse
(*-li* "but," *-ttauq* "also"). Note that morphophonological processes often
change or delete consonants at morpheme boundaries, so that the appearance of a morpheme in a word may be different than its underlying
form given in the glosses here.

MORPHOLOGICAL STRUCTURE

The structure of words in Inuktitut is somewhat more complex than in
English, as might be expected. Word roots in Inuktitut fall into three
main classes—verbs, nouns (including pronouns and demonstratives),
and uninflected particles (including conjunctions, interjections, and
some adverbials). Uninflected particles are independent and appear
without any additional morphology. Verb and noun roots may never
appear alone. Rather, they may be followed by word-internal morphemes and must always be followed by appropriate cross-referencing
inflections.

Each verb or noun root may be followed by up to at least 8 morphemes from among the over 400 word-internal morphemes used productively in this language, including independent verbs, auxiliaries,
adverbials, adjectivals, tense (or time) markers, and the like. As seen

in Example 1, word-internal morphemes may change the class of a word from nominal to verbal or the reverse, and may also change the valency of a verbal word from transitive to intransitive or the reverse.

Each verbal or nominal stem (i.e., root plus word-internal morphemes) must then be followed by 1 of over 900 verbal or over 100 nominal cross-referencing inflections, respectively. Verbal cross-referencing inflections include information about verbal modality (indicative, interrogative, imperative, etc.) as well as the person and number of both the grammatical subject and grammatical object of the verb. Nominal cross-referencing inflections include information about case (absolutive, ergative, locative, etc.) and number of the nominal as well as the person and number of the possessor if relevant. All these inflections are considered portmanteau morphemes in that the total information contained in them is reflected in one indivisible form. Although these inflections were historically separable into their component parts, they are no longer reliably and consistently separable in this manner.

Finally, one or more optional enclitics may be affixed to either verbal or nominal words, as seen in Example 1.

SYNTACTIC STRUCTURE

ERGATIVITY

In terms of case marking, Inuktitut is a morphologically ergative language. In an ergative language, the subjects of intransitive verbs and the objects of transitive verbs group together, both receiving absolutive case marking. The subjects of transitive verbs form a separate group by themselves, receiving ergative case marking. This pattern is illustrated by Examples 2a and 2b.

> (2a) *Jaani nirijuq.*
> Jaani-θ niri-juq
> Johnny-ABS.SG eat-PAR.3sS
> "Johnny is eating."

> (2b) *Jaaniup iqaluk nirijanga.*
> Jaani-up iqaluk-θ niri-janga
> Johnny-ERG.SG fish-ABS.SG eat-PAR.3sS.3sO
> "Johnny is eating the fish."

The ergative system of Inuktitut contrasts with the accusative system in languages like English, in which subjects of both transitive and intransitive verbs group together receiving nominative case marking, with objects of transitive verbs constituting a separate group receiving accusative case marking. This pattern is shown in Example 3, using English pronouns.

(3a) She sleeps.

(3b) She likes her.

Ergativity is only visible in the nominal case marking system in Inuktitut. It is not visible in the verbal cross-referencing inflection system, because the cross-referencing morphemes conflate information about verbal modality as well as person and number of subject and object together into one form that is no longer separable into its individual parts. As it is not possible to tell which part of the cross-referencing inflection indicates subject or object, it is also not possible to determine any pattern of ergativity-related grouping in the cross-referencing inflections.

CLAUSE STRUCTURE

Inuktitut, like English, has two basic clause types—intransitive and transitive—as illustrated in Examples 2a and 2b, respectively. The intransitive clause in 2a contains a verbal root and only one argument, a subject marked with absolutive case, which is cross-referenced in verbal inflection. The transitive clause in 2b contains a verb and two arguments, a subject and a direct object, which are both cross-referenced in verbal inflection. As is typical in ergative languages, the absolutive case on the direct object is the same as that on subjects of intransitive sentences, with the ergative case on the subject unique to that position.

In addition to these basic clause types, Inuktitut allows for several types of derived clauses including antipassives, passives, causatives, and noun incorporation structures, as shown in Examples 4 through 7, respectively. Note that English allows passives and causatives, but not antipassives or noun incorporation structures. Antipassives are typical to ergative languages and noun incorporation structures are often found in polysynthetic languages.

(4) *Jaani iqalummik nirijuq.*
Jaani-θ iqaluk-mik niri-θ-juq
Johnny-ABS.SG fish-MOD.SG eat-ANTP-PAR.3sS
"Johnny is eating a fish."

(5) *Iqaluk Jaanimut nirijaujuq.*
iqaluk-θ Jaani-mut niri-jau-juq
fish-ABS.SG Johnny-ALL.SG eat-PASS-PAR.3sS
"The fish was eaten by Johnny."

(6) *Miajiup Jaani nirititanga.*
Miaji-up Jaani-θ niri-tit-janga
Mary-ERG.SG Johnny-ABS.SG eat-CAUS-PAR.3sS.3sO
"Mary is making Johnny eat."

(7) *Jaani iqaluturtuq.*
Jaani-θ iqaluk-tuq-juq
Johnny-ABS.SG fish-consume-PAR.3sS
"Johnny is eating a/the fish." [cf. "Johnny is fish-eating."]

As the antipassive morpheme is often not overt, as in Example 4, antipassive clauses often look like transitive clauses in which the object is not cross-referenced in verbal inflection. For this reason, they are sometimes referred to as "half-transitive," "semi-transitive," or "accusative" clauses.

WORD ORDER

Basic word order in Inuktitut is generally assumed to be subject-object-verb, in contrast to the subject-verb-object order of English. Deviations from this basic word order in both languages typically indicate a pragmatic or stylistic effect.

One striking aspect of Inuktitut is that subjects and objects are often not represented as independent lexical items, but rather only through verbal cross-referencing inflection. Thus, sentences in Inuktitut tend to be composed primarily of verbal words with relatively few nouns. The prolific ellipsis of independent subjects and objects means that word order is not a particularly useful determinant of syntactic structure in Inuktitut. This pattern contrasts with English in which subjects and objects must typically be obligatorily represented as either full nouns, noun phrases, or pronouns and in which word order is the primary determinant of syntactic structure.

ᛒ

HIGHLIGHTS OF THE ACQUISITION OF
INUKTITUT GRAMMATICAL STRUCTURE

The body of research investigating the acquisition of grammatical structure in Eskimo-Aleut languages is small but growing. Fortescue (1985)
and Fortescue and Lennert Olsen (1992) have documented various aspects of morphological and semantic acquisition in six west Greenlandic children aged 2;2 through 5;2, with Wilman (1988) reporting on
aspects of morphological and syntactic acquisition in a group of kindergarten students in the Northwest Territories in Canada. Finally, Allen (1989, 1995, 1996a), Allen and Crago (1989, 1992, 1996), Allen and
Schröder (in press), Crago (1995), Crago and Allen (1996a, 1996b),
Crago, Allen, and Genesee (1996) and Crago, Allen, et al. (1997) have
documented several aspects of morphological and syntactic acquisition
in eight children aged 1;0 through 3;6 in Northern Quebec.

This section focuses on the latter body of work, in keeping with the
Northern Quebec emphasis. It begins with a discussion about quanti-
fying language abilities in Inuktitut through use of mean length of utterance (MLU) figures. It then gives information about the one- and
two-morpheme stages (including use of baby word vocabulary), representation of subjects and objects, and acquisition of noun incorporation
structures, passives, and causatives. This information is presented in
terms of individual structures rather than by age or MLU because not
enough is yet known to present a comprehensive overall picture of
Inuktitut language development. Finally, this section raises the question of the role of input in acquisition and discusses some contributions
that Inuktitut acquisition research can make to language acquisition
theory.

MEAN LENGTH OF UTTERANCE

Much of the research on language acquisition in general begins with
quantitative measures of children's language at different stages in development. One typical measure used is Brown's (1973) mean length of
utterance (MLU). The length in productive morphemes of a set number
of utterances, minimally 100, is measured and the mean of these utterance lengths constitutes the MLU. Though this measure is known to

TABLE 8–2

Mean length of utterance data (adapted from Allen, 1996).

Subject	Age	Hours of data	No. of utterances	MLU
Elijah	2;0	2.05	805	2.51
	2;5	1.87	621	3.56
	2;9	1.95	731	3.39
Lizzie	2;6	2.05	654	2.81
	2;10	2.03	693	3.24
	3;3	1.00	248	3.39
Louisa	2;10	2.02	288	1.99
	3;2	2.38	643	2.89
	3;6	2.35	632	2.89
Paul	2;6	1.93	310	2.51
	2;11	0.95	220	2.91
	3;3	2.3	460	3.19
Total		**23.28**	**6,305**	

have a number of limitations, it is generally considered the best method available to indicate a child's increasing knowledge of grammar under the logic that a child's utterances will gradually lengthen as a child acquires more grammatical knowledge. Thus, MLU is used as an index of a child's own development as well as a comparison of development across children. This measure has proved useful in Inuktitut child language research to date. It accurately reflects the development of grammatical abilities in the four subjects under study whose language has been analyzed in this regard, as shown in Table 8–2. However, certain cautions must be taken into consideration as indicated below.

Inuktitut presents some unique problems for the calculation of MLU. The primary difficulty lies in determining what constitutes a productive or uniquely analyzed morpheme for the Inuktitut-speaking child. In a language like English in which each word in child language is typically composed of two morphemes at most, productivity is relatively easy to determine as there is relatively little opportunity for fixed forms to occur. However, in a language like Inuktitut in which early multimorphemic utterances almost always consist of two morphemes rather than two separate words and in which words of three and more morphemes appear fairly early in the acquisition process, productivity is not so easy to determine. Inflectional affixes may well not be productively used until some time after they are first produced. Additionally, it is quite conceivable that one morpheme in a word is productive, with the composite of two or more others still constituting a fixed form for the child. A more conservative approach to acquisition may well assume that Inuktitut-speaking children take some time to sort out the analysis of certain morpheme combinations into their separate components.

A thorough approach to the productivity problem might involve assessing each morpheme and morpheme combination for its productivity. Commonly used criteria include presence in the corpus of novel utterances misusing a morpheme in a way indicating productivity, use of the relevant morpheme in contrasting morphological environments, and phonological errors in use of an individual morpheme that indicate a child is not merely parroting a fixed morpheme combination (Allen, 1996a). Creative errors on the part of a child tend to constitute the strongest evidence of productivity, but these are generally rare. The other criteria provide less strong evidence, but are convincing especially when combined. The most important factor in calculating and interpreting MLU is that one be clear about exactly what one is counting as a productive morpheme and about which kinds of utterances are being used in the overall data set.

A final problem in using quantifiable measures such as MLU is determining their comparative value crosslinguistically. It is not at all clear that an MLU of 3.5 means the same thing for an English-speaking child as for an Inuktitut-speaking child. It may well be the case that Inuktitut-speaking children use more morphemes earlier or use more morphemes, in general, since Inuktitut has so much more morphology available than does English and it is so much more focused on morphology. The problem of crosslinguistic comparability of MLU figures is well known; the specifics related to Inuktitut remain to be determined through further research.

THE ONE-MORPHEME STAGE

Inuktitut-speaking children, like English-speaking children, typically begin their production of language by uttering one word at a time. In Inuktitut, these words may be uninflected particles that may freely stand alone (Example 8a), or single noun (Example 8b), or verb (Example 8c) root morphemes that appear without inflection.

(8a) *Auka*
"No" (Tumasi 1;9)[2]

(8b) *Piipi*
"Baby" (Sarah 1;4)

(8c) *Amaama*
"Suckle" (Jini 1;0)

The verbal utterances are particularly non–adult-like, as verb roots can never appear without cross-referencing inflection in adult language. Though noun roots also require case inflection, the most common absolutive singular inflection is not phonetically overt. It is likely that children do not yet realize that at the one-morpheme stage, but nevertheless their nominal words do not differ in appearance from the adult forms.

The range of vocabulary used at this age is typical of child language crosslinguistically (e.g., Nelson, 1973). In addition, many of the verb and noun roots produced are part of the Inuktitut baby word vocabulary, a special vocabulary of words frequent in input to young children, and in the speech of the children, themselves, until about age 3;0. Baby words in Inuktitut tend to be phonologically simpler than, though usually phonologically unrelated to, their adult counterparts. The utterances in Example 9 are typical baby words; their adult counterparts are shown in brackets.

(9a)　　*Apaapa*　　　　[adult: *Nirigumavunga.*]
　　　　　　　　　　　[　　　niri-guma-vunga]
　　　　　　　　　　　[　　　eat-want-IND.1sS]
　　　　"Food / Eat."　[　　　"I want to eat."]　(Jini 1;0)

(9b)　　*Atai*　　　　　[*adult: Anilaurluk.*]
　　　　　　　　　　　[　　　ani-lauq-luk]
　　　　　　　　　　　[　　　go.out-POL-IMP.1dS]
　　　　"Go outside."　[　　　"Let's go outside."]　(Sarah 1;4)

In caregiver input, baby words may appear as unique lexical items as in the child utterances in the examples, but they are very often affixed with the normal range of word-internal and inflectional affixes. Thus, although baby words accommodate to the early phonological abilities

---

[2] Pseudonyms are used to identify all children whose utterances are reported herein, as well as all persons mentioned in these utterances.

of children, adults even in this domain do not try to mask the morphological complexity that is an integral part of Inuktitut (Crago & Allen, 1996b).

EARLY TWO-MORPHEME COMBINATIONS

As soon as English-speaking children graduate from mere single-word utterances, they enter what is commonly known as the two-word stage, or telegraphic stage. For Inuktitut-speaking children, this stage is more a two-morpheme stage because of the highly polysynthetic nature of Inuktitut (Crago, 1995; Crago, Allen, et al., 1996; Crago, Allen, et al., 1997). In addition, it does not appear as telegraphic in comparison to adult language as does English, as nominal ellipsis is very common in adult Inuktitut. Inuktitut-speaking children in this stage typically use either grammatical or lexical two-morpheme constructions. Grammatical constructions are composed primarily of a verb root plus cross-referencing inflection (Example 10a) or a noun root plus possessive marker (Example 10b).

(10a) *Qaigit.*
qai-git
come-IMP.2sS
"(You) come here."   (Jini 1;8)

(10b) *Uiliup.*
Uili-up
Willie-ERG.SG
"Willie's."   (Lucasi 2;8)

Lexical constructions commonly take a number of forms, including a proper noun plus greeting morpheme (Example 11a) and a noun plus adjectival morpheme (Example 11b).

(11a) *Anaanai.*
anaana-ai
mother-greetings
"Hi, mother."   (Tumasi 1;9)

(11b) *Qimmialuk.*
qimmiq-aluk
dog-bad
"Bad dog."   (Lucasi 2;8)

Several two-word utterances also occur, although they are in the minority. Most of these consist of a vocative proper noun plus a noun, location, or relational word in a kind of command structure (Example 12a). It is extremely rare to find a two-word utterance composed of a verb root and either a subject or object (Example 12b).

(12a) *Auka Siasi.*
auka Siasi
no Jessie
"No, Jessie."   (Sarah 1;11)

(12b) *Iqaluk uvaa-.*
iqaluk uvaa
fish bleed
"The fish is bleeding."   (Tumasi 2;1)

The range of semantic groupings found in utterances at this stage in Inuktitut is quite comparable to that reported for typical English acquisition (Brown, 1973; Crago, 1995).

ARGUMENT REPRESENTATION

Once Inuktitut-speaking children move beyond the two-morpheme stage, they begin producing utterances that have subjects and objects represented independently, as nouns (Example 13a) or demonstrative pronouns (Example 13b), as well as in the cross-referencing inflection. However, they are sensitive from a quite young age to the fact that adult Inuktitut exhibits rampant ellipsis of independent subjects and objects (Example 13c). The examples in 13 illustrate each of these three possibilities for an intransitive sentence with a subject.

(13a) *Panik, piarait sinisijuq.*
panik piaraq-it sinik-si-juq
daughter baby-your.ABS.SG sleep-PRES-PAR.3sS
"Daughter, your baby is sleeping."   (Paul 3;3)

(13b) *Una sinisimmat.*
u-na sinik-si-mmat
this.one-ABS.SG sleep-PRES-CSV.3sS
"This one is sleeping."   (Lizzie 2;10)

(13c) *Sinilirmat.*
sinik-liq-mmat
sleep-PRES-CSV.3sS
"(He/she/it) is sleeping."   (Elijah 2;9)

Although English-speaking children aged 2;5 through 2;10 produce independent subjects about 65% of the time and independent objects about 95% of the time (Wang, Lillo-Martin, Best, & Levitt, 1992), Inuktitut-speaking children aged 2;0 through 3;6 produce independent subjects only about 15% of the time and independent objects only about 35% of the time (Allen & Schröder, in press). Although both these groups of children are failing to produce independent subjects and objects some of the time, the difference between the rates at which they do this indicates that each group of children has a great deal of knowledge about their respective target language patterns with respect to argument representation.

The choice of Inuktitut-speaking children to produce or fail to produce independent subjects and objects does not appear to be random. Rather, this choice is related to the pragmatic prominence of the referents that they are representing in their speech. Inuktitut-speaking children produce more independent subjects and objects when talking about referents that are absent from the physical context, referents that have not previously been mentioned in discourse, and referents about which some confusion could arise for discourse or context reasons (Allen & Schröder, in press). This finding is consistent with general discourse theories (Chafe, 1987; Clancy, 1980; DuBois, 1987) and findings for child language in Korean (Clancy, 1993). Thus, Inuktitut-speaking children at a fairly young age demonstrate a large degree of knowledge about what information is shared between the speaker and hearer and what information is not shared and therefore needs to be made explicit.

NOUN INCORPORATION

Noun incorporation is a construction fairly typical of polysynthetic languages in which a noun is incorporated into a verbal word, as illustrated in Example 7. In Inuktitut, the incorporated noun is almost always the object of the sentence. Though this construction is not available at all in English, it is quite common in Inuktitut and begins to appear fairly early in the process of Inuktitut acquisition. A few utterances containing noun incorporation constructions appear at the two-morpheme stage, such as seen in Example 14, although it is not clear that they are yet productive.

(14) *Tiituq.*
    tii-tuq
    tea-consume
    "(I want to) drink tea."   (Sarah 1;11)

By the age of about 2;6 to 3;0, such constructions form approximately 10% of children's utterances containing verbs (Allen, 1996a), including such utterances as those in Example 15.

(15a) *Qangattajuuliaqqauju.*
    qangattajuuq-liaq-qqau-juq
    airplane-go.to-PAST-PAR.3sS
    "She went to the airplane."   (Elijah 2;0)

(15b) *Tuttusiulaaqinuk?*
    tuttu-siuq-laaq-vinuk
    caribou-look.for-FUT-INT.1dS
    "Will we go look for caribou?"   (Paul 2;11)

More advanced forms of this construction begin appearing some months later, including double incorporation (Example 16a) and stranding of elements modifying the incorporated noun (Example 16b). (Note that Elijah is a particularly precocious child in terms of language development, and thus the age at which he produces these utterances is substantially younger than that of his coevals.)

(16a) *Sunaturtuviniuvunga.*
    suna-tuq-juq-viniq-u-vunga
    what-consume-NOM-former-be-IND.1sS
    "What did I have to eat before [= I am one who had what to eat before]."   (Elijah 2;5)

(16b) *Maasiukkut imaittunik saviqarqut.*
    Maasiu-kkut imaittuq-nik savik-qaq-vut
    Matthew-group one.like.this-MOD.PL knife-have-IND.3pS
    "Matthew and his friends have knives like this."   (Elijah 2;9)

The early acquisition of noun incorporation structures indicates that Inuktitut-speaking children are sensitive to and comfortable with the polysynthetic structure of their language from a quite early age—likely from almost as soon as they begin putting two morphemes together.

PASSIVES

The literature on language acquisition typically records that English-speaking children reliably comprehend basic passives only by about age 4;0 and more complex passives only by well into the school-aged years (e.g., Baldie, 1976; Gordon & Chafetz, 1990). In addition, they produce only about 0.4 passives per hour in spontaneous speech before age 5;0 (Pinker, Lebeaux, & Frost, 1987), although there is some disagreement about whether this is because they cannot produce passives early or just because passives are not frequent in English, and thus, do not occur frequently in English child language. Inuktitut-speaking children, on the other hand, produce passives in spontaneous speech approximately 3 times per hour by the age of 3;6 (Allen, 1996a; Allen & Crago, 1996). In addition, they show development in their use of passives over the period between 2;0 and 3;6.

One might well wonder what factors differentiate the time of acquisition of a certain structure crosslinguistically. Interestingly, it is reported that Inuktitut-speaking children hear between three and seven times as many passive structures as English-speaking children in speech directed to them at these ages (Allen, 1996a; Allen & Crago, 1996). It is also the case that the structure of the passive is relatively unusual in terms of syntactic structures common in English, but relatively usual in terms of syntactic structures common in Inuktitut. These facts would seem to indicate caregiver input and language structure as two important factors determining differences in acquisition crosslinguistically. These two factors may well be related, as it is likely that caregivers will more frequently use structures in the input that are common and easy to produce in the target language. Similar findings have been reported for the comparison between passive acquisition in Sesotho and in English (Demuth, 1990).

At the earliest stage, Inuktitut-speaking children are primarily using basic passives with action verbs and without agentive phrases, as shown in the Examples in 17.

(17a) *Kiijautsaruarama.*
     kii-jau-tsaruaq-gama
     bite-PASS-might-CSV.1sS
     "I might be bitten."   (Elijah 2;0)

(17b) *Ilai tuttualuit aijaujuit.*
ilai tuttu-aluk-it ai-jau-juq-it
right caribou-EMPH-ABS.PL get-PASS-NOM-ABS.PL
"The caribou are being gotten, right?"   (Paul 2;11)

At more advanced stages, they use an increasing number of full passives (Example 18a), passives with experiential verbs, passives with nonpatient subjects (Example 18b), and passives of internally complex transitive verb phrases.

(18a) *Ilai patittaukaintu uumunga.*
ilai patik-jau-kainnaq-juq u-munga
right slap-PASS-PAST-PAR.3sS this.one-ALL.SG
"Right, he was slapped by this one."   (Louisa 3;6)

(18b) *Nasaliurtaunngitunga.*
nasaq-liuq-jau-nngit-junga
hat-make-PASS-NEG-PAR.1sS
"I am not being made a hat for."   (Elijah 2;5)

These data indicate that Inuktitut-speaking children's production of passives at various levels of complexity is both earlier and more frequent than that of English-speaking children.

CAUSATIVES

There are generally assumed to be two types of causatives in languages of the world: those that are lexical and those that are expressed through either a bound or independent morpheme. Like English, Inuktitut has both of these types of causatives, as shown in Examples 19 and 20, respectively.

(19) *Jaaniup puvirtajuuq qaartanga.*
Jaani-up puvirtajuuq-θ qaaq-janga
Johnny-ERG.SG balloon-ABS.SG burst-PAR.3sS.3sO
"Johnny burst [= caused to burst] the balloon."

(20) *Jaaniup piaraq qiatitanga.*
Jaani-up piaraq-θ qia-tit-janga
Johnny-ERG.SG baby-ABS.SG cry-make-PAR.3sS.3sO
"Johnny is making the baby cry."

Inuktitut-speaking children, like English-speaking children, use lexical causatives from quite early ages, as shown in the Examples in 21.

(21a) *Una ukkualangajara.*
u-na ukkuaq-langa-jara
this.one-ABS.SG close-FUT-PAR.3sS.3sO
"I'm going to close [= make close] this one." (Lizzie 2;6)

(21b) Ataata, una aarqilauruk.
ataata u-na aarqik-lauq-guk
father this.one-ABS.SG fix-POL-IMP.2sS.3sO
"Dad, fix [= make be fixed] this one." (Paul 2;6)

In fact, approximately 6% of utterances with verbs in the speech of four Inuktitut-speaking children aged 2;0 through 3;6 contained lexical causatives (Allen, 1995, 1996a). However, it is not clear for either English- or Inuktitut-speaking children that the causative sense of these verbs has been productively acquired (Allen, 1995, 1996a; Bowerman, 1974).

Children learning both English and Inuktitut tend to start producing analytic causatives such as in Example 20 by around age 2;6. In Inuktitut, the earliest uses of analytic causatives tend to be in fixed forms involving a politeness marker and a small selection of imperative affixes, with or without a verb root. Examples such as those in 22 are typical.

(22a) *Tilauruk.*
tit-lauq-guk
CAUS-POL-IMP.2sS.3sO
"(You) make it do X." (Lizzie 2;6)
(e.g., asking father to remove her sock)

(22b) *Takutilaunnga.*
taku-tit-lauq-nnga
see-CAUS-POL-IMP.2sS.1sO
"(You) make me see." (Elijah 2;0)
(e.g., wanting to be lifted up to the window to see outside)

By slightly older ages, children begin using causative morphology in declarative structures such as those in Example 23.

(23a) *Uqrutillagu?*
uqru-tit-lagu
fall-CAUS-IMP.1sS.3sO

"Should I make it fall over?"   (Elijah 2;5)
(threatening to tip over a chair that he has been rocking)

(23b) *Panik, itsivatitait.*
panik itsiva-tit-jait
daughter sit-CAUS-PAR.2sS.3sO
"Daughter, you made it sit."   (Paul 3;3)
(telling his playmate that she made a doll sit down)

One of the most interesting findings about the acquisition of causatives crosslinguistically is that children in many languages tend to overgeneralize their use of the lexical causative to verbs that do not permit a lexical causative use (e.g., Bowerman, 1974). Inuktitut-speaking children also seem to do this, as indicated in Example 24.

(24) *Kutsuniarakkit.*
kutsuk-niaq-gakkit
chew.gum-FUT-CSV.1sS.2sO
"I will chew you after." [= I will make you chew after.]
    (Louisa 3;3)
(offering to give her playmate some gum that she could
    later chew)

One child also seemed to go through a stage in which she overgeneralized the lexical causative in some instances with a certain verb root (Example 25a) and correctly produced that same verb root with a causative morpheme in other instances (Example 25b).

(25a) *Ijukkasijara.*
ijukkaq-si-jara
fall-PRES-PAR.1sS.3sO
"I'll fall it." [= "I'll make it fall."]   (Louisa 3;2)

(25b) *Ijukkatilauruk.*
ijukkaq-tit-lauq-guk
fall-CAUS-POL-IMP.2sS.3sO
"(You) make it fall."   (Louisa 3;2)

It is interesting to note that the use of the causative morpheme in fixed forms as well as the correct use of the causative morpheme with verb roots sometimes involved in overgeneralizations are all structures in which an imperative command is involved. By contrast, utterances in which the causative morpheme fails to appear are not commands. These observations lead to the hypothesis that in early Inuktitut the causative morpheme is integrally related to command contexts, and that only later do children learn that the causative morpheme can be used in other contexts including declaratives and interrogatives. Such an hypothesis would explain the lexical causative overgeneralizations found in the data as instances of incorrect omission of the causative morpheme in nonimperative contexts (Allen, 1995, 1996a). Interestingly, the children at the most advanced ages in our sample are no longer using causative morphology in any imperative structures, but rather only in declarative and interrogative structures. This phenomenon is unusual in comparison with adult language, as adults do use causative morphology in imperative structures as well as other structure types. This pattern may be a result of children overcompensating for their earlier use of causatives exclusively with imperatives or may simply be an artefact of the data set.

┗┓

SIGNIFICANCE OF INUKTITUT ACQUISITION RESEARCH TO LANGUAGE ACQUISITION THEORY

The information presented concerning Inuktitut language acquisition indicates that children learning Inuktitut follow a pattern of acquisition that is similar in many ways to patterns reported for the acquisition of English, the language to which it is being compared in this chapter. However, it also indicates that certain aspects of Inuktitut acquisition are different from those in English. Finally, certain patterns occur in Inuktitut that are either not relevant to or not found in English. This three-way result will likely occur with every pair of languages across which one compares acquisition patterns. However, it also reveals one of the most crucial aspects affecting the timing and patterning of language acquisition—the structure of the language in question. Much seminal work by Slobin (1973, 1982) and many others has already revealed language structure as an important influence in acquisition. Inuktitut is particularly significant in this regard, because it exhibits a number of features rare in languages on which acquisition research has been conducted. The most striking of these are rich inflection, polysynthesis, and ergativity. The relevance of each of these features is described next.

As discussed, both verbal and nominal inflectional paradigms in Inuktitut are extremely rich, giving information about each of case, modality, person, and number. Inflections are also required for a wider range of elements than is typical in most languages, including both subjects and objects of verbs and both unpossessed and possessed nouns. This richness of inflection provides fertile ground for a detailed study of the acquisition of inflection in Inuktitut. Early presence of inflection could be interpreted as strong evidence for the early existence of functional categories in this language, adding to crosslinguistic evidence pointing in this direction (e.g., Deprez & Pierce, 1994; Hyams, 1992). Research on the two-morpheme stage in Inuktitut described here is a step in this direction. An additional interest about argument structure is the way in which children use verbal inflection to determine the argument structure of verbs in Inuktitut. Given the prevalent ellipsis of full NP and demonstrative overt arguments in Inuktitut, children must make much more use of inflections to determine argument structure in comparison with children learning English, for example, to the extent that they use morphosyntactic rather than semantic means to determine argument structure (Pinker, 1989). Finally, research on specific language impairment in Inuktitut indicates that verbal inflection is an area of particular vulnerability for at least one child with language impairment (Crago & Allen, 1996a).

Polysynthetic languages offer a rich and almost totally unexplored source of data relevant to language acquisition. Relatively little is known about the acquisition of word-internal morphology and even less about the effect of this type of morphological structure on the timing of acquisition of grammatical elements expressed in this way. Research on the acquisition of passives in Inuktitut indicates that polysynthetic structure may facilitate acquisition in certain ways, as passives are learned earlier in Inuktitut than in English. On the other hand, no such facilitating effect is apparent for the the acquisition of causatives. Further revealing work might be in the domain of negation or tense, both of which are primarily expressed morphologically in Inuktitut. Also of interest would be the acquisition of structures surrounding some verbs taking clausal complements which are expressed as word-internal morphemes in Inuktitut but as independent verbs in English. One might hypothesize that such verbs expressed as bound morphemes in Inuktitut may be interpreted by children differently than in languages in which hierarchical clausal structure is more visible. Finally, any polysynthetic language would provide data for research on morpheme segmentation abilities in the language learner (Allen, 1996b; Peters, 1983, 1985). Research in Mohawk, another polysynthetic language, suggests that segmentation in that language occurs initially on a syllabic rather than morphemic basis (Mithun, 1989), although this pattern has not been observed in Inuktitut to date.

A final potential contribution of Inuktitut acquisition data is in the area of the acquisition of ergativity. Though relatively little research has been reported about the acquisition of ergative languages, such research could reveal a great deal about the way children are able to use the case system of a language to derive further information about that language. It will be intriguing to discover how children learn to group subjects and objects in ergative or accusative patterns and whether learners make revealing errors at the earliest stages. Inuktitut is particularly interesting for this, because the ergative pattern is only really visible in the nominal case system; the verbal cross-referencing inflections constitute portmanteau morphemes that reveal little of the ergative structure. To date, no research explicitly addressing the effect of ergativity on language acquisition has been undertaken in Inuktitut.

ᓕ

CHARTING A FUTURE COURSE

Despite the enormous social and theoretical importance of a language such as Inuktitut, the future for its acquisition is not easy to discern. Dorais (1992b) predicted that the percentage of speakers of Inuit languages in Canada would drop from 74% in 1981 to 55% in 1992. This continuing process of erosion is due to the long-term effects of second-language exposure, reduced geographic isolation, and the profound effects of second-language media. As the percentage of speakers drop, the percentage of children acquiring a language also decreases. Even if schools and institutions create strong educational language policies, these cannot correct for homes and/or daycare centers where adults cannot or do not systematically expose their preschool children to their indigenous language. There are also indications that parents in Inuit communities can be complacent and overly optimistic about the future of their language (Crago, Genesee, & Allen, 1996; Taylor & Wright, 1989).

Finally, as Arctic communities become more ethnically and linguistically mixed, there are increasing numbers of Inuit children acquiring two languages, both sequentially and simultaneously. Their acquisitional patterns and the language use patterns in their homes and communities have become important to document for both theoretical and practical purposes (Crago, Allen, et al., 1996; Crago, Genesee, et al., 1996). In some Inuit communities, code switching and code mixing become the norm among children who grow up with blended identities, both linguistically and ethnically. Language shifts such as these are a part of a complex process of cultural evolution, a process that can imply creative change as well as loss (Duranti, Ochs, & Ta'ase, 1995; Heath, 1994; Kulick, 1992). Charting a course into the next century will be challenging for speakers of the Inuit languages. Close documentation of the process should help to inform the choices to be made and the directions to be taken.

⌐ᴸ

ACKNOWLEDGMENTS

As in all our work, our greatest debt is to the Inuit children, their families, and teachers who participated in our research. In addition we thank our colleagues, Lizzie Ningiuruvik, Betsy Annahatak, Doris Winkler, Alice Eriks-Brophy, Diane Pesco, and Wendy Hough-Eyamie for their good counsel and collaboration. The research reported here was funded by the Kativik School Board, the Social Sciences and Humanities Research Council of Canada, and the Toronto Hospital for Sick Children.

⌐ᴸ

REFERENCES

Allen, S. E. M. (1989). Preschool language acquisition of Inuktitut: A case study of one Inuk boy. In J. F. Basinger & W. O. Kupsch (Eds.), *Student research in Canada's North: Proceedings of the Second National Student Conference on Northern Studies. Musk-Ox, 37,* 159–167.

Allen, S. E. M. (1995). Acquisition of causatives in Inuktitut. In E. V. Clark (Ed.), *Proceedings of the 27th Stanford Child Language Research Forum* (pp. 51–60). Stanford, CA: Center for Study of Language and Information.

Allen, S. E. M. (1996a). *Aspects of argument structure acquisition in Inuktitut.* Amsterdam: John Benjamins.

Allen, S. E. M. (1996b). *Assessing productivity in acquisition data from polysynthetic languages.* Paper presented at the Seventh International Congress on the Study of Child Language, Istanbul, Turkey.

Allen, S. E. M., & Crago, M. B. (1989). Acquisition of noun incorporation in Inuktitut. *Papers and Reports on Child Language Development, 28,* 49–56.

Allen, S. E. M., & Crago, M. B. (1992). First language acquisition of Inuktitut. In M. J. Dufour & F. Therien (Eds.), *Looking to the future: Papers from the Seventh Inuit Studies Conference* [Inuit Studies Occasional Papers 4] (pp. 273–281). Quebec, QC: Association Inuksiutiit Katimajiit.

Allen, S. E. M., & Crago, M. B. (1996). Early passive acquisition in Inuktitut. *Journal of Child Language, 23,* 129–155.

Allen, S. E. M., & Schröder, H. (in press). Preferred argument structure in early Inuktitut spontaneous speech data. In J. W. Du Bois, L. E. Kumpf, & W. J. Ashby (Eds.), *Preferred argument structure: Grammar as architecture for function.* Amsterdam: John Benjamins.

Baldie, B. J. (1976). The acquisition of the passive voice. *Journal of Child Language, 3,* 331–348.

Bowerman, M. (1974). Learning the structure of causative verbs: A study in the relationship of cognitive, semantic and syntactic development. *Papers and Reports on Child Language Development, 8,* 142–178.

Brown, R. (1973). *A first language: The early stages.* Cambridge: Harvard University Press.

Chafe, W. L. (1987). Cognitive constraints on information flow. In R. Tomlin (Ed.), *Coherence and grounding in discourse* (pp. 21–51). Amsterdam: John Benjamins.

Clancy, P. (1980). Referential choice in English and Japanese narrative discourse. In W. L. Chafe (Ed.), *The Pear stories: Cognitive, cultural, and linguistic aspects of narrative production* (pp. 127–202). Norwood, NJ: Ablex.

Clancy, P. (1993). Preferred argument structure in Korean acquisition. In E. V. Clark (Ed.), *Proceedings of the 25th Annual Child Language Research Forum* (pp. 307–314). Stanford, CA: Center for Study of Language and Information.

Crago, M. B. (1988). *Cultural context in communicative interaction of Inuit children.* Unpublished doctoral dissertation, McGill University, Montreal, QC.

Crago, M. B. (1992). Communicative interaction and second language acquisition: An Inuit example. *TESOL Quarterly, 26,* 487–505.

Crago, M. B. (1995). *From two morphemes to passive constructions in Inuktitut: Issues of variability in acquisition.* Colloquium presented at the Linguistics Department, Lund University, Lund, Sweden.

Crago, M. B., & Allen, S. E. M. (1996a). Building the case for impairment in linguistic representation. In M. L. Rice (Ed.), *Toward a genetics of language* (pp. 261–289). Mahwah, NJ: Lawrence Erlbaum.

Crago, M. B., & Allen, S. E. M. (1996b). *Linguistic and cultural aspects of simplicity and complexity in Inuktitut (Eskimo) child-directed speech.* Paper presented at the Twenty-First Annual Boston University Conference on Language Development, Boston.

Crago, M. B., Allen, S. E. M., & Genesee, F. H. (1996). *Two languages, two morphemes: Bilingual acquisition as a source of information about early language development.* Paper presented at the Tenth Biennial International Conference on Infant Studies, Brown University, Providence, RI.

Crago, M. B., Allen, S. E. M., & Hough-Eyamie, W. P. (1997). Exploring innateness through cultural and linguistic variation. In M. Gopnik (Ed.), *The inheritance and innateness of grammars.* Oxford: Oxford University Press.

Crago, M. B., Annahatak, B., & Ningiuruvik, L. (1993). Changing patterns of language socialization in Inuit homes. *Anthropology and Education Quarterly, 24*, 205–223.

Crago, M. B., & Eriks-Brophy, A. (1993a). Culture, conversation and the co-construction of interaction: Implications and applications for intervention. In J. Duchan, L. Hewitt, C. Reynolds, & R. Sonnenmeier (Eds.), *Pragmatics: From theory to therapy* (pp. 43–58). Englewood Cliffs, NJ: Prentice-Hall.

Crago, M. B., & Eriks-Brophy, A. (1993b). Feeling right: Approaches to a family's culture. *Volta Review, 95*(5), 123–129.

Crago, M., Eriks-Brophy, A., Pesco, D., & McAlpine, L. (1997). Culturally-based miscommunication in classroom interaction. *Language, Speech and Hearing Services in the Schools, 28*, 245–254.

Crago, M. B., Genesee, F. H., & Allen, S. E. M. (1996). *Decision making and dilemmas in bilingual Inuit homes.* Paper presented at the Tenth Inuit Studies Conference, Memorial University, St. John's, NF.

Demuth, K. (1990). Subject, topic and Sesotho passive. *Journal of Child Language, 17*(1), 67–84.

Deprez, V., & Pierce, A. (1994). Crosslinguistic evidence for functional projections in early child grammar. In T. Hoekstra & B. Schwartz (Eds.), *Language acquisition studies in generative grammar* (pp. 57–84). Amsterdam: John Benjamins.

Dorais, L. J. (1988). *Tukilik: An Inuktitut grammar for all.* Quebec, QC: Association Inuksiutiit Katimajiit.

Dorais, L. J. (1990). *Inuit uqausiqatigiit: Inuit languages and dialects.* Iqaluit, NWT: Arctic College (Nunatta Campus).

Dorais, L. J. (1992a). Les langues autochtones d'hier à aujourd'hui. In J. Maurais (Ed.). *Les langues autochtones du Québec* (pp. 63–113). Québec, QC: Publications du Québec.

Dorais, L. J. (1992b). La situation linguistique dans l'arctique. *Inuit Studies, 16*, 237–255.

DuBois, J. W. (1987). The discourse basis of ergativity. *Language, 63*, 805–855.

Duranti, A., Ochs, E., & Ta'ase, E. K. (1995). Change and tradition in literacy instruction in a Samoan American community. *Educational Foundations, 3,* 57–74.

Eriks-Brophy, A. (1992). *The transformation of classroom discourse: An Inuit example.* Unpublished master's thesis, McGill University, Montreal, QC.

Eriks-Brophy, A. (1997). *Instructional discourse of Inuit and non-Inuit teachers of Nunavik.* Unpublished doctoral dissertation, McGill University, Montreal, QC.

Eriks-Brophy, A., & Crago, M. B. (1993). Inuit efforts to maintaining face: Elements from classroom discourse with Inuit children. *American Speech-Language and Hearing Association Monographs, 30,* 10–16.

Eriks-Brophy, A., & Crago, M. B. (1994). Transforming classroom discourse: An Inuit example. *Language and Education, 8*(3), 105–122.

Fortescue, M. (1985). Learning to speak Greenlandic: A case study of a two-year-old's morphology in a polysynthetic language. *First Language, 5,* 101–114.

Fortescue, M., & Lennert Olsen, L. (1992). The acquisition of West Greenlandic. In D. I. Slobin (Ed.), *The crosslinguistic study of language acquisition* (Vol. 3, pp. 111–220). Hillsdale, NJ: Lawrence Erlbaum.

Foster, M. (1982). Indigenous languages: Present and future. *Language and Society, 7,* 7–14.

Gordon, P., & Chafetz, J. (1990). Verb-based versus class-based accounts of actionality effects in children's comprehension of passives. *Cognition, 36,* 227–254.

Heath, S. B. (1983). *Ways with words: Language, life and work in communities and classrooms.* Cambridge, UK: Cambridge University Press.

Heath, S. B. (1994). *Cracks in the mirror: Class, gender, and ethnicity in multicultural education.* Paper presented at the annual meeting of the American Educational Research Association, New Orleans.

Hough-Eyamie, W. P. (1993). *A microanalytic analysis of caregiver-child interaction: An Inuit example.* Unpublished master's thesis, McGill University, Montreal, QC.

Hough-Eyamie, W. P., Pan, B., Crago, M. B., & Snow, C. (in preparation). A cross-cultural comparison of caregiver-child interaction.

Hyams, N. (1992). The genesis of clausal structure. In J. M. Meisel (Ed.), *The acquisition of verb placement: Functional categories and V2 phenomena in language acquisition* (pp. 371–400). Dordrecht: Kluwer.

Kulick, D. (1992). *Language shift and cultural reproduction: Socialization, self, and syncretism in a Papua New Guinean village.* Cambridge, UK: Cambridge University Press.

Mehan, H. (1979). *Learning lessons.* Cambridge, MA: Harvard University Press.

Mithun, M. (1989). The acquisition of polysynthesis. *Journal of Child Language, 16,* 285–312.

Nelson, K. (1973). Structure and strategy in learning to talk. *Monographs of the Society for Research in Child Development, 38.*

Peters, A. M. (1983). *The units of language acquisition.* New York: Cambridge University Press.

Peters, A. M. (1985). Language segmentation: Operating principles for the perception and analysis of language. In D. I. Slobin (Ed.), *The crosslinguistic study of language acquisition* (Vol. 2, pp. 1029–1067). Hillsdale, NJ: Lawrence Erlbaum.

Pinker, S. (1989). *Learnability and cognition: The acquisition of argument structure.* Cambridge, MA: MIT Press.

Pinker, S., Lebeaux, D., & Frost, L. A. (1987). Productivity and constraints in the acquisition of the passive. *Cognition, 26,* 195–267.

Schieffelin, B. B., & Eisenberg, A. (1984). Cultural variation in children's conversations. In R. L. Schiefelbusch & J. Pickar (Eds.), *The acquisition of communicative competence* (pp. 377–422). Baltimore: University Park Press.

Slobin, D. I. (1973). Cognitive prerequisites for the development of grammar. In C. A. Ferguson & D. I. Slobin (Eds.), *Studies of child language development.* New York: Holt, Rinehart & Winston.

Slobin, D. I. (1982). Universal and particular in the acquisition of language. In E. Wanner & L. R. Gleitman (Eds.), *Language acquisition: The state of the art* (pp. 128–172). Cambridge, UK: Cambridge University Press.

Taylor, D., & Wright, S. (1989). Language attitudes in a multilingual northern community. *The Canadian Journal of Native Studies, 9,* 85–119.

Wang, Q., Lillo-Martin, D., Best, C. T., & Levitt, A. (1992). Null subject versus null object: Some evidence from the acquisition of Chinese and English. *Language Acquisition, 2,* 221–254.

Wilman, D. (1988). *The natural language of Inuit children: The key to Inuktitut literacy.* Unpublished doctoral dissertation, University of New Mexico, Albuquerque.

MARTHA B. CRAGO, Ph.D.

Martha B. Crago, Ph.D., is an Associate Professor in Communication Sciences and Disorders and the Associate Vice-Principal (Graduate Studies) at McGill University. Her research and publications span a variety of issues in child language development, including language socialization, language acquisition, and language impairment. Dr. Crago's research includes work with monolingual, bilingual, typically developing children and children with language impairment who speak English and/or French or Inuktitut. Her work appears in a number of journal articles and book chapters.

SHANLEY E. M. ALLEN, Ph.D.

Shanley E. M. Allen, Ph.D., received her bachelor's degree in Hispanic Studies and her doctorate in Linguistics from McGill University. She is currently a Research Fellow at the Max Planck Institute for Psycholinguistics in the Netherlands. Dr. Allen's primary research interests include the language learning of monolingual and bilingual Inuit children, with a focus on morphology, syntax, and argument structure.

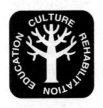

CHAPTER 9

ACQUISITION OF KOREAN

SOONJA CHOI, Ph.D.

Recent surveys show that the Korean immigrant population in the United States has grown steadily during the past 10 years—about half a million now—and that Koreans now occupy a significant portion (about 17%) of the Asian/Pacific population in this country (Cheng & Chang, 1995; Park, 1983; U.S. Bureau of Census, 1997). As many Korean families come to work and reside in this country, the number of young children who speak Korean in this country also grows. In fact, the Korean language is reported to be one of the top 10 languages spoken in the school system in several major cities (Cheng & Chang, 1995; U.S. Bureau of Census, 1997).

Korean immigrant families in the U.S. tend to live in clusters and form rather closed monolingual communities. Most of their social life stays within the Korean community: They interact with other Korean families most of the time and many of them go to Korean churches on Sundays (Chu, 1993; E. Kim, 1984). In these communities, immigrant parents raise their children monolingually, using only Korean in the home. In these families, it is also likely that children have more social contacts with Korean-speaking peers than English-speaking peers. Thus, even though Korean children in immigrant homes may be born in the United States, they may acquire the Korean grammar as their first language (L1) during the first 3 or 4 years of their life (until they go to an English-speaking school). Even when they go to an English-speaking school and learn English at a fast rate, their parents continue to speak Korean at home. Thus, these children are exposed to the Korean language and culture consistently in their home and community.

Chu (1993) pointed out that, although Korean children of immigrant parents get exposure to English mainly through media such as television, radio, and magazines, such exposure may not lead to an adequate development of communicative competence. He recommends that teachers be sensitive to these environmental factors in assessing the English skills of Korean children. In particular, Chu states that the English language skills of Korean students should be carefully assessed given linguistic and cultural differences between English-speaking and Korean-speaking children (p. 30).

This chapter reports some aspects of the acquisition of Korean as L1 and compares them, whenever possible, with the acquisition of English. It is hoped that this report will contribute to a better understanding of similarities and differences between the acquisition of English and Korean and that it provides useful information to both educators and clinicians in assessing the language development of children from a Korean background.

⊐

THEORIES OF THE RELATIONS BETWEEN LANGUAGE AND COGNITION

Learning a language means learning systematic relations between form and meaning at all levels of grammar: phonology, morphology, semantics, syntax, and discourse. To the extent that grammars differ significantly across languages (cf. Bowerman & Pederson, 1992; Whorf, 1956), learning a language includes discovering the kinds of meaning the target language systematically encodes and the particular forms it uses to express them. For example, the child needs to discover what kinds of temporal notions are systematically encoded in the target language. Thus, a child acquiring English must discover that it encodes past and present in a systematic way and that the notion of past is expressed by the suffix -ed (e.g., I want-ed), whereas the notion of present is expressed by a zero morpheme (e.g., I want-0). Although the task seems enormous, it is well known that normal children complete a significant portion of this task within a few years from birth: Children start saying their first words at around 12 to 18 months, and by 3 or 4 years of age, they have acquired the basic grammar of the language. How do children accomplish this task within such a short period of time?

Over the last few decades, largely influenced by Chomsky (1965), language acquisition research has largely been directed toward the discovery of universals of language acquisition. More specifically, the view has been that much of the linguistic structure (called the language acquisition device, or LAD) is prewired in an infant's brain before exposure to language-specific input. An earlier version of the LAD theory was that a particular linguistic structure was innate and thus shared by all children. Research in the 1970s focused on identifying the precise nature of that innate structure. However, as more and more syntactic and morphological variations across languages were reported, a new version of the LAD, namely, parameter setting theory has been proposed to accommodate such variations (Hyams, 1986; Roeper & Williams, 1987). According to parameter setting theory, children are born with the capacity to set the correct parameter of the language they are learning after minimal exposure to language input. For example, children learning Italian must set the parameter to the "pro-drop" setting (indicating that subject pronouns can be deleted), whereas children learning English must set the parameter to the non-pro-drop setting (indicating that subject pronouns cannot be deleted) (Hyams, 1986).

Such a universalist approach to language acquisition has also been predominant in research on the relation between language and cognition. Following a Piagetian view, the hypothesis has been that language development is guided and also constrained by universal cognitive development. More specifically, during the first year of life before children begin to produce language, children develop a number of important nonlinguistic concepts, such as agency, causality, and various spatial relations. According to this view, the initial stage of learning a language involves mapping linguistic forms onto these nonlinguistic cognitive concepts. For example, in acquiring words, such as in and on in English, children simply map the words onto the conceptual categories of containment and support that are nonlinguistically established (Clark, 1973; Johnston & Slobin, 1979). According to this view, language is acquired rapidly, because the foundations for the acquisition of the semantic system is already in place when children are ready to acquire language.

Following this tradition, several lexical-learning principles have been proposed in recent years to account for the rapid growth of vocabulary learning in the early years (i.e., five words a day between 2 and 7 years of age [Carey, 1978]). For example, according to the whole-object constraint (Markman, 1989), children are constrained to interpret words as referring to a whole object and not to any of its parts. This constraint would help children identify the referent of a word in an efficient way. Another constraint that gained much attention in recent years is the shape-bias theory (Landau, Smith, & Jones, 1988). According to this theory, children are constrained to consider shape as the critical semantic feature of object words.

In some sense, all of these proposals supporting "the cognitive primacy view" consider children to be rather passive learners, as they are constrained in making hypotheses and they simply need to link linguistic forms to concepts that have been established prelinguistically. Such a universalist view also predicts that children learning different languages show similarities during the initial stage of language learning, as they start language learning with prelinguistically determined cognitive concepts.

However, a serious weakness in many of the mentioned studies is that they are based on data from one language, namely English. To test the universality of the claims made, then, crosslinguistic studies are needed. During the past few years, several studies have been conducted examining early lexical and morphosyntactic development in different languages (Choi & Bowerman, 1991; Choi & Gopnik, 1995; Clancy, 1996; de Leon, 1996; Tardif, 1996). These studies showed evidence that children are sensitive to the language-specific properties of the L1 grammar from the beginning of language acquisition. These studies also suggested that children are sensitive to language-specific input at a much earlier age than previously thought, and that the acquisition of the L1 grammar is accomplished through children's interactions with caregivers.

To understand the extent to which language-specific input and universal cognition contribute to language acquisition, one must conduct systematic comparisons of children learning very different grammars. Korean is a good language to study, because its grammar is significantly different from English in several ways. In the following, I first describe some basic grammatical aspects of Korean, focusing on those that differ significantly from English. Then, in the remainder of the chapter, I present acquisition data for Korean.

ᄀ

KOREAN GRAMMAR

WORD ORDER AND CASE MARKERS

The word order of a language is an important grammatical aspect that determines the type of language to which it belongs. In English, the word order is subject-verb-object (SVO) as shown in Example 1.

(1) *Mary pushed Paul.*
   subject-verb-object

In English, the SVO word order is strictly observed in both spoken and written forms. Thus, a change in word order will result in ungrammaticality or incorrect interpretation. For example, placing the verb before the subject, as in *Pushed Mary Paul* is ungrammatical. Also, a change in the positions of noun arguments results in different meanings. That is, *Paul pushed Mary* means something quite different from *Mary pushed Paul:* In the former sentence, *Paul* is the agent of the action whereas in the latter sentence, *Mary* is the agent.

   Korean differs from English in three ways: the word order, degree of its flexibility, and case marking system. First, Korean is a verb-final language: The main verb typically occurs at the end of a sentence as in Example 2.

(2) *Mary-ka Paul-ul mil-ess-ta.*
   Mary-NOM Paul-ACC push-PAST-DECL[1]
   "Mary pushed Paul."

As shown in Example 2, the canonical word order in Korean is subject-object-verb (SOV). However, Korean allows flexibility in word order, particularly in informal speech. For example, one can highlight or emphasize a noun argument by putting it in either the beginning or the final position in the sentence, as in Example 3, or by repeating it after the verb as in Example 4.

---

[1] The following abbreviations are used in this chapter: ACC: accusative case; CONN: connective; DECL: declarative ending; DO: direct object; GL: goal; HON: honorific; IO: indirect object; LOC: locative; NOM: nominative case; PAST: past; PRES: present; POSS: possessive; MOD: modal; SUBJ: subject; and TOP: topic.

TABLE 9–1

Major casemarkers and their grammatical functions in Korean.

Casemarkers	Function
-i/ka	Subject
-un/nun	Topic
-ul/lul	Direct object
-eykey	Indirect object, goal/animate
-ey	Goal/Inanimate, location (with stative verbs)
-eyse	Source, location (with activity verbs)
-ulo	Instrument
-uy	Possession

(3) *Paul-ul Mary-ka mil-ess-e.*
Paul-ACC Mary-NOM push-PAST-DECL
"Mary pushed Paul."

(4) *Mary-ka Paul-ul mil-ess-e Mary-ka.*
Mary-NOM Paul-ACC push-PAST-DECL Mary-NOM
"Mary pushed Paul."

The differences among sentences in Examples 2 through 4 lie in the pragmatic information about the noun arguments: whether they are given or new or foregrounded versus backgrounded in discourse. However, the semantic roles of the arguments (e.g., the agent, patient) remain the same in all three sentences. This is largely because noun arguments carry case markers that provide information about their grammatical relation to the verb. The subject of the sentence typically takes the nominative casemarker, -ka (or -i if the noun ends with a consonant), and the direct object takes the accusative casemarker -lul (or -ul after a consonant). As shown in Table 9–1, distinct case markers are used to indicate indirect object, goal, source, location, and so on. Some of these markers also distinguish between animate and inanimate nouns, and between activity and stative verbs (Choi, 1993). Notice that, unlike the case marking system in Indo-European languages, the case markers in Korean do not mark gender or number of the noun.

In informal spoken discourse, some of these case markers are optional. Clancy (1995) and Y. Kim (1997) reported that among the case markers, the accusative case marker *-lul* is one of the most often deleted. Probably because of the lower frequency of this form in the input, Korean children acquire the accusative marker later than the nominative marker (Clancy, 1995).

Although Korean allows flexibility in word order, the predominant order in spoken form is verb-final. For example, in caregivers' speech to children, 90% of Korean mothers' utterances are verb-final (Choi, 1996; Y. Kim 1997). Thus, children hear verbs in sentence-final position most of the time. According to Slobin's operating principles (1973), this position is perceptually the most salient in the sentence, and children acquire the items occurring in this position earlier than those occurring elsewhere in a sentence.

VERB MORPHOLOGY

As we will see, many of the characteristic features of Korean relate to verbs. In Korean, the grammatical morphemes on the verb are suffixed in an agglutinative fashion, and, thus, are easily segmentable. These morphemes encode deference, tense, aspect, and modality as shown in Example 5.

(5) *Sensayngnim-i haksayng-eykey chayk-ul cwu-si-ess-ta.*
teacher-SUBJ student-IO book-DO give-HON-PAST-MOD
"The teacher gave a book to the student."

These inflections occur in a particular order. The verb stem (e.g., *cwu-* "give") is first followed by the honorific marker *-si-*, if the subject is older and/or of a higher rank than the speaker. The honorific marker is then followed by a tense/aspectual marker. In Example 5, *-ess-* is the past tense morpheme. The last morpheme is a sentence-ending (SE) suffix that expresses mood and modality of various kinds (H. Lee, 1991). About 20 different SE suffixes are freely used in this position in spontaneous speech. Appropriate uses of these suffixes require attention to the discourse pragmatics such as new or old information, shared or inferred information. (See the section on early acquisition of modality.) Sentences in Example 6 show the most frequently used SE modal suffixes along with the corresponding modal meaning.

(Modal meanings)
(6) *halmeni-ka aki-lul anu-si-ess-e.*   (well-established info.)
    "   "   *-ta.*   (new noteworthy info.)

"	"	"	*-ci.*	(certain/shared info.)
"	"	"	*-tay.*	(hearsay)
"	"	"	*-ney.*	(witnessed info.)

grandmother-SUBJ baby-DO hold-HON-PAST-MOD
"The grandmother held the baby."

The suffix *-e* occurs most frequently, expressing that the information conveyed is well-established in the speaker's mind. In H. Lee's (1991) speech sample of adult speakers, *-e* occurs in 58% of utterances. Thus, it is considered as an unmarked form. Other suffixes are used to denote more specific epistemic/evidential meanings. For example, *-ta* is used to convey that the information is newly perceived and noteworthy (H. Lee, 1993). The suffix *-ci* expresses that the information is certain and/or shared with the listener. These modal suffixes occur with all types of verbs: Activity verbs like *mek-*"eat," and stative/adjectival verbs like *coh-*"like."

It should be pointed out that the kinds of notions that the verb morphology encodes in Korean are distinct from those in Romance languages, such as Spanish and Italian. Whereas in Romance languages, verb morphology carries information about the person and number of the subject, in Korean it does not. Rather, Korean verb morphology encodes the relationship between the speaker and the subject of the sentence (i.e., presence or absence of the honorifics) and the discourse status of information expressed by the sentence.

SYNTAX AND DISCOURSE STRUCTURE

Discourse plays an important role in Korean in at least two ways. First, unlike English, which is a subject-prominant language, Korean is a topic-prominant language. It has a distinct marker, namely *-un/-nun* (cf. Table 9–1), that specifies the discourse topic at the sentential level. In Korean, sentences in discourse are typically organized in terms of discourse topic (H. Kim, 1989). That is, discourse topic predominantly serves as the subject of the sentence. Second, noun arguments (e.g., subject and object of a sentence) can be deleted if they are retrievable from prior discourse. The presence or absence of a noun argument is governed by various discourse factors, such as givenness and topic continuity (Clancy, 1997; H. Kim, 1989). Kim's (1989) analysis on spoken narratives in Korean shows that the discourse topic is typically a human character and it occupies the subject position of the sentence. Once a human referent is introduced as topic with a full noun phrase in discourse, subsequent mentions of the referent is realized by ellipsis (i.e., zero anaphora) as shown in Example 7.

(7) *(7)Younghi-nun hakkyo-ey ka-taka, ton-ul kil-eyse palkyenha-ko, kyungchalse-ey kotpalo ka- ss-ta.*
Younghi-TOP school-GL go-while, money-DO street-LOC discover-CON, police-GL directly go-PAST-DECL
"While Younghi was on the way to school, (she) saw money on the street, and so (she) directly went to the police."

Studies show that Korean children are sensitive to these discourse characteristics from a very young age: Clancy (1997), who studied young Korean children's discourse patterns during interaction with their caregivers, found that 2-year-olds use noun ellipsis in a systematic way that is motivated by discourse pragmatic factors such as givenness and topic continuity. (See the section on transitive and intransitive verbs for more detail.)

So far, I have described a number of characteristic aspects of Korean grammar that differ from English. The developmental patterns of these grammatical aspects will give us some information about how language-specific features influence the early acquisition of Korean.

卐

ACQUISITION OF KOREAN

The present discussion of the acquisition of Korean focuses on verbs, as they represent a grammatical area that differs from English in a significant and interesting way. Furthermore, recent studies in linguistics show that verbs play a central role in child and adult grammars (Gleitman, 1990; Levin, 1985). Here, I examine four aspects of verb acquisition in Korean: verbs versus nouns in early lexicons, development of verb semantics, morphology, and syntax.

In examining the developmental patterns in the acquisition of Korean, I bring up several issues currently being actively debated in the language acquisition literature and present relevant Korean acquisition data. In particular, I critically evaluate the theories that claim universality by examining whether Korean data are compatible with such theories.

EARLY LEXICONS

THEORIES OF THE ACQUISITION OF NOUNS AND VERBS

Over the last two decades, a number of studies on early words in English acquisition have supported the view that nouns are acquired earlier than verbs. This view is based on two types of data: (1) At around 18 months, many children go through a period of vocabulary spurt and the majority of the lexical items involved in this spurt are nouns (Goldfield & Reznick, 1990; Halliday, 1975; McShane, 1980; Nelson, 1973), and (2) nouns represent the predominant category in early lexicons (e.g., the first 100 words; Bates et al., 1994).

In 1982, Gentner wrote an influential paper showing that the phenomenon of noun primacy in early lexicons is not restricted to English, but is universal. She concluded this on the basis of a crosslinguistic survey of previously collected data (acquired between 12 and 30 months of age). The crosslinguistic data came from various sources, data collected from different researchers who used different methods for recording children's early words. Also, the children were at varying developmental stages, with ages ranging from 14 to 29 months. The survey showed that nouns formed the majority of words in early lexicons (50–85%), whereas verbs/predicates represented only only a small portion (0–35%). Gentner (1982) thus proposed that nouns are universally acquired earlier than verbs. She provided some possible explanations for such universality, such as concrete nouns refer to cohesive perceptual entities that typically belong to natural categories. That is, categories such as apples and bananas for fruits, and cats and dogs for animals, form natural categories that are universal at the basic level. Furthermore, these nouns usually refer to whole objects that children have previously isolated perceptually from their surroundings. On the other hand, verb meanings are not so obvious by mere perception. For example, the verb *run* in English refers to only certain aspects of an action, namely the manner of motion. On the other hand, the verb *enter* refers to the path of motion and not to its manner. Furthermore, languages differ in the kinds of aspects they encode in the main verb. For example, English considers manner of motion to be an important aspect for encoding the main verb, as in *John ran into the room,* whereas Spanish considers its path to be the important aspect to encode in the main verb, as in *Juan entró al cuarto.* According to Gentner, as noun categories are universal and natural, children do not have to rely much on language-specific input to acquire these categories. Thus, nouns are quite accessible early. On the other hand, verbs are language-specific—therefore, children need a certain amount of language-specific input to acquire their meanings. Thus, learning verbs is posited as taking more time than learning nouns.

The phenomenon of early acquisition of nouns found in English, also known as the "noun bias," motivated several researchers to investigate the underlying principles of lexical learning. As mentioned earlier, several proposals have been made to date: Markman (1989) has proposed that when young children hear a word, they infer that it refers to the object and not to events and, furthermore, that it refers to the whole object and not to its parts. On the other hand, Landau and her colleagues (Landau et al., 1988) proposed that children attend to the shape of objects when they learn object names.

Several recent studies, however, have challenged the assumption that children universally begin language learning by naming objects (Bloom, Tinker, & Margulis, 1993; Lieven, Pine, & Dresner Barnes, 1992; Nelson, Hampson, & Kessler Shaw, 1993). These studies have carefully examined the kinds of nouns English-speaking children acquire and have shown that some of the words counted as nouns in previous studies were ambiguous as to whether they refer to entities. For example, previous studies have included nonobject nouns, such as those referring to time (e.g., *birthday*) and place (e.g., *farm*), in the noun category. The recent studies that have distinguished such nouns from object nouns (i.e., words encoding basic-level object categories) showed that object nouns occupy less than 40% of the lexicon and, therefore, are not as predominant in early lexicons as previously thought (Bloom et al., 1993; Lieven et al., 1992; Nelson et al., 1993).

There is also evidence in the literature that children acquire relational words early. Bloom (1973) and Gopnik (1982, 1988) reported that children learning English produce non-nominal words that express various types of relational concepts (e.g., nonexistence, recurrence, success) from a very early stage. For example, 15- to 18-month-old English learners say *gone* when something has disappeared and *down* to encode downward motion (Gopnik, 1982). Furthermore, Gopnik reported that at this early stage children produce non-nominal words frequently and consistently when the appropriate context arises.

These studies on the acquisition of English suggested that object nouns are not as predominant in children's early words as previously thought and that a set of relational words are acquired from the one-word stage. It is important to note, however, that most of these early non-nominal/relational words in English are not verbs, but belong to a variety of grammatical categories, such as particles (*up, down*) and adverbs and adjectives (*there, more*). Indeed, when adult morphological criteria are applied, English-learners seem to acquire verbs later than nouns. But, the late acquisition of verbs in English may be the result of the specific grammar a child is learning. That is, in English, many of the early relational concepts are in fact encoded by a variety of grammatical categories.

The hypothesis that the late acquisition of verbs in English is a language-specific phenomenon is supported by a growing number of studies with children acquiring other languages. Tardif (1996) reported that children learning Mandarin Chinese acquire more verbs (i.e., action words) than nouns (i.e., object labels) during their single-word period. De León (1996) and Brown (1996) also reported that children learning Mayan languages, Tzotzil and Tzeltal, acquire a number of specific verbs with appropriate morphological endings from an early age. In my own studies with Gopnik (Choi & Gopnik, 1995; Gopnik & Choi, 1995), we found that Korean children start acquiring verbs as early as nouns.

EARLY LEXICAL DEVELOPMENT IN KOREAN

As discussed in the section on Korean grammar, the morphosyntax of verbs in Korean grammar is interestingly different from English. In particular, verbs in Korean have the following features that can promote saliency in the input: (1) Verbs typically occupy the salient sentence-final position in Korean; (2) verbs can occur alone as complete utterances, even in declarative sentences, as nominal arguments are often deleted when these are given/old information in discourse; and (3) verbs have a morphological unity in that they all occur with a modal suffix at the end of a sentence.[2] All of these features may facilitate the acquisition of verbs in Korean.

DATA SOURCES AND CODING. In collaboration with Alison Gopnik (at the University of California at Berkeley), I conducted a longitudinal study of lexical development in Korean. For the Korean study, I followed five monolingual subjects raised in Korean immigrant homes in the San Diego, CA, area. The parents of all five children were first-generation Korean immigrants and they spoke only Korean at home.

---

[2] This morphological transparency contrasts with English in which verbs often occur in bare forms, and depending on the type, different aspectual suffixes are attached to the verb. For example, whereas activity verbs (e.g., *play, eat*) occur with the progressive marker *-ing*, state verbs (e.g., *like, be*) do not.

The parents' social contacts (largely through Korean churches) were restricted to Korean families. All five mothers had graduated from college and were of lower-to-mid middle class. They worked in the home fulltime taking care of the children. At the time of the study, the children did not show any apparent hearing or cognitive disorders.

The language development of the five children was followed regularly from their first word (average age: 13 months) until they had acquired at least 150 words (average age: 24 months). During the study period, the children were visited once every 3 or 4 weeks for approximately 1 hour. At each visit, the mother reported on the child's language development by filling out a standardized questionnaire about the child's words acquired since the last visit. In addition, the child's spontaneous speech during his or her free play with the mother or the investigator was videorecorded for about 15 minutes (see Choi & Gopnik, 1995, for more detail). This combination of questionnaire and spontaneous speech was designed to elicit as much accurate information about the child's early language as possible (cf. Pine, Lieven, & Rowland, 1997).

In determining the lexical category of newly acquired words, both formal (i.e., morphosyntactic) and semantic criteria were considered. This largely follows Lieven et al. (1992) procedures (and also Bloom et al., 1993) for measuring lexical development in English. For nouns, the formal criterion was that the child's word form approximated the adults' conventional noun form. The semantic criterion was that the word referred to objects or people. One difference between Lieven et al. (1992, and also Bloom et al., 1993) and the present study was that, whereas Lieven and associates excluded kinship terms from their noun measures in the present study on Korean, kinship terms such as *emma* "mommy" and *appa* "daddy" were included. This is because, in Korean, kinship terms are readily generalizable to other nonrelated people. For example, *halmeni* "grandmother" is not only used for a child's own grandmother, but also for any elderly woman. However, following Lieven et al. (1992), proper names, such as *Mary* were excluded, as these refer to one specific individual and, thus, are not generalizable to other entities. Also, pronouns (e.g., *ike* "this") and onomatopoeic words (e.g., *ccaykccayk* "tweet tweet") were excluded. For verbs, the formal criteria were that they represented main verbs, and occurred with a sentence-ending (SE) modal suffix. As discussed in the section on Korean grammar (and also the section on early grammar), modal suffixes are characteristic and obligatory in Korean sentence-final verbs. The semantic criterion for verbs was that the word referred to an action/activity (e.g., *mekta* "to eat"), change of location (e.g., *kata* "to go"),

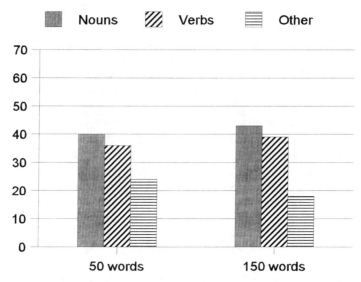

FIGURE 9–1
Proportions of nouns and verbs in Korean children in their first 50
and 150 words (*N* = 5).

change of state (e.g., *kkayta* "to wake up"), or state (e.g., *ipputa* "to be
pretty," *issta* "to be located/to exist") (*-ta* is a citation form). The stative/
adjectival verbs are morphosyntactically verbs in Korean as they inflect
in tense (past and future) and modality. The copula verb *-i-* and auxiliary verbs were excluded.

EARLY ACQUISITION OF VERBS IN KOREAN. The lexical development
data of the five children are shown in Figure 9–1. It shows the proportions of nouns and verbs in the children's lexicon at two different times:
(1) when they had acquired approximately 50 words (mean age: 19
months, 7 days), and (2) when they had acquired approximately 150
words (mean age: 24 months, 3 days). The figure shows that in the
children's first 50 words, on average, verbs constitute 36% and nouns
40% of their lexicons. At the 150-word mark, verbs represent 39% and
nouns 43% of the children's lexicons. These data show that verbs occupy a prominent position in the children's lexical development **along**

with nouns from at least the 50-word mark, and that the proportions of nouns and verbs are consistent over time.

Comparisons of these data with recent studies on English development show that, whereas the proportions of object nouns in early lexicons are similar between the two languages, those of verbs are not. More specifically, if we follow the noun criteria used in Lieven et al. (1992) by excluding kinship terms from the children's noun lexicons in Korean, the percentage of object nouns are 34% and 37% for the 50-word mark and the 150-word mark, respectively. These percentages are remarkably similar to those reported in recent studies for English learners (Bloom et al., 1993; Lieven et al., 1992; Nelson et al., 1993), which is between 33 and 39%. Thus, both Korean- and English-speaking children acquire object nouns to a similar degree. What is different in Korean from English, however, is that the majority of the non-nominal words are **verbs** in Korean, whereas in English they belong to a variety of grammatical classes (e.g., particles, prepositions, adjectives, adverbs). Bates et al. (1994) reported that in English verbs are almost nonexistent at the beginning (less than 10%) and increase only after the acquisition of 100 words. In contrast, the present Korean data show that verb is a predominant category (36–38% of the lexicon) from the beginning and it maintains the same proportion throughout the single-word period.[3]

Another striking difference between nouns and verbs in English and Korean is that all five Korean children showed a **verb spurt** about a month before their first noun spurt, that is acquisition of 10 new verbs during the 3–4-week interval between sessions. This type of verb spurt has never been reported in research on the acquisition of English.[4]

---

[3] Even if we exclude stative/adjectival verbs (which in English may be expressed by a copula and an adjective, e.g., "be pretty") from the Korean verb lexicon, the percentages do not change much: 35% and 33% at the 50 and 150 word marks, respectively. These percentages show that almost all the verbs during the first period were action or change of state/location verbs and that stative verbs gradually increased during the second period.

[4] The five children reported in this chapter are from a larger study whose goal was to follow children's development and track their cognitive development until their first noun spurt (Choi & Gopnik, 1995; Gopnik & Choi, 1995). The five children were observed for a longer period of time for our further investigation on language development beyond the first noun spurt period. Some of the children in the larger study did not show a verb spurt during the observation period (which ended when they first showed a noun spurt) or showed it one session after their first noun spurt. Thus, we found some individual differences in the timing of the verb spurt phenomenon.

In summary, early lexical development in Korean shows a significant difference from English in that, in Korean, verbs develop in parallel with nouns from the single-word period. Thus, these data do not support the claim that verbs are universally learned later than nouns and that they are less accessible than nouns to young children. Rather, my Korean data suggested that the late acquisition of verbs in English may be a language-specific phenomenon. In the next section, I examine caregivers' speech to children to identify possible sources of variation in the acquisition of verbs in Korean and English.

RELATION BETWEEN CAREGIVERS' INPUT AND THE EARLY ACQUISITION OF VERBS

As pointed out in the section on early lexical development of Korean, Korean grammar provides several morphosyntactic and perceptual advantages to learners for acquiring verbs early. For example, verbs occur at the ends of sentences or alone without nominal arguments. Studies of caregiver speech in Korean have shown that caregivers do, in fact, use verbs in these ways. Choi (1996) and also Y. Kim (1997) found that verbs occur sentence-finally in 90% of caregivers' speech, and Clancy (1996) found that the two Korean mothers in her study, on average, did not mention subject and object nouns about 30% of the time in their utterances with frequently-occurring verbs.

In addition to structural advantages, Korean caregivers may also provide semantic and pragmatic advantages helping Korean learners acquire verbs early. Choi and Gopnik (1995) and Gopnik & Choi (1995) compared semantic and pragmatic aspects of caregivers' speech in English and Korean. In that study, Korean-speaking and English-speaking mothers were asked to interact with their children (aged between 17 and 19 months) for 5 minutes with a set of toys and for another 5 minutes with two wordless books.

We conducted both lexical and pragmatic analyses on the caregivers' input. In our lexical analysis, we were interested not only in the overall frequency of nouns and verbs, but also the kinds of nouns and verbs the caregivers used. Adapting Maratsos' (1991) categories, we subcategorized nouns into object (e.g., *bed, car*) and nonobject (e.g., *way, household*) nouns, and verbs into action (e.g., *run*) and nonaction (e.g., *know*) verbs. The results are shown in Table 9–2. We found that English-speaking mothers produced significantly more object nouns (both in type and token) per utterance than Korean mothers. The pattern was reversed for action verbs: Korean mothers produced more action verb types and tokens per utterance than English-speaking

TABLE 9–2
Average number of nouns and verbs per 100 utterances in English-
and Korean-speaking caregivers' speech.

	Object Nouns		Non-Object Nouns		Total	
	Type*	**Token***	**Type**	**Token**	**type***	**token**
English	22.6	44.9	2.1	2.6	24.7	47.5
Korean	9.7	29.6	1.7	3.1	11.4	32.7
	Action Verbs		**Non-Action Verbs**		**Total**	
	Type**	**Token***	**Type***	**Token***	**type**	**token***
English	10.8	22.3	13.1	30.3	23.9	52.6
Korean	15.7	48.9	3.6	13.6	19.3	62.5

*p<.05, **p<.01, ***p<.001
(Statistical data relate to differences between English and Korean-speaking caregivers.)
Notes: Object Nouns refer to specific objects or people (e.g., ball, baby).
Non-Object Nouns include abstract nouns (e.g., opportunity), locative nouns (e.g.,
front), and nonspecific nouns (e.g., thing).
Action Verbs refer to specific action/activity (e.g., eat, put X in Y).
Non-Action Verbs include stative verbs (e.g., like, feel), mental verbs (e.g., think, know),
and attention-getting verbs (e.g., look, watch). Attention-getting verbs were used to
direct the child's attention either to an action or an object.

mothers. (This difference was consistent across caregivers.) However,
English-speaking mothers produced more nonaction verbs than Korean
mothers—specifically, they used significantly more attention-getting
verbs (e.g., see, look), and mental verbs such as know, think, guess.

A pragmatic analysis also shows a significant difference between
the two groups of mothers. In this analysis, utterances are coded as
naming or activity-oriented utterances. Utterances are coded as naming-
oriented when they encourage the child to name an object, such as
What is it? or label the object explicitly, such as That's a ball. Utterances
are coded as activity-oriented when they encourage the child to do
something, What are you doing? or explicitly describe the impending or
completed action, You put the car in the garage. We found that Korean
mothers produced activity-oriented utterances (48%) significantly more
often than naming-oriented ones (10%). They also did this significantly more often than English-speaking caregivers. In contrast, English-
speaking mothers produced naming-oriented utterances (21%) as often

as activity-oriented ones (25%) and they produced them significantly more often than the Korean mothers.

In summary, Korean learners receive different types of input than do English learners. Korean children hear verbs in a salient position, and they hear more action verbs and are more prompted to talk about action than English learners. These differential aspects of the input probably explain the differences in the acquisition of nouns and verbs in the two languages. The relation between input and early acquisition of verbs is also found in a recent crosslinguistic study of English, Italian, and Mandarin Chinese by Tardif, Shatz, and Naigles (1996) (see also Tardif, 1996). In their systematic analysis of both the structures of the three languages and the actual caregiver input data, Tardif et al. found a higher saliency for verbs in Chinese compared to either English or Italian. They suggested that structural differences among languages affect input emphases on nouns and verbs and that this explains the early acquisition of verbs in Chinese.

SEMANTIC DEVELOPMENT OF SPATIAL WORDS

We now turn to the meanings of early verbs in Korean. The semantic domains of the early verbs in Korean appear to be similar to those of the early relational words reported for English (Bloom, 1973; Gopnik, 1982; Gopnik & Meltzoff, 1986; Nelson, 1973; Tomasello, 1992): They encoded success/failure, disappearance, locative action, state, or change of state. Among these, the Korean subjects produced a significant number of verbs expressing change of location and change of state, such as *kkita* "put in/on tightly" and *ppwulecita* "break." A detailed analysis of the meanings of these verbs shows that while the Korean children talked about the same semantic domains of actions and relations as English-speaking children, they made finer and different distinctions within each domain. For example, the Korean children acquired several different verbs pertaining to the notion of breaking, and used them appropriately: *kkayta* "break into pieces"; *ppwulecita* "a long stick-like thing is broken"; *kocangnata* "something doesn't function properly"(e.g., radio); *mangacita* "something has fallen apart" (e.g., toy).

These Korean children also produced specific verbs of locative action that related to different body parts and different types of figure-ground relations. For example, they produced *ipta* "put clothes on the trunk of the body" and *kkita* "put a figure object tightly in/on a ground object." Notice that the meanings of these locative verbs in Korean do not have single-word translation equivalents in English. Indeed, as is shown later, the way the Korean semantic system divides up spatial relations is considerably and significantly different from English. Given the crosslinguistic differences in semantic categorization, a question arises as to when and how children acquire the specific categorization system of their language.

A traditional Piagetian view on the issue has been that, at an early stage, children's spatial words map directly onto nonlinguistic concepts that have been already established (Bloom, 1973; McCune-Nicholich, 1981; Nelson, 1974). For example, based on the early acquisition of *up* and *down* by English-speaking children and their speed in generalizing the words across diverse contexts, these researchers have proposed that vertical motion is a nonlinguistic concept that children develop early. Several researchers have also proposed that the early acquisition of *in* and *on* in English reflect pre-established nonlinguistic understanding of containment and support relations among objects (Clark, 1973; Johnston 1984). Such a view, which we can call a "cognitive primacy view," has gained support from a number of studies on the development of spatial concepts in infancy as well as from crosslinguistic studies (Baillargeon, 1995; Johnston & Slobin, 1979; Needham & Baillargeon, 1993; Spelke, 1989). In particular, Johnston and Slobin (1979) found that children learning different languages acquire spatial words in a consistent order: *In, on,* and *under* are acquired before *between* and *behind*. These studies suggested that, at least at the initial stage of language acquisition, children are constrained by the universal developmental sequence of spatial cognition. According to this cognitive primacy view, language-specific meanings would be acquired later (Slobin, 1985). However, it is important to point out that in these studies the spatial words in different languages have simply been equated with their "translation equivalents" in English. In other words, these studies ignored detailed but significant semantic differences between the spatial words of different languages.

As will be shown, when the semantic systems of spatial words in English and Korean are examined in detail, actions of "putting on," "taking off," and the like are categorized significantly differently by the two languages. These differences provide us with good test cases. If it is nonlinguistic concept rather than language-specific input that guides children's generalization of early spatial words, we would see that the situations in which English learners say *on*, for example, should correspond closely to the situations in which Korean children say a roughly equivalent word. On the other hand, if language-specfic input guides at least in part children's acquistion of word meaning from the beginning, we would find language-specific properties in children's semantic learning from the beginning.

In the following, I first analyze the semantic categorization of spatial relations in English and Korean and then investigate acquisition. The analyses reported in this section are the results of a collaborative work with Melissa Bowerman at the Max Planck Institute for Psycholinguistics in Nijmegen, the Netherlands.

SEMANTIC CATEGORIES OF SPATIAL RELATIONS IN ENGLISH AND KOREAN

In English, words such as *in, out, on,* and *off* are part of a larger, closed-class system of spatial morphemes that encode what Talmy (1975, 1985) termed the path of motion. It encodes the path along which the figure (i.e., the moving object) moves to the ground object (i.e., reference object). In English, these particles are used regardless of whether the action is spontaneous or caused by an agent (e.g., *put IN* versus *go IN*) and regardless of the specific manner by which the figure moved to the ground (e.g., *take/pull/push OFF; go/run/crawl IN*). This English pattern is also found in other Indo-European languages, although not in Romance languages. In Romance languages, such as Spanish, path meanings are not singled out as particles in the grammar, but are incorporated in the main verb. For example, in Spanish, verbs such as *entrar* "go IN" and *meter* "put IN" incorporate path information and are typically used as main verbs in sentences expressing a motion event (Talmy, 1985). For example, in expressing John putting a ball in a box, a Spanish speaker would typically say, *Juan metí la pelota en la caja* "John put.in the ball in the box." Korean presents a somewhat mixed picture, but it patterns in the Romance way for verbs specifying caused motion. That is, in Korean, the path meaning of a caused motion is expressed by the main verb, as in Spanish. (See the section on early grammar for spatial expressions and Choi & Bowerman, 1991.)

In English, the choice among path particles is governed by what we might loosely call the "geometry" of the spatial relationship. Thus, if the figure is moving toward the ground ending completely or partially contained by the ground, *in* is used (e.g., *put the candle in the candle holder or put the doll in the bathtub*). In contrast, *on* is used when the figure ends up in contact with or attached to the surface of the ground (*put the suitcase on the table/ put one Lego piece on another*) or when it completely or partially covers or encircles the ground object (*put the*

pillowcase **on** *the pillow/the ring* **on** *your finger*). *On* is also used for putting clothes on the body, regardless of the specific bodypart involved
(*put hat/shirt/pants* **on**). English has another frequently used particle:
together. It is used when two objects are similar in size and are both
moved relative to each other. In this case, the contrast between *on* and
in is lost, as in *put two magnets/two pop-beads* **together**. (The encoding of
the converse actions of taking things *out*, *off*, and *apart* are governed by
similar considerations.)

The Korean semantic system divides up spatial relations (i.e., different paths) in quite different ways. First, as mentioned earlier, these
notions are expressed by verbs in Korean. Second, the categories associated with everyday Korean path verbs cross-cut the contrasts drawn
by the English particles. The verb *kkita* (and the opposite *ppayta*) is a
case in point. The path denoted by *kkita* "fit the figure tightly in/on the
ground" is a tight fit/three-dimensional meshing. Specifically, it is used
for actions in which the figure object is brought into a relationship of
tight fit or attachment with the ground object. And as long as the condition of tight fit is met, there is no difference as to whether the figure
goes **into, onto, over**, or **together** with the ground. Thus, it is routinely
used to express putting earplugs into ears, one Lego piece onto or together with another, and the top of a pen onto (= over) the pen. *Kkita* is
also used for both putting a ring onto a finger and putting a finger into
a ring, because both involve a tight fitting relationship. Different verbs
are used for loose containment (*nehta* "put in a loose containment") and
surface contact (*nohta* "put something loosely on a surface"/*cipta* "pick
something up"). Figure 9–2 shows schematically how the semantic category of *kkita* cross-cuts the categories of *put in*, *put on*, and *put together*
in English.

Korean path verbs of joining (and separation) also incorporate aspects of figure and ground. For example, distinct verbs are used for
solid veusus liquid figures (e.g., *nehta* "put.in loosely" versus *pwusta*
"pour in"), and for flat versus elongated figures (e.g., *pwuthita* versus
kkocta). Distinctions are also made when the human body is the ground
object: Different verbs are used for putting clothing onto different body
parts and also for putting people or objects into/onto different body
parts for support or carrying. For example, *ipta* is used for putting
clothes onto the trunk of the body; *sinta* is used for putting shoes/socks
on feet; *anta* is used for putting something in arms. Acts of putting a
figure onto the back are distinguished between whether the figure is
animate (*epta*) or inanimate (*cita*). Thus, many Korean path verbs have
a narrower range of uses than the English path markers that translate
them.

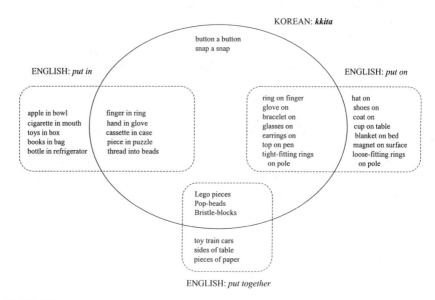

FIGURE 9-2
The category of *kkita* "put into relationship of tight fit or attachment" compared to English *put in/on/together*.

DEVELOPMENT OF THE SEMANTIC CATEGORIES OF SPATIAL RELATIONS

Bowerman and I (Bowerman & Choi, 1994; Choi & Bowerman, 1991) investigated how English and Korean children develop spatial semantic categories. We first examined the development of spatial words in our longitudinal spontaneous speech data of two English-speaking and nine Korean-speaking children from their first words until about 3 years of age.

We found some similarities between the two groups in their development of spatial words. But the similarities were at a rather general level. First, the onset ages of production of spatial words were similar in the two groups. All children began to produce spatial words sometime before 2 years of age, ranging from 14 to 21 months. Second, there was a remarkable similarity between the two sets of children in the kinds of events that they were interested in talking about. For example, they talked about wanting to go outside; they asked caregivers to pick up or carry them; and they referred to donning and doffing clothing and to object manipulations of many kinds, such as putting things into a bag and taking them out and putting Lego pieces or Popbeads together and taking them apart. These similarities in onset age and general content of spatial expressions probably reflect children's general cognitive development (Gopnik & Choi, 1990; Gopnik & Meltzoff, 1986).

Although the topics referred to by the two sets of children were remarkably similar, the patterns of linguistic expressions of learners of the two languages differed systematically. Our analysis of the differences showed a clear influence of language-specific properties, both morphological and semantic, on children's early expressions of motion events.

For joining and separating objects, the Korean children used *kkita* "put onto/into a tight-fitting ground" and *ppayta* "take off/out from a tight-fitting ground," respectively for figure and ground objects that have tight-fitting relationships regardless of whether the relationship involved containment, support or attachment, such as putting Lego pieces together and taking them apart or putting plastic shapes into matching holes and taking them out. Interestingly, the children often overextended the two verbs for situations that, although involving tight fit, would be encoded with different verbs by adults. For example, they overextended the verb *ppayta* to taking a T-shirt or shoes off before learning the appropriate verb, *pesta* "take clothes off." One child also said *ppayta* when asking his mother to release him when she was holding him tight in her arms. This is not an appropriate use of *ppayta* for adult speakers. Adult speakers would use the verb phrase *noh-a cwuta*, release give, "release" for this situation, as the mother does not take the child out from her arms surrounding him, but rather lets go of the child by releasing her arms from a holding position.

For putting objects loosely into a container such as putting toys into a basket or putting an object into a plastic bag, the children used either *nehta* "put.in loosely," or *tamta* "put relatively small things loosely in a container." For putting objects loosely on a surface, such as a table or the floor, children appropriately used *nohta* "put something loosely on surface."

As discussed earlier, many spatial verbs of Korean incorporate information about ground and sometimes figure. From the beginning of lexical development, the studied children's use of these verbs was generally appropriate, showing that they were sensitive to the incorporation of these elements. Between 17 and 20 months, the children distinguished two verbs for supporting/carrying according to the body part that serves as ground (*anta* "put into arms to support/carry" versus *epta* "put on back to support/carry"). They began to use appropriate clothing verbs according to the body part: *ipta* "put clothes on trunk" and *sinta* "put shoes or socks on feet." They also began to use the verb for removal of clothes, *pesta* "take clothes off."

Learners of English also use path particles according to the adult system of their language. In their spontaneous speech, our two subjects systematically distinguished between *in/out* and *on/off* on the basis of whether the figure goes into/out of a container or onto/off of a surface. Their use of the two path particles was indifferent to whether the figure fit the ground object tightly or loosely, or—in the case of clothing— what part of the body the figure ended up on. For example, they used *in* both for putting books into a fitted container and a piece into a puzzle (tight fit) and for dropping a key into a glasses case and putting blocks into a pan (loose fit). They used *on* for all types of attachment (e.g., putting tops on pens, lids on jars, magnets on surfaces) as well as for putting on clothes, regardless of the involved body part.

This analysis of spontaneous speech data in English and Korean revealed that the children in the study understood the language-specific meanings of the spatial words they were learning. Moreover, the data suggested that such language-specificity starts very early: from the one-word stage (i.e., before 2 years of age). But it is difficult to make systematic comparisons using such data because there is much variation in contexts in which children spontaneously produce words.

Bowerman and I (Bowerman & Choi, 1994), therefore, conducted a controlled elicitation experiment with young children learning English or Korean as their first language. On the basis of our spontaneous data, we selected a standardized set of actions of joining and separating two objects, for example, putting a cassette in a case (tight containment relationship), putting toys in a bag (loose containment relationship), and donning and doffing clothing of different kinds (carried out with a doll). The experimenter presented the two objects in either a joined or separated state (e.g., cassette presented in a fitted case or cassette in one hand and a case in the other) and asked the child to prompt her about what to do with them. Overall, there were 43 and 44 joining and separation actions. Our goal was to see whether children would categorize the actions similarly across languages as the cognitive primacy view would predict or in a language-specific way. For each language, there were 40 subjects: 10 adults and 30 children, 10 each in the age ranges 2;0–2;5, 2;6–2;11, and 3;0–3;5. Even the children in the youngest group responded well to our procedure. In this chapter, I report only the results of joining actions for which the children in both groups made several semantic distinctions.

The results of our elicitation study support our findings of the spontaneous speech data: From at least the age of 2 (i.e., the youngest children in our study), children's semantic categorization is already being shaped by the language-specific system to which they are exposed. But their sensitivity to the language-specific system interacts with nonlinguistic strategies of categorizing spatial relations in a complex way. Figures 9–3 and 9–4 show the semantic categorization of 2-year-olds in Korean and English (Figures 9–3B and 9–4B) in comparison with the adult system in the respective language (9–3A and 9–4A). The following summarizes the major findings.

The semantic categories of the youngest age group in each language are significantly more similar to those of the adult group of the corresponding language than to the same-age group learning the other language. That is, the categories of Korean 2-year-olds are significantly more similar to those of adult Koreans than to English-speaking 2-year-olds.

Patterns of categorization in 2-year-old Korean- and English-speaking children are, in fact, quite different. For example, Korean children appropriately distinguish clothing verbs: *ipta* for trunk of body, *ssuta* for head, and *sinta* for feet. Also, Korean children say *kkita* for tight-fitting relations, regardless of whether the figure ends up being contained in the ground (e.g., piece in jigsaw puzzle) or supported by the ground (e.g., one Bristle block on top of another). The word is indifferent to whether there is a symmetrical or asymmetrical movement between the figure and the ground (e.g., putting two magnetic train cars together versus adding one Popbead to a string of Popbeads).

The 2-year-old Korean subjects distinguish between tight fit and loose fit relations. For example, they say *kkita* for putting a ring on a pole that just fits the ring's hole, whereas they say *nehta* for putting toys into a suitcase. Also, whereas they say *kkita* for putting one Lego piece tightly on another, they say *nohta* for a loose-support relation, such as putting a suitcase on a table.

In contrast to the several categories distinguished by Korean 2-year-olds for these actions, English-speaking 2-year-olds distinguish only two major categories, *in* and *on*. The 2-year-old learners of English use *in* only for containment relationship whether it is tight or loose, such as putting a piece in a jigsaw puzzle and toys into a suitcase. Unlike the Korean 2-year-olds' *nehta* category, the *in* category formed by the English-speaking children of the same age exclude relations in

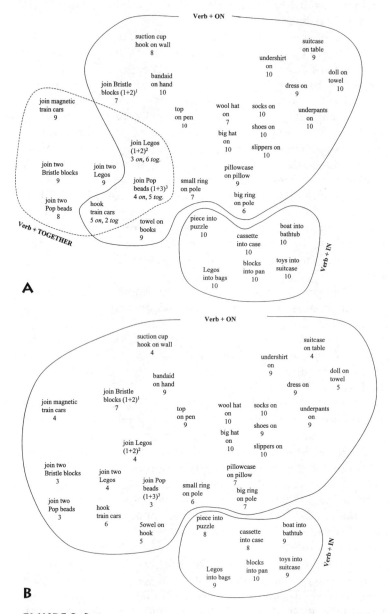

FIGURE 9-3

A. Categorization of joining actions by Korean adults. **B.** Categorization of joining actions by Korean children age 2;0–2;5.

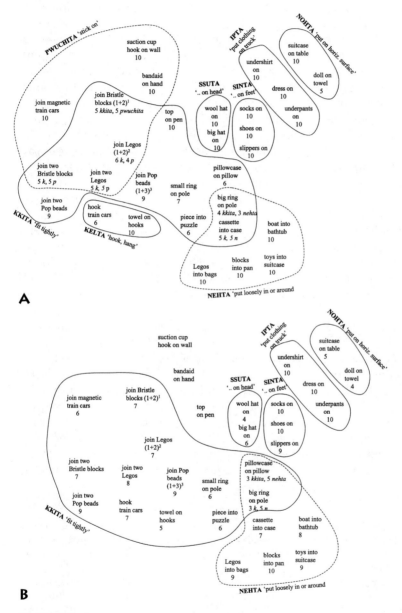

A

B

FIGURE 9–4

A. Categorization of joining actions by English-speaking adults. B. Categorization of joining actions by English-speaking children age 2;0–2;5.

which the figure encircles or covers the ground, such as putting a big ring on a pole and putting a pillowcase on a pillow.[5]

Unlike the way Korean-children use *kkita*, English-speaking children use *on* for all types of attachment (e.g., putting a top on a pen), encirclement (e.g., putting a small/big ring on a pole), and covering (e.g., putting a pillowcase on a pillow), including putting clothes on all parts of the body. Interestingly, they do not readily use *on* for what adults would think of as prototypical instances of the meaning of *on*— putting something down on a surface (e.g., a suitcase on a table). The majority of the children simply said *here* or didn't know what to say, although they probably recognized the anticipated spatial relation between the suitcase and the table.

The actions that could be considered as central members (those actions for which eight or more children said a given word) of the 2-year-olds' *on* category have some specific attachment or contact relationship between figure and ground. The figure and ground in these cases are perceptually distinct from each other, such as putting clothes on a part of the body and putting a top on a pen, (see Gopnik & Meltzoff, 1986, for an insightful discussion of the early uses of *on* in English).

Although the category of *kkita* for Korean 2-year-olds overlaps somewhat with the *on* category in English, the two categories differ in what can be considered their central members. The central members of the *kkita* category for Korean 2-year-olds are the figure-ground objects that are similar in size and shape, and that have natural tight fit relations, such as putting magnets,[6] Bristle blocks, and Legos together. However, for English-speaking 2-year-olds, these actions do not form a clear category; only three or four children said *on*. The children's unwillingness to use *on* for these actions suggests their sensitivity to the adult system: English-speaking adults do not use *on* for the symmetric

---

[5] Two-year-old Koreans' use of *nehta* for putting a pillowcase on pillow is an overextension. In Choi (1997), I provided a detailed analysis of this overextension and showed that it reflects children's hypothesis based on their understanding of the overall Korean semantic system of spatial categories.

[6] Korean makes a semantic distinction between two types of tight fit: the verb *kkita* for a three-dimensional tight fit (e.f., putting a Lego piece on another or putting a ring on a finger) and *pwuthita* for a two-dimensional tight fit (e.g., putting a Band Aid™ on hand or putting a magnet on the refrigerator). Thus, for putting magnets together, the appropriate word in the adult grammar would be *pwuthita*. However, 2-year-old Korean children overextended *kkita* to this context. This suggests that they understand the tight fit aspect of the word *kkita* but not the three-dimensional aspect.

joining of two objects that are similar in size and shape, but rather use *together.*

Our data also showed some similarities between English and Korean learners. First, children in both groups respond very consistently to the situations that involve loose containment. That is, in both languages, the response patterns are clear for situations such as putting a boat into a bathtub and putting toys into a suitcase. These actions form the central members of the categories *in* and *nehta* "put.in loosely." However, the peripheral uses of these words show that the children in each language group overextend them in a way that conforms to the language-specific principles of spatial categorizations (See Choi, 1997 for more details).

Second, in both language groups, the categorizations of the 3-year-olds are closer to the categorizations of the adult system than are those of the 2-year-olds. In other words, there is a progression toward the adult categorization from the youngest to the oldest age group of children. In both languages, 3-year-olds make finer categorizations than 2-year-olds, more closely approaching the adult system of categorization. For example, the development of the category *pwuthita* (typically used for two-dimensional attachments such as putting a Band Aid™ on hand) emerged between 2;6 and 3;0: two-year-olds either overextended the word *kkita* (a word for three-dimensional tight fit relations) to two-dimensional attachments or said nothing, whereas most of the 3-year-olds used the specific word *pwuthita* for two-dimensional attachments.

In English, a major difference between 2- and 3-year-olds is the treatment of symmetric and asymmetric movement. For symmetrical actions like putting two magnets or two Lego pieces together, the youngest group in English either overextended the word *on* or did not respond. The distinction between the two types of movement began to develop between 2;6 and 3;0, with half of the 3-year-olds distinguishing the two types of joining actions. These developmental orders can be attributed to the degree of perceptual and cognitive complexity.

SUMMARY

Korean and English-speaking children talk about similar locative events and situations at about the same age. But a closer examination of the children's language shows that the two groups of children differ systematically in their early semantic structure and that these differences reflect language-specific patterns of the adult language. Our data show that children attend to a number of critical features in the adult system that distinguish one semantic category from another. English-

and Korean-speaking children are able to extract these language-specific features and use them productively from virtually the beginning of language development. These data significantly weaken the claim that children initially map pre-established nonlinguistic spatial concepts directly onto spatial words. Rather, our data showed evidence that from the beginning of productive language, children construct spatial semantic categories that are significantly in accordance with language-specific input.

EARLY GRAMMAR

So far, I have examined the development of Korean at the single-word level. But how does syntax develop in Korean? In particular, what kinds of patterns do Korean children show in their early word combinations and in what way is the early grammar of Korean different from the development of English? In answering these questions, I focus on two areas: (1) early syntactic expressions of motion events and (2) argument structures of transitive and intransitive verbs in early word combinations.

SPATIAL EXPRESSIONS

Recall that in English, in expressing motion events, English uses a combination of a main verb and a particle: The main verb typically expresses manner, and the particle expresses path (cf. the section on semantic categories of spatial relations in both languages). This combinatory principle is consistently used in both intransitive clauses expressing spontaneous motion (e.g., *John walked/ran/ into the room*) and transitive clauses expressing caused motion (e.g., *John pushed/kicked the keg into the storeroom*).

Bowerman's data (1994) showed that her two English-speaking subjects used this combinatory rule productively from an early age (19–21 months). That is, the children began to combine path particles with a variety of verbs specifying the manner of motion regardless of whether the event was spontaneous or caused. For example, Bowerman's subjects produced the following combinations of manner (or cause) and path between 21 and 24 months, among many others (Bowerman, 1994, p. 40):

Utterance	Context
step up	(As the child steps on a stool.)
pull up	(As mother pulls up her pants.)
put down	(Asking mother to put a train on the floor.)

push down	(Asking mother to push a jack-in-the-box down in its box.)
close in	(Trying to close the lid on the jack-in-the-box.)
fall off	(As the doll balanced on a tiny staircase falls off.)

Many of the children's verb-particle combinations are also common in adult speech, but there is evidence that they understood the underlying combinatorial principle and were not simply imitating. First, they produced novel combinations such as *carry up* (picking up and righting a fallen-over stool), *close in* (trying to stuff a jack-in-the-box down into box and shut the lid), and *catch in* (asking M to go capture her between two boxes). Second, they freely combined particles and manner verbs with each other as independent components. For example, they used *out* to express a figure's exit from containment and combined it freely with different manner verbs as in *run/come out* (for spontaneous motion) or *pull/get out* (for caused motion), also combining the various manner verbs such as *run* appropriately with different path particles to express different trajectories, such as *run up, run down, run out.*

The Korean children in my study differed from English-speaking children in significant ways. Recall that in the section on semantic categories of spatial relations, I have mentioned that the syntax of spatial expressions in Korean is rather complex. The complexity is based on its distinct syntactic patterns used for caused and spontaneous motion. In Korean, caused motion is expressed in a way similar to Romance languages: path is encoded in the main verb (e.g., *kkita* "put.in/on tightly," *nehta* "put.in loosely") and manner is optionally encoded preceding the main verb. An example is shown in 8. The brackets denote optional elements.

(8) *John-i kong-ul sangca-ey [kwulli-e] neh-ess-ta.*
John-SUBJ ball-DO box-GL [roll-CONN] put.in-PAST-DECL
"John put the ball in the box [(by) rolling (it)]."

Expressions for spontaneous motions are distinct from caused motions in that deixis of motion (equivalent to *come/go* in English) is obligatorily specified after the path verb (see Example 9).

(9) John-i pang-ey [ttwui-e] tul-e ka-ss-ta.
John-SUBJ room-GL [run-CONN] enter-CONN go-PAST-DECL
"John entered the room [by running]."

In Example 9, the final verb *ka-* "go" denotes that the speaker is outside the room and John's entering the room resulted in John being farther away from the speaker.

To summarize, in Korean, for caused motion a path verb is required whereas for spontaneous motion both path and deictic verbs are required. In both cases, manner verbs are optional. That is, in Korean, manner does not have to be specified in talking about a motion event. All of these characteristics are distinct from English.

The first observation to be made for the development of spatial expressions in Korean is that children used distinct types of combinations for spontaneous and caused motions from the two-word combination period. For spontaneous motion, the productive pattern was a path verb followed by a deictic verb, *o-* "come" or *ka-* "go." This pattern conforms to the adult grammar for expressing spontaneous motion (Choi & Bowerman, 1991). The children in my study productively said the following combinations from about 20 months.

olla + *ka-/o-*	ascend go/come	"go/come up"
naylie + *ka-/o-*	descend go/come	"go/come down"
na + *ka-/o-*	exit go/come	"go/come out"
tule + *ka-/o-*	enter go/come	"go/come in"

For example, one child said *tule ka*, enter go, "go in," to ask the father to go into the shower. Another child said *na o-ass-e*, exit come-PAST-DECL, "came out," as she saw an owl come out in the show about Muppets.

For caused motion, children produced a distinct syntactic pattern: they used path verbs alone and did not combine them with deictic verbs. For example, as they took off a Popbead from a string of Popbeads, they said the transitive path verb, *ppay* "take off." When children combined a path verb with another verb, the other verb was typically an auxiliary verb. The auxiliary verbs used most often in these contexts were *cwu-ta* "do something for somebody" used to ask help from the caregiver, or *po-ta* "try, attempt" used to ask the caregiver to perform the action. Here are some examples:

Utterance	Gloss	Context
ppay cwu-e.	"take.off help"	(Asking investigator to take Popbeads off.)
kki-e cwu-e.	"put.in help"	(Asking caregiver to put a Lego piece on.)

kka cwu-e.	"unwrap/peel.off help"	(Asking caregiver to take off the wrapping of candy bars.)
ppay po-a.[7]	"take.off try"	(Asking investigator to take Bristle blocks off.)

Children's use of auxiliary verbs in spatial expressions was restricted to caused motions: It did not occur in expressions for spontaneous motion. The Korean children in my study thus used distinct combination patterns for spontaneous and caused motions. And, compared to English-speaking children, Korean children were much slower in acquiring manner verbs. Furthermore, unlike English-speaking children who productively combined manner verbs with path particles from an early age, Korean children rarely combined manner and path verbs for either spontaneous or caused motion. The late acquisition of manner verbs is probably due to the input grammar in which they are only optional.

TRANSITIVE AND INTRANSITIVE VERBS

A further analysis of children's early grammar in Korean revealed that the use of distinct syntactic patterns for spontaneous and caused motions is not restricted to spatial expressions. In more recent work, I examined the development of argument structures of early sentences in two of my longitudinal subjects. More specifically, I conducted a syntactic analysis of early verbs and examined the kinds of arguments (e.g., subject, direct object) that co-occur with these verbs in multiword utterances produced by the two children between 16 and 25 months. The database consisted of more than 200 multiword utterances for each child. Results of the analysis showed that (1) children went through three distinct periods of development of increasing the number of multiword utterances in their speech, and (2) children developed distinct argument structures, depending on the syntactic type of the verb.

For this analysis, all of the multiword utterances in the data were categorized according to the syntactic type of the main verb: transitive or intransitive. Such syntactic categories are based on the adult grammar. That is, if the verb takes a direct object in the adult grammar, then

[7] -*E* and -*a* are allomorphs. Generally, -*a* is used when the preceding vowel is a mid-back or low vowel, and -*e* is used in all other environments. This rule applies when the verb is in present tense.

TABLE 9–3
Development of verb types and argument structure: Frequency of uses of different arguments structures during three developmental periods between 16 and 25 months for two Korean children.

Child I Period (Age in months)	Transitive			Intransitive	
	DO+Vtr	S+Vtr	S+DO+Vtr	S+Vi	S+Loc+Vi
I (16–19)	2	1	–	–	–
II (20–23)	28	7	10	12	3
III (24–25)	35	14	24	12	14

Child II Period (Age in months)	Transitive			Intransitive	
	DO+Vtr	S+Vtr	S+DO+Vtr	S+Vi	S+Loc+Vi
I (16–19)	3	–	–	1	–
II (20–23)	26	2	2	6	2
III (24–25)	34	14	8	20	4

Notes: Vtr: Transitive verb; Vi: Intransitive verb; S: Subject; DO: Direct object; and Loc: Locative.

the verb is considered a transitive verb. The transitive verbs in the children's data were mostly transitive agentive verbs that typically expressed caused events. These verbs denoted change of state or change of location/possession caused by an agent, such as *kkuta* "turn:on," *pesta* "take-off (clothing)," *ipta* "put-on (dress, shirt)," *sinta* "put-on (shoes, socks)," *ppayta* "take off (object)," *cwuta* "give." The intransitive verbs are mostly spontaneous change of location/posture verbs, such as *kata* "go," *ota* "come," *ancta* "sit down," and a few activity verbs, such as *mekta* "eat" and *nolta* "play."

Once the syntactic type of each verb was identified, I then examined the kinds of arguments that co-occurred with each type of verb. The results are in Table 9–3. In this table, only the frequency of core arguments (subject (S), direct object (DO), and location (Loc)) occurring with transitive and intransitive verbs are shown.

The patterns shown in Table 9–3 include Period I, with transitive verbs appearing first with a direct object. This structure progressively predominated during the two subsequent periods. Furthermore, during Period II, almost all transitive verbs occurred with a direct object. Thus, the pattern [DO + Vtr (= transitive verb)] seemed to be the basic structure for transitive verbs. Some examples are: *son chap-a,* hand hold, "hold (my) hand," *pap cwu-e,* rice give, "give (me) rice," *ike neh-e,* this put.in, "put this in." Adding the subject to the basic pattern, [S + DO + Vtr], was less frequent and a later development. [S + Vtr] seemed only an optional structure: Some of the verbs that occurred in [DO + Vtr] also occurred in the [S + Vtr] frame, but not the reverse. This overall pattern for transitive verbs continued through Period III. All of these data suggest that [DO + Vtr] is the predominant pattern for transitive verbs in early grammar.

The syntax of intransitive verbs could not be observed until Period II (except for one utterance by Child II). Thus, syntactic constructions involving these verbs developed more slowly compared to the syntactic development of transitive verbs. Also, the predominant syntactic frames for intransitive verbs were different from transitive verbs. With intransitive verbs, it was the subject argument that predominantly co-occurred with the verbs, [S + Vi (= intransitive verb)]. In some cases, the locative argument was added to the structure, [S + Loc + Vi]. Some examples are *emma anc-e,* mommy sit.down "Mommy sat down," *beybi nemeci-ess-e,* baby fell.down, "Baby fell down," *appa hakkyo ka-ss-e,* daddy school went, "Daddy went to school."

Thus, my data suggested that Korean children distinguish two types of verbs with distinct argument structure: With transitive verbs the predominantly co-occuring argument was the direct object, whereas with intransitive verbs it was the subject. These data are in accord with Clancy's (1993, 1997) findings on Korean acquisition. Her analysis of two Korean subjects' spontaneous speech produced between age 1;10 and 2;3 showed essentially the same pattern: transitive verbs occurred predominantly with direct objects and intransitive verbs occurred pre-dominantly with subjects. What these data mean is that when Korean 2-year-olds talk, they systematically delete the subject of the sentence when the verb is transitive, whereas they preserve it when it is intransitive.

What motivates such patterns? Clancy's (1993, 1997) analysis from a discourse-pragmatic perspective provides an explanation. Clancy convincingly showed that these "preferred argument structures" (Du Bois, 1985) for transitive and intransitive verbs in Korean reflect chil-dren's early sensitivity to discourse functions of the noun arguments in the sentence. More specifically, Clancy found a very strong tendency for subjects of transitive sentences to convey given information. That is, the referents that are mentioned in prior discourse are predominantly assigned to the subject role of the transitive sentence. And children systematically opted not to overtly mention given information. That is, they used ellipsis (zero anaphora) for given information. The result is that subjects of transitive sentences were systematically ellipted. Clancy (1993, 1997) also found that such relations between discourse and grammar present in the children's speech was also evident in the caregivers' speech. That is, the preferred argument structures of transitive and intransitive sentences were also characteristic of the caregivers' input. Based on these data, Clancy proposed that the acquisition of grammar in children develop from their sensitivity to discourse functions of noun arguments provided by their caregivers. Clancy's data showed that sensitivity to discourse-pragmatic factors starts at a very early age, around 1;10.

It is not yet clear whether English learners show similar preferred argument structures. However, a detailed diary study of one American child conducted by Tomasello (1992) suggested that at an early stage (comparable to the ages in Clancy's study and my own studies), English learners do not show such pronounced differences between transitive and intransitive verbs. In fact, Tomasello could not find any predominant syntactic patterns for either transitive or intransitive verbs. It seems, then, that the particular patterns that Clancy and I observed independently on early Korean syntax come from children's sensitivity to language-specific input.

MODALITY

In this last section, I report perhaps the most striking evidence that children attend to language-specific meanings: The acquisition of the modal system in Korean. As described in the section on verb morphology, Korean has a class of morphemes that express epistemic modality (varying degrees of the truth of a proposition) and evidentiality (the source of information). For example, these morphemes encode notions such as possibility or probability of the truth of the proposition, somewhat similar to the modal auxiliary *might* in *John might be right* or *must* in *John must be right.* They also encoded whether the information was a hearsay or directly witnessed by the speaker.

In previous research (primarily on English), epistemic modality was found to be learned quite late, around 4 or 5 years. For example, Moore, Pure, and Furrow (1990) found that English learners do not distinguish between *may* and *must* until 4 years of age. However, as is shown, Korean children acquire several SE modal suffixes by 2 years of age (Choi, 1990, 1995). In this chapter, I discuss the kinds of modal meanings Korean children acquire early and investigate some possible explanations. But, first, a brief description of the Korean modal system is necessary.

THE MODAL SYSTEM IN KOREAN

Sentence-ending (SE) modal suffixes form an obligatory grammatical category and occupy the final position among the inflections on the predicate (verb or adjective). As Korean is a verb final (SOV) language, the suffixes occur typically at the end of a sentence, as in Example 10.

(10) *Younghi-ka Seoul-ul ttena-ss-e.*
Younghi-SUBJ Seoul-OBJ leave-PAST-MOD
"Younghi left Seoul."

As noted in the section on verb morphology, the Korean speaker must make a choice about a particular SE form each time he/she produces a sentence. The meanings denoted by these morphemes are quite abstract. Several recent studies (Choi 1991; H. Lee 1991; K. Lee 1986) have suggested that many of the SE suffixes code the differential status of information in the speaker's knowledge system. H. Lee (1991) states the functions of SE suffixes as follows:

> What is differentiated by sentence-terminal suffixes is various epistemic modality categories, including the speaker's knowledge status, background expectation, evidentiary sources of the information conveyed, and the speaker's assumption about the addressee's point of view. (H. Lee 1991, p. 471)

According to H. Lee (1991), one of the distinctions that SE suffixes make relates to degrees of integration of information in the speaker's mind. The contrasts among the two suffixes, -*ta* and -*e*, illustrate this point. The suffix -*ta* is often used by the speaker when he or she has just perceived something noteworthy in the present context, "either because it is about the accomplishment of awaited events or states of affairs at the very moment of speaking" (H. Lee, 1993, p. 157). Consider the context: John is watching a basketball game and is cheering for Team A. Team A is ahead, but John is not sure that it will win, as it's a close game. Finally, hearing the buzzer signaling the end of the game, John says:

(11) *iki-ess-ta!*
    win-PAST-MOD   "(They) won!"

The use of *-ta* is appropriate in this context in which John has just recognized what happened and registers the information in his mind for the first time. Comments made with *-ta* need not be directed to the listener; they can be noteworthy self-remarks to the speaker. Once the speaker has registered this new information, in subsequent conversations, for example, when the speaker repeats the information to a friend, or when telling the result of the game later to another friend, John would use the SE form *-e*:

(12) *iki-ess-e.*
    win-PAST-MOD   "(They) won."

In this latter context, the use of *-ta,* in *iki-ess-ta** would be ungrammatical.

The use of *-ta* is not restricted to perception of the external world. It can also occur with an internal state of mind. For example, adult Koreans often say *al-ass-ta,* know-PAST-MOD "(I)'ve got (it)" when they have just come to an understanding of something. It should be noted that *-ta* is not an aspectual marker denoting perfective aspect. One can use *-ta* when describing a state of affairs as well as an on-going activity if it draws the speaker's attention for the first time, such as, *ippu-ta* pretty-MOD "(she's) pretty," or *o-n-ta* come-PRES-MOD "(They) are coming."

In contrast to *-ta, -e* is used when information has been assimilated into a speaker's knowledge system, that is, when the speaker acquired the information in the past and has known it for some time. As mentioned, once newly perceived information is encoded with *-ta, -e* must be used in subsequent mentions of the information. In H. Lee's survey (1991), *-e* is the most frequent suffix (58%) in spontaneous discourse interactions. This is not surprising, as in conversations participants often contribute to the topic by offering information that they already have about the topic. Indeed, one can conclude that *-e* is the unmarked suffix in conversations.

All of these suffixes are used only in informal conversational interactions where participants, familiar with one another, freely and spontaneously exchange information about a current topic. The choice of the SE form is intimately related to a current discourse context. Probably due to this characteristic, the meanings of many suffixes incorporate a speaker's assumption about how much the listener knows. That is, a speaker's choice of a specific SE suffix reflects an assumption about the listener's status of knowledge of the proposition (H. Lee 1991). For example, the suffix -*ci* is used when a speaker self-commits to the truth of the proposition: It, therefore, expresses certainty whether the information is from direct experience or from inference. At the same time, -*ci* denotes that the information is also known to the listener or can be readily inferred by the listener. This analysis is confirmed by the use of -*ci* in questions. The suffix -*ci?* is used in a question when the speaker is certain about the truth of a proposition and at the same time wants to confirm that the listener also believes (or knows) it to be true. Thus, in the case of Example 13, the mother is certain of her inference, and therefore she can use -*ci*.

(13) (The mother, seeing her daughter, notices that her eyes are red. The mother says,)
   ne wul-ess-ci?
   you cry-PAST-MOD
   "You cried, didn't you?"

I have discussed several examples to show that a number of SE modal suffixes in Korean express evidentiality and different statuses of knowledge that involve a speaker's and listener's beliefs about an event or state. Probably because of the requirement of incorporating what the listener believes about a particular situation in using modal suffixes, they are neither used in formal situations (e.g., a formal speech), nor in contexts where the speaker/writer does not have a particular listener/ reader in mind, such as newspapers. In other words, these suffixes are used only in interactive contexts (e.g., a conversation or personal letter) in which the speaker knows what the listener knows.

DEVELOPMENT OF SE SUFFIXES IN KOREAN CHILDREN

I followed the development of SE modal suffixes in two Korean children from age 1;8 to 3;0. As is shown, the Korean acquisition data for modal suffixes suggest that the discourse-interactional features and nonverbal contextual cues that accompany them facilitate and enhance the acquisition of SE modal suffixes.

TABLE 9–4
Verbs that initially occur with the modal suffix -*ta*
and contexts in which the verbs are used.

Verbs	Events/States
iss-ta "exist" *eps-ta* "not-exist"	Existence/disappearance
twayss-ta "have become"	Success
can-ta "sleeping" *kath-ta* "be same"	State
hayss-ta "done" *ollakass-ta* "went up"	Completed action

ACQUISITION OF THE SUFFIXES -*TA* AND -*E*: DISTINCTION BETWEEN NEWLY PERCEIVED AND OLD INFORMATION

The first two suffixes that the children used contrastively were -*ta* and -*e* at around 1;8. At this early period of language development, -*ta* was suffixed to just a few verbs that reflected the child's cognitive interests about the world (see Table 9–4). The kinds of events and states of affairs that the children described with -*ta* were about the here-and-now and closely related to cognitive concepts that children acquire at the early developmental stage. Those concepts could be categorized into four types as shown in Table 9–4: existence/disappearance of an entity, success/failure, state, and change of state/location (Gopnik & Choi, 1990; Gopnik & Meltzoff, 1986; Slobin, 1985). That is, statements made by the children with the suffix -*ta* at this stage reflected the kinds of concepts they were trying to assimilate into their general cognitive system. This probably explains why Korean children acquire the form -*ta* early, even though the relative frequency of the input for this form is much lower than suffixes such as -*e* (Choi, 1990).

The children expressed all four types of events/states with the suffix -*ta* repeatedly (whenever these contexts occurred) during the first few weeks of its use, typically using the specific verbs shown in Table 9–4. Some examples are shown in 14 and 15.

(14) TJ: (1;11)

M: *Mickey eti iss-ni?*
Mickey where exist-MOD
"Where is Mickey?"
(TJ pointing to the picture of a Mickey Mouse on her doll house)

→ TJ: *Mickey yeki iss-ta.*
Mickey here exist-MOD
"Mickey is here."

(15) HS: (1;10)
(HS puts a Lego person in a chair.)

→ HS: *tway-ss-ta.*
become-PAST-MOD
"Done."

In Example 14, TJ says *iss-ta* "exist" as she sees the picture of Mickey, and in Example 15, HS marks the change of state as she completes her goal of putting a Lego person in a chair. Thus the events described in Examples 14 and 15 occur in the children's immediate context and are newly registered in their minds.

The suffix *-e* was used contrastively with *-ta* to encode higher degree of assimilation of the proposition (i.e., event or state to be encoded in language) in the child's knowledge system. Specifically, whereas the children used *-ta* for newly perceived information not fully assimilated into their knowledge system, they used *-e* for information that had been integrated into their system.

Whereas *-ta* was used typically to express new events/states that the child had just observed or accomplished, the suffix *-e* was used typically to talk about past events/states or to negate presupposed events/states. Let's look at Examples 16 and 17.

(16) TJ (2;1)
(At the beginning of the recording session, TJ shows the investigator a cushion that her mother made a few days ago.)

→ *emma mantul-ess-e.*
mommy make-PAST-MOD
"Mommy made (it)."

(17) TJ (1;11)
(TJ is in another room. M asks TJ to bring a color book.)

M: *ppalli kac-ko o-a. illwu o-a.*
quickly take-and come-MOD here come-MOD
"Bring (it) quickly. Come here."

→   TJ: *an ka(-e)*. (*-e* is deleted after the vowel /a/.)
      not go (-MOD)
      "(I'm) not going."

In Example 16, TJ states a past event that is well known to her. In Example 17, M has asked TJ to return to the living room, and TJ negates the proposition. In both examples, the information that the child conveys has been established in her mind before actually saying it. In addition, *-e* was used to talk about an event/state that was not occurring at the time of speech, such as for actions that the child was about to perform or make-believe events while playing with a doll or a toy. It was also used in questions to verify the truth of a proposition. Thus, the functional distribution of *-e* was clearly different from that of *-ta* (see Choi, 1985, for a more detailed analysis).

Another systematic difference between *-ta* and *-e* related to discourse contingency, that is, whether or not the utterance maintains the current topic and adds new information to it (Bloom, Rocissano, & Hood, 1976). If the function of *-ta* is to register a new and noteworthy event/state that draws a child's cognitive interest, the form would be used in introducing new topics. On the other hand, *-e* would be used more frequently in exchanging information about an established topic, as it conveys information that has become part of a speaker's knowledge system. The analysis of discourse contingency confirms this hypothesis. The children used *-e* more often than *-ta* as they responded to adult utterances giving more information about a topic. The children used *-ta* 83% of the time on average as they shifted to a new topic that drew their attention. An example is shown in 18 in which TJ uses *-ta* abruptly interrupting the topic of coloring to talk about a baby's crying.

(18) TJ (2;0)
      (Investigator points to the girl that she colored)
      Inv: *i salam ippu-ci?*
            this person pretty-MOD?
            "Isn't this person pretty?"

      TJ: *ippu-ci.*
            pretty-MOD
            "pretty."

      Inv: *i salam ippu-ci?*
            this person pretty-MOD?
            "Isn't this person pretty?"
      (TJ hears a baby cry upstairs.)

→   TJ: *aka u(l)-n-ta.*
            baby cry-PRES-MOD.
            "A baby is crying."

     Inv: *aka ul-e?*
            baby cry-MOD
            "Is baby crying?"

In contrast, the propositions with *-e* showed a much lower frequency of noncontingency (35% on average). In fact, more than half of
the time, the propositions with *-e* maintained the current topic. More
specifically, *-e* was used to respond to or comment on the preceding
adult question or statement as shown in the next examples.

(19) TJ (2;4)
      (Investigator and TJ are looking at a picture of a boy on a
      dog's back.)
      Inv: *yay-nun eti iss-ni?*
             this.child-TOP where be-MOD?
             "Where is this child?"
→   TJ: *oll-a ka-ss-e.*
             move.up-CONN go-PAST-MOD
             "(He) went up."

ACQUISITION OF *-CI*: SHARED KNOWLEDGE AND CERTAINTY OF THE TRUTH OF THE PROPOSITION

The third modal suffix to be acquired by the children (around 2;0) was
-ci, the suffix that encodes certainty and shared knowledge in the adult
grammar. From early on, the three children's use of *-ci* reflected sensitivity to those features as they used it spontaneously in the contexts (a)
when reiterating a proposition in the preceding utterance produced
either by the child or by the interactant (see Example 20), or (b) when
redescribing an event or state that had been described several times
before (see Example 21).

(20) TJ (2;2)
      (TJ touches Investigator's record player.)
      Inv: *ike manci-ci ma. acwumma-kke-ya.*
             this touch-CONN NEG. aunt-POSS-MOD.
             "Don't touch this. This is aunt's." (referring to Inv.)

→ TJ: *acuwmma-kke-ci.*
aunt-POSS-MOD.
"This is aunt's."

(21) TJ (2;3)
(TJ is telling a story looking at the picture of a teddy bear fallen down on the floor. In many previous sessions, TJ talked about the same picture in the same way.)
→ TJ: *khwung nemecy-ess-ci.*
Boom fall.down-PAST-MOD
"Boom, (it) fell down."

Inv: *ung?*
What
"What?"

→ TJ: *khwung nemecy-ess-cyana.*
Boom fall.down-PAST-MOD
"Boom, (it) fell down."
(Note: *-cyana* is a strong form of *-ci*)

In Example 20, *-ci* is used when repeating the adult's statement, and in Example 21 it is used for information that the child said several times before. The characteristic uses of *-ci* suggest that children pay attention to preceding discourse and also remember conversations that took place in the past. The repetition of the proposition with *-ci* in this way allows the child to be certain that information contained in a proposition is shared with the caregiver.

Later in development, *-ci* was extended to encode certainty of information. For example, HS at 2;9 expressed that her cash register toy was broken with the verb *kocangna-* "break" (i.e., *kocangna-ss-ci* "broke") as she was trying it several times and it didn't work. Still later, *-ci* also began to be used for events that were normally expected in a given situation, for example routine activities in a bathing situation (e.g., taking off clothes before taking a bath). All of these uses of *-ci* provide evidence that children use it to code certain and shared information.

In summary, children's early uses of SE suffixes show a developmental pattern. First, *-ta* is acquired to denote newly perceived information at the moment of speech that attracts the child's cognitive interest. This use of *-ta* contrasts with *-e* or *-ci* in that the information it codes is unrelated to the preceding discourse. Soon, *-e* is acquired to exchange old information in discourse interaction. Next, the modal form *-ci* is acquired that specifically codes the sharing of information with the listener. The characteristic developmental pattern for *-ci* is that it starts as an imitation of the caregiver's immediately preceding use of the modal form. Later, children use it to confirm that the information is shared with the caregiver, or to code certainty of information.

FACTORS CONTRIBUTING TO THE EARLY DEVELOPMENT OF MODAL SUFFIXES

In these data, we have observed that before 3 years of age, Korean children acquire a variety of epistemic meanings relating to different degrees of assimilation of knowledge in their minds, different sources of information, and the knowledge status of the listener. Explanation for this probably has to do with several factors, which include cognitive and pragmatic aspects and input.

First, children acquire SE suffixes initally to express their own knowledge status (-ta and -e) and subsequently to incorporate the listener's knowledge status (-ci). This conforms to the general view that children's use of language reflects gradual decentration, that is, from more self-centered to less (Piaget, 1955). Also, children acquire a suffix (-ta) first to convey information in the immediate context and later to convey information about past events (-e and -ci). This is in line with children's general cognitive development that progresses from an understanding of present events to an understanding of events that are removed from the present. Not only across suffixes, but also within a single suffix, the development of functions reflects underlying cognitive capacity at the time of acquisition. For example, the use of -ci was first limited to repetitions of the immediately preceding propositions and later was expanded to include events in the past.

Within these cognitive limitations, however, Korean children acquire a number of epistemic modals. Such early acquisition of epistemic modal functions in Korean is interesting because crosslinguistic research has shown that epistemic modality is acquired later than agent-oriented modality (Stephany, 1986). In addition, a number of experimental studies investigating the development of epistemic modality in English have shown that an understanding of different degrees of certainty about a proposition develops after 4 years (Byrnes & Duff, 1989; Hirst & Weil, 1982; Moore, et al., 1990). But the epistemic meanings of modal auxiliaries in English relate to the status of knowledge that is relatively independent of a particular discourse-interactional context. For example, the distinction between *must* and *may* in English in *He must/may be home by 5 o'clock* has little to do with the speaker's assumption about how much other participants know about the proposition. In fact, in most of the experimental studies on the acquisition of epistemic modality, tests have been designed to understand such context-independent reasoning. For example, in Moore et al. (1990), children (between 3 and 6 years of age) were asked to guess the location of an object hidden in a box solely on the basis of one-sentence cues that varied in epistemic modal auxiliaries, such as *It must be in the red box* or *it might be in the blue box*. Moore et al. found that the ability to find the hidden object on the basis of the modal meaning was apparent in children older than 4 years. The results of these studies, however, give little indication of how and when children understand modal forms that incorporate discourse-interactional meanings.

One distinct feature of the SE modal suffixes in Korean is that their meanings are intimately related to discourse interaction. That is, the primary function of the modal suffixes is to exchange information and construct shared knowledge among conversation participants. In the research of the development of communicative competence, it is well known that children learn to be good participants in conversations from a young age. Several studies (Pellegrini, Brody & Stoneman 1987; Shatz 1983, 1984) have shown that even 2-year-olds are capable of giv-ing enough information and keeping their linguistic contributions truthful and relevant to the topic of discourse. Bloom et al. (1976) have also shown that before children reach 2 years, they have learned a basic rule of discourse, that of conversational turns, and that between 2 and 3 years, children increase the amount of information they contribute to the shared topic. The data presented here on Korean modal suffixes suggests that such an ability in young children, namely, to follow the progression of discourse toward more and more shared knowledge between the speaker and the listener, is instrumental to the early acqui-sition of SE modal suffixes.

Furthermore, there are several characteristic morphological fea-tures of SE suffixes that may facilitate early acquisition of SE suffixes in Korean, particularly when we consider Slobin's (1973) operating prin-ciples of language development. First, SE suffixes occur at the ends of sentences (most often with one syllable consisting of a consonant and a vowel) and, therefore, are perceptually salient. Second, the SE suffixes constitute an obligatory category in that all sentences in discourse inter-actions must end with a SE suffix. During interactions with children, the caregiver provides a variety of SE suffixes appropriate to specific discourse contexts (Choi, 1996). From the acquisition perspective, this means that children hear different SE suffixes frequently from their caregivers.

Thus, the discourse interactional functions of the suffixes coupled with perceptual saliency of the morphemes probably explain the early acquisition of SE modal suffixes in Korean. The data also suggest that the ability in young children to follow the progression of discourse toward shared knowledge between themselves and the caregivers is instrumental to the early acquisition of SE modal suffixes. But, whatever their source, the modal functions of SE suffixes in Korean seem to be within children's cognitive grasp and linguistic capacity at an early age.

ㅓ

CONCLUSION

In this chapter, I have reviewed some aspects of the acquisition of Korean. The focus was on the early stages of grammatical development related to verbs. A larger goal was to investigate how young Korean children are sensitive to language-specific properties of the grammar they are learning. For this goal, systematic crosslinguistic comparisons in English and Korean were made whenever possible. These crosslinguistic investigations allowed me to evaluate universalist views, such as the cognitive primacy view that children's language is initially guided by universal cognitive principles.

The data presented in this chapter provide evidence that from the beginning of language production, children's grammar is influenced by language-specific characteristics. First, at the single-word level, Korean learners acquire a significant number of verbs from the beginning of the one-word stage, whereas English learners do not. The development of modal suffixes showed that Korean children acquire verbs as a morphologically coherent class. Furthermore, the semantic development of modal suffixes and the syntactic development of transitive and intransitive sentences show that Korean children attend to differences in discourse pragmatics and are able to extract those features that have grammatical consequences in their language. In the case of modal suffixes, we have seen that 2-year-old Korean children can systematically encode notions such as newly-perceived information and shared information on their verb morphology. In learning the syntax of the input language, Korean children can attend to discourse fuctions such as given and new information and can consistently apply the functions to their grammar.

Our investigation of children's semantic categorization of spatial relations shows that they categorize relations according to language-specific principles from at least 2 years of age. These studies suggested that language-specific aspects of grammar influence children's language from an early age, perhaps even before language production begins. In fact, a comprehension study we are currently conducting shows evidence that 18-month-olds who do not yet have words, such as *kkita* (for Korean-speaking children) and *in* (for English-speaking children) in their productive vocabulary, understand the words according to the language-specific principles of semantic organization (Choi, McDonough, Bowerman, & Mandler, in preparation).

In recent crosslinguistic acquisition research, an increasing number of studies have reported data suggesting an influence of language-specific input in language acquisition (Hoff-Ginsberg, 1986; Sera, Rettinger, & Castillo-Pintado, 1991; Shatz, 1991; Tardif, 1996; Weist, Wysocka, & Lyytinen, 1991). For example, Hoff-Ginsberg (1986) reported that mothers' communicative styles and their structural characterstics can influence 2-year-olds' language development. Weist et al. (1991) showed that specific temporal properties of individual languages can influence young children's tense systems.

To the extent that children's early grammar is molded by language-specific grammatical patterns, children's nonlinguistic cognitive systems and possible innate linguistic structure that underlie the acquisition of grammar must be flexible (Bowerman, 1985, 1989). The data presented in this chapter suggest that from a remarkably early age, children actively extract relevant meaning components of a word by attending to what is consistently present across all the contexts in which a given word is used. For example, the child discovers that in all the contexts in which *kkita* "put in/on tightly" is used, there is a consistent aspect of tight fit between figure and ground. Given the significant number of crosslinguistic differences in the way languages categorize the world, the identification of a particular feature (e.g., tight fit) as a critical aspect of word meaning may be an insight on a child's part after having observed a number of contexts in the input that are referred to by the same expression, and may not be something that is derived directly from a set of available nonlinguistic concepts. As Gopnik and Meltzoff (1997) discussed, this insight by a child is undoubtedly within his or her cognitive capacity at a particular developmental stage. In this way, there is an intimate bidirectional relation between language-specific input and cognitive development.

The findings discussed in this chapter, then, do not support a strong form of the cognitive primacy view, namely, that regardless of the language children are learning, they are initially guided by universal cognitive development. Rather, the chapter shows that from the beginning of language development (including the comprehension stage) children acquire a **language-specific** grammar.

For professionals whose work involves assessment and intervention of children's language, the present Korean data suggest that an assumption should not be made that a child learning (or exposed to) language other than English will show the same developmental patterns as a child learning English. In this respect, a language measure primarily designed for English-speaking children may not be appropriate for assessing development of children whose primary language is significantly different from English. For example, pre-established checklists or questionnaires that are translations from English would not be appropriate for measuring language development in languages such as Korean. Word-for-word translations are likely to miss many early words or constructions that Korean children productively use (Choi & Gopnik, 1995). Given significant differences in the way children acquire grammar in different languages, ideally, specific language measures should be constructed that can correctly assess the linguistic competence of the learners of a particular language.

Our future task is to conduct extensive and detailed research on the acquisition of grammar in different languages. We also need to know more about the linguistic input that caregivers provide to children in different linguistic communities and about the precise relationship between input and language development in each language. A thorough database will no doubt require considerable time. Until then, it would be helpful, at least for clinicians and educators working with children whose primary language is not English, to understand that language development patterns that deviate from English may potentially be normal paths for those learners.

⏚

REFERENCES

Baillargeon, R. (1995). A model of physical reasoning in infancy. In C. Rovee-Collier & L. P. Lipsitt (Eds.), *Advances in Infancy Research, 9,* 305–371.

Bates, E., Marchman, V., Thal, D., Fenson, L., Dale, P., Reznick, J. S., Reilly, J., & Hartung, J. (1994). Developmental and stylistic variation in the composition of early vocabulary. *Journal of Child Language, 21,* 85–124.

Bloom, L. (1973). *One word at a time.* The Hague: Mouton.

Bloom, Lois, Rocissano, L., & Hood, L. (1976). Adult-child discourse: Developmental interaction between information processing and linguistic knowldge. *Cognitive Psychology, 8,* 521–552

Bloom, L., Tinker, E., & Margulis, C. (1993). The words children learn: Evidence against a noun bias in early vocabularies. *Cognitive Development, 8,* 431–450.

Bowerman, M. (1985). What shapes children's grammars? In D. I. Slobin (Ed.), *The crosslinguistic study of language acquisition: Vol. 2. Theoretical issues* (pp. 1257–1319). Hillsdale, NJ: Lawrence Erlbaum Associates.

Bowerman, M. (1989). Learning a semantic system: What role do cognitive predispositions play? In M. L. Rice & R. L. Schiefelbusch (Eds.), *The teachability of language* (pp. 133–169). Baltimore: Paul H. Brooks.

Bowerman, M. (1994). From universal to language-specific in early grammatical development. *Philosophical Transactions of the Royal Society of London B, 346,* 37–45.

Bowerman, M., & Choi, S. (1994, January). *Linguistics and nonlinguistic determinants of spatial semantic development: A crosslinguistic study of English, Korean, and Dutch.* Paper presented at Boston University Conference on Language Development, Boston.

Bowerman, M., & Pederson, E. (1992, December). *Cross-linguistic perspectives on topological spatial relationships.* Paper presented at the annual meeting of the American Anthropological Association, San Francisco.

Brown, P. (1996). Isolating the CVC root in Tzeltal Mayan: A study of children's first verbs. In E. Clark (Ed.), *The Proceedings of the 27th Annual Child Language Research Forum* (pp 1–12). Stanford, CA: Stanford University, Center for the Study of Language and Information.

Byrnes, J. P., & Duff, M. A. (1989). Young children's comprehension of modal expressions. *Cognitive Development, 4,* 369–387.

Carey, S. (1978). The child as word learner. In M. Halle, J. Bresnan, & G. A. Milled (Eds.), *Linguistic theory and psychological reality* (pp. 264–293). Cambridge, MA: MIT Press.

Cheng, L., & Chang, J. (1995). Asian/Pacific islander students in need of effective services. In L. Cheng (Ed.), *Integrating language and learning for inclusion* (pp. 3–27). San Diego: Singular Publishing Group.

Choi, S. (1991). Early acquisition of epistemic meanings in Korean: A study of sentence-ending suffixes in the spontaneous speech of three children. *First Language, 11,* 93–119.

Choi, S. (1993). Development of locative case markers in Korean. In P. Clancy (Ed.), *Japanese/Korean linguistics* (Vol. 2, pp. 205–221). Stanford, CA: CSLI Publications.

Choi, S. (1995). Early acquisition of epistemic sentence-ending modal forms and functions in Korean children. In J. Bybee & S. Fleischman (Eds.), *Modality in grammar and discourse* (pp. 165–204). Amsterdam: John Benjamins.

Choi, S. (1996, July). *Development of verbs in Korean.* Paper presented at the International Congress for the Study of Child Language, Istanbul, Turkey.

Choi, S. (1997). Language-specific input and early semantic development: Evidence from children learning Korean. In D. I. Slobin (Ed.), *The crosslinguistic study of language acquisition: Vol. 5. Expanding the contexts* (pp. 41–133). Mahwah, NJ: Lawrence Erlbaum.

Choi, S., & Bowerman, M. (1991). Learning to express motion events in English and Korean: The influence of language-specific lexicalization patterns. *Cognition, 41,* 83–121.

Choi, S., & Gopnik, A. (1995). Early acquisition of verbs in Korean: A crosslinguistic study. *Journal of Child Language, 22,* 497–530.

Choi, S., McDonough, L., Bowerman, M., & Mandler, J. (in preparation). Early sensitivity to language-specific spatial categories in English and Korean.

Chomsky, N. (1965). *Aspects of the theory of syntax.* Cambridge, MA: MIT Press.

Chu, H. (1993). *The Korean Americans.* Montgomery County Public Schools, Department of Human Relations, Rockville, MD.

Clancy, P. (1993). Preferred argument structure in Korean acquisition. In E. Clark (Ed.), *The Proceedings of the 25th Annual Child Language Research Forum* (pp. 307–316). Stanford, CA: Stanford University, Center for the Study of Language and Information.

Clancy, P. (1995). Subject and object in Korean acquisition: Surface expression and casemarking. *Harvard Studies in Korean Linguistics, 6,* 3–17.

Clancy, P. (1996). Referential strategies and the co-construction of argument structure in Korean acquisition. In B. Fox (Ed.), *Studies in anaphora* (pp. 33–68). Amsterdam: John Benjamins.

Clancy, P. (1997). Discourse motivations for referential choice in Korean acquisition. In H. Sohn & J. Haig (Eds.), *Japanese/Korean linguistics* (Vol. 6, pp. 639–659). Stanford, CA: CSLI Publications.

Clark, E. (1973). Non-linguistic strategies and the acquisition of word meanings. *Cognition, 2,* 161–182.

de Leon, L. (1996). Vertical path in Tzotzil (Mayan) early acquisition: Linguistic vs. cognitive determinants. In E. Clark (Ed.), *The Proceedings of the 27th Annual Child Language Research Forum* (pp. 183–197). Stanford: CA: Stanford University, Center for the Study of Language and Information.

Du Bois, J. (1985). Competing motivations. In J. Haiman (Ed.), *Iconicity in syntax.* Amsterdam: John Benjamins.

Gentner, D. (1982). Why nouns are learned before verbs: Linguistic relativity versus natural partitioning. In S. A. Kuczaj II (Ed.), *Language development: Vol. 2. Language, thought, and culture* (pp. 301–334). Hillsdale, NJ: Lawrence Earlbaum.

Gleitman, L. R. (1990). The structural sources of verb meanings. *Language Acquisition, 1,* 1–27.

Goldfield, B., & Reznick, J. S. (1990). Early lexical acquisition: Rate, content, and the vocabulary spurt. *Journal of Child Language, 17,* 171–183.

Gopnik, A. (1982). Words and plans: Early language and the development of intelligent actions. *Journal of Child Language, 9,* 303–318.

Gopnik, A. (1988). Three types of early words: The emergence of social words, names, and cognitive-relational words in the one-word stage and their relation to cognitive development. *First Language, 8,* 49–69.

Gopnik, A., & Choi, S. (1990). Do linguistic differences lead to cognitive differences?: A crosslinguistic study of semantic and cognitive development. *First Language, 10,* 199–215.

Gopnik, A., & Choi, S. (1995). Names, relational words, and cognitive development in English and Korean-speakers: Nouns are not always learned before verbs. In M. Tomasello & W. Merriman (Eds.), *Beyond names for things: Young children's acquisition of verbs* (pp. 63–80). Hillsdale, NJ: Lawrence Erlbaum.

Gopnik, A., & Meltzoff, A. (1984). Semantic and cognitive development in 15- to 21-month-old children. *Journal of Child Language, 11,* 495–513.

Gopnik, A., & Meltzoff, A. (1986). Relations between semantic and cognitive development in the one-word stage: The specificity hypothesis. *Child Development, 57,* 1040–1053.

Gopnik, A., & Meltzoff, A. (1997). *Words, thoughts and theories.* Cambridge, MA: MIT Press.

Halliday, M. A. K. (1975). *Learning how to mean: Explorations in the development of language.* London: Edward Arnold.

Hirst, W., & Weil, J. (1982). Acquisition of epistemic and deontic meaning of modals. *Journal of Child Language, 9,* 659–666.

Hoff-Ginsberg, E. (1986). Function and structure in maternal speech: Their relation to the child's development of syntax. *Developmental Psychology, 22,* 155–163.

Hyams, N. (1986). *Language acquisition and the theory of parameters.* Dordrecht, Holland: D. Reidel.

Johnston, J. (1984). Acquisition of locative meanings: "Behind" and "in front of." *Journal of Child Language, 11,* 407–422.

Johnston, J., & Slobin, D. I. (1979). The development of locative expressions in English, Italian, Serbo-Croatian, and Turkish. *Journal of Child Language, 16,* 531–547.

Kim, E. (1984, January). *Korean Americans in the United States: Problems and alternatives.* Paper presented at the Annual Conference of Ethnic and Minority Studies, Kansas City, MO.

Kim, H. (1989). Nominal reference in discourse: Introducing and tracking referents in Korean spoken narratives. *Harvard Studies in Korean Linguistics, 3,* 431–444.

Kim, Y. J. (1997). The acquisition of Korean. In D. I. Slobin (Ed.), *The crosslinguistic study of language acquisition* (Vol. 4, pp. 335–444). Mahwah, NJ: Lawrence Erlbaum Associates.

Landau, S., Smith, L., & Jones, S. (1988). The importance of shape in early lexical learning. *Cognitive Development, 3,* 299–321.

Lee, H. S. (1991). *Tense, aspect, and modality: A discourse-pragmatic analysis of verbal affixes in Korean from a typological perspective.* Unpublished doctoral dissertation, University of California at Los Angeles.

Lee, H. S. (1993). Cognitive constraints on expressing newly perceived information: With reference to epistemic modal suffixes in Korean. *Cognitive
Linguistics, 4*, 135–167.

Lee, K. (1986). Pragmatic function of sentence enders. *Inmunkwahak (Humanities), 56*, 41–59.

Levin, B. (1985). Lexical semantics in review: An introduction. In. B. Levin (Ed.),
Lexical semantics in review: Lexicon Project Working Papers, No. 1. Cambridge,
MA: MIT Center for Cognitive Science.

Lieven, E., Pine, J., & Dresner Barnes, H. (1992). Individual differences in early
vocabulary development: Redefining the referential-expressive distinction.
Journal of Child Language, 19, 287–310.

Maratsos, M. (1991). How the acquisition of nouns may be different from that
of verbs. In N. Krasnegor, D. Rumbaugh, R. Schiefelbusch, & M. Studdert-
Kennedy (Eds.), *Biological and behavioral determinants of language development*
(pp. 67–88). Hillsdale, NJ: Lawrence Erlbaum Associates.

Markman, E. (1989). Constraints children place on word meanings. *Cognitive
Science, 14*, 57–77.

McCune-Nicolich, L. (1981). The cognitive bases of relational words in the single-word period. *Journal of Child Language, 8*, 15–34.

McShane, J. (1980). *Learning to Talk.* Cambridge, UK: Cambridge University
Press.

Moore, C., Pure, K., & Furrow, D. (1990). Children's understanding of the modal
expression of speaker certainty and uncertainty and its relation to the development of a representational theory of mind. *Child Development, 61*,
722–730.

Needham, A., & Baillargeon, R. (1993). Intuitions about support in 4.5-month-
old infants. *Cognition, 47*, 121–148.

Nelson, K. (1973). Structure and strategy in learning to talk. *Monographs of the
Society for Research in Child Development, 38*(Nos. 1–2), 1–136.

Nelson, K. (1974). Concept, word, and sentence: Interrelations in acquisition
and development. *Psychological Review, 81*, 267–285.

Nelson, K., Hampson, J., & Kessler Shaw, L. (1993). Nouns in early lexicons:
Evidence, explanations and implications. *Journal of Child Language, 20*, 61–84.

Park, C. K. (1983). *A handbook for teaching Korean-speaking students.* California
State Departmen of Education. Evaluation, Dissemination and Assessment
Center, CSU, Los Angeles.

Pellegrini, A., Brody, G., & Stoneman, Z. (1987). Children's conversational competence with their parents. *Discourse Processes, 10*, 93–106.

Piaget, J. (1955). *The Language and thought of the child* (M. Gabin, Trans.). New
York: Meridian Books. (Original work published 1926).

Pine, J., Lieven, E., & Rowland, C. (1997). Observational and checklist measures
of vocabulary composition: What do they mean? *Journal of Child Language,
23*, 573–590.

Roeper, T., & Williams, E. (Eds.). (1987). *Parameter setting.* Dordrecht, Holland:
D. Reidel.

Sera, M., Rettinger, E., & Castillo-Pintado, J. (1991). Developing definitions of objects and events in English and Spanish speakers. *Cognitive Development, 6,* 119–143.

Shatz, M. (1983). Communication. In P. H. Mussen (Series Ed.), J. Flavell & E. Markman (Vol. Eds.), *Handbook of child psychology: Vol. 3. Cognitive development* (pp. 841–890). New York: John Wiley.

Shatz, M. (1991). Using cross-cultural research to inform us about the role of language in development: Comparisons of Japanese, Korean, and English, and of German, American English and British English. In M. H. Bornstein (Ed.), *Cultural approaches to parenting* (pp. 139–153). Hillsdale, NJ: Laurence Erlbaum.

Slobin, D. I. (1973). Cognitive prerequisites for the development of grammar. In C. A. Ferguson & D. I. Slobin (Eds.), *Studies of child language development* (pp. 175–208). New York: Holt, Rinehart, & Winston.

Slobin, D. I. (1985). Crosslinguistic evidence for the language-making capacity. In D. I. Slobin (Ed.), *The crosslinguistic study of language acquisition: Vol. 2. Theoretical Issues* (pp. 1157–1256). Hillsdale, NJ: Lawrence Erlbaum Associates.

Spelke, E. S. (1989). Object perception in infancy: Interaction of spatial and kinetic information for object boundaries. *Developmental Psychology, 25,* 185–196.

Stephany, U. (1986). Modality. In P. Fletcher & M. Garman (Eds.), *Language acquisition* (2nd ed., pp. 375–400). Cambridge, MA: Cambridge University Press.

Talmy, L. (1975). Semantics and syntax of motion. In J. Kimball (Ed.), *Syntax and semantics* (pp. 181–238). New York: Academic Press.

Talmy, L. (1985). Lexicalization patterns: Semantic structure in lexical forms. In T. Shopen (Ed.) *Language typology and syntactic description: Vol. III. Grammatical categories and the lexicon* (pp. 57–149). Cambridge: Cambridge University Press.

Tardif, T. (1996). Nouns are not always learned before verbs: Evidence from Mandarin speakers' early vocabularies. *Developmental Psychology, 32,* 492–504.

Tardif, T., Shatz, M., & Naigles, L. (1996, July). *The influence of caregiver speech on children's use of nouns and verbs: A comparison of English, Italian, and Mandarin.* Paper presented at the VII International Congress for the International Association for the Study of Child Language, Istanbul, Turkey.

Tomasello, M. (1992). *First verbs.* Cambridge UK: Cambridge University Press.

U.S. Bureau of Census. (1997). *The Official Statistics: National Population.* Washington, DC: Government Printing Office.

Weist, R., Wysocka, H., & Lyytinen, P. (1991). A cross-linguistic perspective on the development of temporal systems. *Journal of Child Language, 18,* 67–92.

Whorf, B. L. (1956). In J. B. Carroll (Ed.), *Language, thought, and reality: Selected writings of Benjamin Lee Whorf.* Cambridge, MA: MIT Press.

SOONJA CHOI, PH.D.

Soonja Choi, Ph.D., is an Associate Professor in the Department of Linguistics and Oriental Languages at San Diego State University. Since her doctoral dissertation (SUNY at Buffalo) on cross-linguistic similarities and differences in the acquisition of English, Korean, and French, Dr. Choi's primary research interest has been in the relations between language-specific input and semantic development in young children. Dr. Choi has conducted several cross-linguistic studies with Korean- and English-speaking children in the areas of negation, modality, and spatial expressions. Her studies suggest that children are sensitive to language-specific semantic categories and that there is a dynamic interaction between language and cognition from early on.

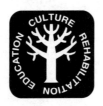

INDEX

K

Kalaallisut, 247, 248
Kalaallit, 247
K'iche', prosody in, 15
Korean
  case markers of, 285–287
  discourse factors of, 288–289
  grammar of, 285–288
  honorifics in, 8, 287–288
  independent subject or object
    production, 265
  inflectional morphology of,
    agglutinating, 5
  modality in, 317–319
  noun ellipsis in, 315–316
  path verbs of, 301
  spatial relations, syntactical
    expression of, 62, 310–313
  verb features, 292–294
  verb morphology of, 287–288
  word order of, 285–287
Korean children, exposure to English,
  282
Korean language acquisition, 281–329
  of case markers, 287
  and discourse factors, sensitivity
    to, 289
  grammar development, early, 310–317
  lexical development, 292–296
  of modal system, 316–317
  of nouns, 285–296
  of sentence-ending suffixes, 319–327
  spatial relations, semantic
    development of, 298–310
  of verbs, 289–292, 294–296
  verbs, semantic development of,
    298–299
  verbs, transitive and intransitive,
    syntactic patterns of, 313–316

L

Language
  and cognition, relationship of,
    282–284

  as socially situated cultural form,
    27
  standard variety versus dialects,
    29
Language acquisition
  culturally specific variations of,
    27
  versus development, 122–144
  inflections, understanding of,
    4–5
  innate faculty for, 22, 115–117
  positive versus negative evidence
    for, 119–122
  of prefixes versus suffixes, 13
  stimulus for, lack of, 118–122
  theories on, 21–22
  time frame of, 54–55
  of two or more languages, 30
  and Universal Grammar, 113–115
  universals of, 15, 21, 22, 282
Language acquisition device (LAD),
    22–23, 116, 118, 283
  dialects, application to, 29
  speech community impact on,
    28–29
  triggering experience of, 116–117
Language assimilation, 210, 213
Language content, 48
  of African American children,
    48–49
Language delay
  crosscultural identification of,
    91–94
  and invisible presence of forms,
    129
  ROWPVT identification of, 89
Language development
  versus acquisition, 122–144
  and inflectional morphology, 4–5
  early syntax of, 134–136
  stages of, 132–134
Language erosion, 247–248
  of Inuit languages, 273
Language evolution, 124–125
  and innovations, 67–69